"Finally, a map that women can use to chart their voyage through menopause the natural way."

—Marilyn Linton, author of *Taking Charge by
Taking Care: A Canadian Guide to Women's Health*

"Leslie Beck has written the first book that specifically outlines the relationship between nutrition and certain symptoms associated with the peri- and post-menopausal years. This book can help alleviate stressful side effects of menopause and lower the risk of disease through diet and nutrition."

—Rose Reisman, bestselling author of *The Balance of Living Well*

"*Leslie Beck's 10 Steps to Healthy Eating* contains everything you need to know to get healthy and stay healthy by eating right. The 'Getting Ready' section is especially impressive and helpful!"

—Christiane Northrup, MD, author of *Women's
Wisdom* and *The Wisdom of Menopause*

"If you are looking for a comprehensive resource *Leslie Beck's Nutrition Guide to a Healthy Pregnancy* is a must read."

—*Toronto Sun*

"If you're not sure where to start to improve your diet, get your hands on a copy of nutritionist Leslie Beck's ... *Foods That Fight Disease*. The book is a mini-course on nutrition."

—*The Province* (Vancouver)

PENGUIN CANADA

HEART HEALTHY FOODS FOR LIFE

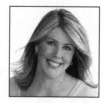

LESLIE BECK, a registered dietitian, is a leading Canadian nutritionist and the bestselling author of nine nutrition books. Leslie writes a weekly nutrition column in *The Globe and Mail*, is a regular contributor to CTV's *Canada AM*, and can be heard one morning a week on CJAD Radio's *The Andrew Carter Show* in Montreal.

Leslie has worked with many of Canada's leading businesses and international food companies and runs a thriving private practice at the Medcan Clinic in Toronto. She also regularly delivers nutrition workshops to corporate groups across North America.

Visit Leslie Beck's website at **www.lesliebeck.com**.

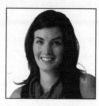

MICHELLE GELOK is a registered dietitian who completed her degree in food and nutrition at Ryerson University and her dietetic internship at the University Health Network in Toronto. Michelle has worked extensively with Leslie Beck since 2004. In that time, she developed recipes for four of Leslie's books, *The No-Fail Diet, Foods That Fight Disease, Heart Healthy Foods for Life,* and *Leslie Beck's Longevity Diet.*

Visit Michelle's website at **www.michellegelok.com**.

Also by Leslie Beck

Leslie Beck's Nutrition Encyclopedia

Leslie Beck's Nutrition Guide for Women

10 Steps to Healthy Eating

Leslie Beck's Nutrition Guide to a Healthy Pregnancy

Healthy Eating for Preteens and Teens

The Complete Nutrition Guide to Menopause

The No-Fail Diet

Foods That Fight Disease

The Complete A–Z Nutrition Encyclopedia

The Complete Nutrition Guide for Women

Leslie Beck's Longevity Diet

HEART HEALTHY FOODS FOR LIFE

Preventing Heart Disease through Diet and Nutrition

Leslie Beck, RD

Michelle Gelok, RD
Recipe development and nutritional analysis

PENGUIN
CANADA

PENGUIN CANADA

Published by the Penguin Group

Penguin Group (Canada), 90 Eglinton Avenue East, Suite 700, Toronto, Ontario, Canada M4P 2Y3
(a division of Pearson Canada Inc.)

Penguin Group (USA) Inc., 375 Hudson Street, New York, New York 10014, U.S.A.
Penguin Books Ltd, 80 Strand, London WC2R 0RL, England
Penguin Ireland, 25 St Stephen's Green, Dublin 2, Ireland (a division of Penguin Books Ltd)
Penguin Group (Australia), 250 Camberwell Road, Camberwell, Victoria 3124, Australia
(a division of Pearson Australia Group Pty Ltd)
Penguin Books India Pvt Ltd, 11 Community Centre, Panchsheel Park, New Delhi – 110 017, India
Penguin Group (NZ), 67 Apollo Drive, Rosedale, North Shore 0632, New Zealand
(a division of Pearson New Zealand Ltd)
Penguin Books (South Africa) (Pty) Ltd, 24 Sturdee Avenue, Rosebank,
Johannesburg 2196, South Africa

Penguin Books Ltd, Registered Offices: 80 Strand, London WC2R 0RL, England

First published in a Penguin Canada paperback by Penguin Group (Canada),
a division of Pearson Canada Inc., 2009

Published in this edition, 2011

1 2 3 4 5 6 7 8 9 10   (WEB)

Copyright © Leslie Beck Nutrition Consulting Inc., 2009
Foreword copyright © Rob Myers, 2009
Recipe development and nutritional analysis: Michelle Gelok, RD

Manufactured in Canada.

Library and Archives Canada Cataloguing in Publication data available
upon request to the publisher.

ISBN: 978-0-14-305690-4

Visit the Penguin Group (Canada) website at **www.penguin.ca**

Special and corporate bulk purchase rates available; please see
www.penguin.ca/corporatesales or call 1-800-810-3104, ext. 2477 or 2474

*This book is dedicated to
the Canadians living with heart disease
and their family members*

Contents

Foreword xv
Acknowledgments xix
Introduction xxi

PART 1 UNDERSTANDING HEART DISEASE 1

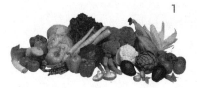

1   What is heart disease? 3
Your heart and circulatory system 4
The process of heart disease 6
Blood tests 13
Screening procedures 21

2   Are you at risk for heart disease? 29
Major risk factors 30
Contributing risk factors 52

PART 2 PREVENTING HEART DISEASE WITH DIET AND NUTRITION 55

3   Foods and nutrients to limit or avoid 57
Saturated fat 59
Trans fats 64
Dietary cholesterol 67
Added sugars 71
Sodium 74
Alcoholic beverages 79

4 Heart healthy foods 83
Omega-3 fats 84
Monounsaturated fats 93
Whole grains 98
Legumes and soy 104
Nuts 111
Fruit and vegetables 116
Tea: green and black 122
Dark chocolate 125

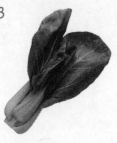

5 Heart healthy vitamins, minerals, and supplements 131
Antioxidant nutrients 132
B vitamins: folate (folic acid), B6, and B12 138
Vitamin D 143
Magnesium 145
Coenzyme Q10 150
Garlic 152

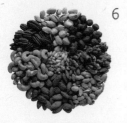

6 Diet plans to help prevent heart disease 157
The DASH (Dietary Approaches to Stop Hypertension) diet 159
The OmniHeart diets 163
The portfolio diet 168

7 Shopping for heart healthy foods 173
Before you grocery shop 174
What healthy food symbols do and don't tell you 175
Deciphering the Nutrition Facts box 178
Understanding nutrition and health claims 182
Making healthy choices in the grocery store 183

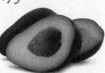

8　Heart healthy dining out　189
　　Calories, fat, and sodium in restaurant meals　190
　　Tips for ordering in restaurants　194
　　Choosing healthy ethnic cuisine　197
　　Tips for ordering a heart healthy breakfast　202

9　Maintaining a healthy weight　205
　　How healthy is your weight?　206
　　10 strategies for losing weight　210
　　Tips for maintaining your weight over the years　216

10　Exercise for preventing heart disease　221
　　Cardiovascular exercises, 4 to 7 days per week　223
　　Strength exercises, 2 to 4 days per week　225
　　Flexibility exercises, 4 to 7 days per week　227
　　Tips to build in lifestyle activity　228
　　Tips for sticking with exercise　228
　　When to check with your doctor first　230

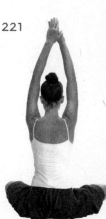

PART 3　RECIPES THAT PREVENT HEART DISEASE　231
　　Breakfasts　245
　　Salads and dressings　256
　　Soups　269
　　Side dishes (vegetables and grains)　283
　　Pasta and stir-fries　293
　　Meatless main dishes　307
　　Fish and seafood　320
　　Poultry and meat　330
　　Quick breads and muffins　342
　　Desserts　362

　　Appendix: Internet resources for consumers　379
　　References　384
　　General index　399
　　Recipe index　410

Foreword

Heart disease kills more Canadians than any other disease. In fact, every 7 minutes, someone dies from heart disease or stroke. Cardiovascular disease—which encompasses diseases of the blood vessels and stroke—accounts for at least 34% of all deaths among women and 32% among men. Roughly one-half of these deaths (54%) are due to coronary heart disease, the very topic of this book.

Coronary heart disease—also referred to as ischemic heart disease—is a progressive disease that reduces blood flow through the arteries that supply the heart with blood and oxygen. The disease, caused by atherosclerosis or the buildup of fatty plaques on the inner lining of the coronary arteries, can lead to angina (chest pain), heart attack, heart failure, heart rhythm disorders, and sudden cardiac arrest.

According to the Heart and Stroke Foundation of Canada, there are at least 70,000 heart attacks each year in this country. Sadly, it's estimated that 19,000 Canadians die each year as a result of suffering a heart attack and, in most cases, these deaths occur outside of the hospital.

Encouragingly, the prevalence and death rate from heart disease has fallen over the past 40 years. Since 1956, the rate of dying as a result of having heart disease has dropped by 70%. Reduction in cigarette smoking—a major risk factor for heart disease—and improvements in survival due to advances in medical care have contributed to lower mortality rates.

Yet, this downward trend is likely to come to an end. According to some researchers it already has with the prevalence of heart disease beginning to shift upwards in 2000. The reason remains unclear, but more than likely the epidemics of obesity and type 2 diabetes play a role. Indeed, the number of Canadians living with coronary heart disease remains high and increases with age. According to the 2003 Canadian Community Health Survey, 5 million Canadians say they are affected by heart disease, high blood pressure, and stroke.

The notion that heart disease is a man's disease is far from reality. While men are more likely to develop heart disease early in life, women catch up around menopause. And the gap between men and women in the number of deaths from heart disease has narrowed. In 2003, the number of female deaths from heart disease and stroke was equivalent to male deaths.

Children are also at risk for developing heart disease—and likely at a younger age than their parents' generation. With risk factors such as high cholesterol, hypertension, obesity, and type 2 diabetes increasingly being diagnosed in kids and teenagers, children today are expected to be the first generation in modern memory to have a shorter life expectancy than their parents.

Despite these grim statistics, coronary heart disease is not inevitable. It is highly preventable by making healthy lifestyle choices. And if you've been diagnosed with heart disease or have suffered a heart attack, lifestyle modifications can greatly improve the quality of your life.

The first step in reducing your personal risk for heart disease is understanding its risk factors and taking action to change, or manage, the ones that affect you. Cigarette smoking, high blood pressure, high cholesterol, diabetes, overweight, and physical inactivity are all major risk factors for coronary heart disease. And unlike your family history or age, they're risk factors that you have control over.

Following a healthy diet and exercising regularly are vital to preventing heart disease. Eating the right foods—and limiting your intake of those that can harm your blood vessels—can lower blood pressure and LDL (bad) cholesterol, control weight, and help manage your blood sugar level. If your physician has prescribed medication to help you reduce blood pressure, lower cholesterol, or prevent type 2 diabetes, following a heart healthy diet will further benefit your cardiovascular health. And in some cases, making dietary changes and losing excess weight can reduce the need for medication.

I encourage you to read *Heart Healthy Foods for Life* and incorporate Leslie's nutrition advice into your family's meals. Her book offers plenty of sound nutrition information and evidence-based diet strategies that can help protect you from coronary heart disease. It's all about implementing a sustainable, heart healthy lifestyle. The tools in this book will help you achieve this.

Dr. Rob Myers, MD FRCPC FACC
Division of Cardiology
Sunnybrook Health Sciences Centre
Toronto, Canada
Director of Cardiology, Medcan Clinic, Toronto
Assistant Professor of Medicine, University of Toronto

Acknowledgments

No book is written through the efforts of a single person, and this one is no exception. The support and diligent work of a number of people brought this book to life. The following people deserve a special thank you for their important contributions to *Heart Healthy Foods for Life*.

Michelle Gelok, a registered dietitian who created, tested, and analyzed all 102 recipes in this book. I've had the pleasure of working with Michelle for the past four years and am always inspired by her passion for food and health. Her meticulous work on recipe development and nutritional review along with her creative culinary skills have resulted in recipes that deliver as much taste as they do heart healthy nutrients. As well, thank you to her mother, Gia Gelok, for lending her kitchen and her time to test each and every recipe.

Dr. James Aw, Medical Director of the Medcan Clinic in Toronto, for taking the time to review the medical chapters of the book. His attention to detail and accuracy and suggested revisions were greatly appreciated.

Dr. Rob Myers, Director of Cardiology at the Medcan Clinic, for providing his expert overview on the state of heart disease in Canada in the foreword to this book.

Rosemary Chubb, Emily Kennedy, Dawn Bone, Renee Hughes, and Michelle Onlock, my support team at the Medcan Clinic whose dedication and hard work in managing my busy private practice allowed me to write this book.

My private practice clients, who keep inspiring me to continue learning and honing my skills as a nutrition professional.

The team at Penguin Canada for their ongoing and unwavering support of my work.

Darrell Ball, whose patience, cheerleading, and optimism never faltered during the months I spent researching and writing this book. Thank you for believing in me.

Introduction

- Every 7 minutes in Canada, someone dies from heart disease or stroke.
- Cardiovascular disease accounts for 32% of all deaths in Canada, more than any other disease.
- Eight out of 10 deaths from cardiovascular disease are a result of coronary heart disease and heart attack.
- There are an estimated 70,000 heart attacks every year in Canada.
- Heart attacks kill approximately 19,000 Canadians each year.
- Eight in 10 Canadians have at least one risk factor for heart disease.
- About 40% of Canadians have high blood cholesterol.
- One in five (22%) Canadians have high blood pressure and as many as 42% may be unaware their blood pressure is too high. Only 16% of people with high blood pressure have it treated and under control.
- Nearly six out of 10 (59%) Canadian adults are overweight or obese.
- One-quarter of Canadian children are overweight or obese.
- At least 1.3 million Canadians are living with diabetes and the vast majority (90%) has type 2 diabetes, which is largely preventable.
- A woman with diabetes has an 8-fold greater risk of heart disease than a woman without diabetes.
- Nearly half (48%) of Canadians aged 12 and over report being physically inactive.
- More than one-quarter of Canadians aged 31 to 50 get more than 35% of their calories from fat, the threshold beyond which health risks increase.
- Almost two-thirds (64%) of adults eat fewer than 5 servings of fruit and vegetables each day. Seven out of 10 kids aged 4 to 8 consume less than 5 servings per day.

These statistics from the Heart and Stroke Foundation of Canada certainly don't paint a pretty picture of our nation's heart health. After reading this list, it probably seems obvious why heart disease is the number one killer of Canadians. In addition to an aging population, many of the "big" risk factors for heart disease—high blood pressure, obesity, type 2 diabetes, and physical inactivity—are on the rise in adults and children.

As a registered dietitian in private practice, I help people every day take control of their risk factors for heart disease. I offer nutrition advice and develop customized meal plans that allow clients to lower their blood cholesterol and blood pressure, reduce triglycerides, prevent type 2 diabetes, and lose weight. People often consult me in an effort to avoid taking medication to treat high cholesterol or elevated blood sugar. By making specific dietary changes, many people are successful in improving their blood test results and staying away from prescription drugs. Some clients, who are already taking medication, are able to reduce their dose or stop taking their pills altogether.

If you have one or more risk factors for heart disease—be it family history, high blood pressure, elevated cholesterol, overweight, or impaired fasting glucose—adopting a heart healthy diet can help reduce your risk of being diagnosed with heart disease and experiencing a heart attack.

Eating to guard against heart disease means more than limiting, or avoiding, certain foods and nutrients that can damage your arteries, such as saturated fat, trans fat, sodium, and excessive alcohol. While that's certainly a good start to adopting a heart healthy diet, eating to prevent heart disease also requires adding foods to your diet that offer protection. Foods rich in soluble fibre, omega-3 fatty acids, and monounsaturated fats help reduce LDL cholesterol in your bloodstream. When it comes to lowering your blood pressure—or warding off hypertension—you need to consume foods with plenty of magnesium, calcium, and potassium. A diet that contains whole grains and foods with a low glycemic index can help manage blood sugar and lower the odds of developing type 2 diabetes. And of course managing portion size in combination with regular exercise is essential for controlling your weight.

How to use *Heart Healthy Foods for Life*

This book is intended to educate you about the link between foods and heart disease and to help you control the disease's diet-related risk factors through scientifically sound and sustainable nutrition principles. In Part I, *Understanding Heart Disease*, you'll learn how coronary heart disease develops and progresses and which factors greatly increase the odds of succumbing to the disease. You'll also read about various blood and screening tests that doctors and cardiologists use to determine a patient's risk for heart disease and, in some cases, detect its presence.

Part II, *Preventing Heart Disease with Diet and Nutrition*, offers everything you need to know in order to adopt the heart-healthiest diet possible. In these chapters, I discuss the science behind diet—how certain foods and nutrients work in your body to increase or decrease heart disease risk—along with appropriate serving sizes and plenty of practical tips for improving your diet. You'll learn how to shop for heart healthy foods by deciphering nutrition labels and how to order heart healthy from a restaurant menu when dining out.

If you're the type of person who likes to follow a structured meal plan, I've provided details about three diets, each one scientifically proven to help fight heart disease: the DASH diet, the OmniHeart diet, and the portfolio diet. I have also included important strategies to help you control your weight and increase physical activity, key factors in maintaining cardiovascular health.

Over 100 recipes that guard against heart disease

Of course, nutrition information is only useful if you're able to apply it to your lifestyle. In Part III, *Recipes that Prevent Heart Disease*, I've transformed heart healthy foods into tasty meals you and your family will enjoy. Each and every recipe in this book was developed, tested, and analyzed by Michelle Gelok, a nutritionist who worked with me to develop the delicious recipes in my previous two books—*Foods That Fight Disease* and *The No-Fail Diet*. Recently, Michelle completed her dietetic internship in Toronto and is now a full-fledged registered dietitian!

In *Heart Healthy Foods for Life*, Michelle has translated the scientific research to 102 tasty recipes that are low in saturated fat, sodium, and refined sugars. You'll find mouth-watering recipes that are excellent sources of omega-3 fatty acids, monounsaturated fat, soluble fibre, magnesium, and folate. Along with my tips to add heart healthy foods to your meals and snacks, these delicious and easy to prepare recipes will help you introduce a variety of healthy meals to your family menus.

To help you find a recipe that suits your needs, I've listed them by heart healthy food (i.e., fish, nuts, legumes, soy, whole grains, etc.) as well as by type of dish (i.e., soup, salad, fish and seafood, poultry and meat, etc.). Each recipe is accompanied by a per serving nutrient analysis, a breakdown of its calories, fat, protein, fibre, sodium, and so on.

Preventing heart disease through diet, weight control, and regular physical activity is important for every age group and should begin in childhood. As parents, we need to steer our children towards a healthy adulthood by helping them make positive lifestyle choices. We need to be good role models for our children by practicing what we preach. Kids will follow your lead if they see you eating a variety of heart healthy foods and being physically active.

It's never too late to make positive changes to your diet. By implementing many of the strategies discussed on the pages that follow—nutrition tips that are based on current scientific knowledge—you'll not only guard against coronary heart disease, you'll increase your energy level and improve your overall sense of well-being. I hope you find *Heart Healthy Foods for Life* an invaluable resource to help pave the way to a healthier lifestyle and, of course, a healthier heart.

Leslie Beck, RD
The Medcan Clinic
Toronto, 2009

PART 1

UNDERSTANDING HEART DISEASE

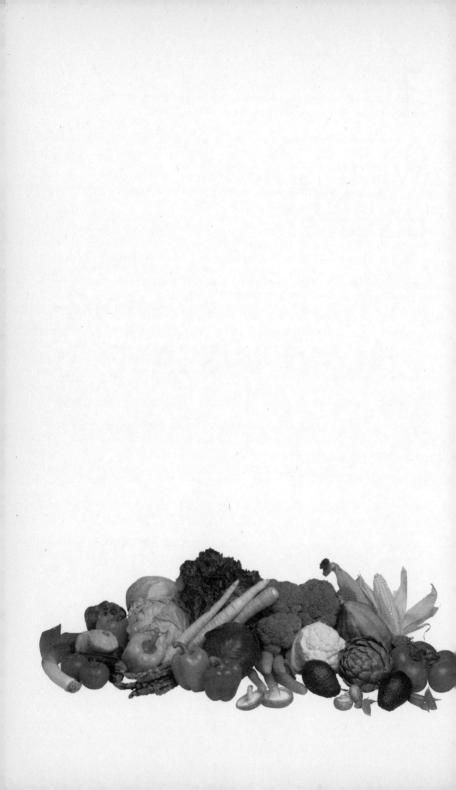

1

What is heart disease?

Heart disease isn't just one condition. Many types of cardio-vascular disease affect the heart's ability to function properly. In fact, this group of diseases affects the blood vessels throughout the entire body, including those in the heart, brain, lungs, and legs. Coronary artery disease, heart valve disease, heart rhythm disorders, heart failure, hypertension, peripheral vascular disease, and congenital heart disease all come under the umbrella term *cardiovascular disease*.

The most common type of cardiovascular disease is *coronary artery disease*, often referred to as coronary heart disease or simply heart disease. This progressive condition reduces blood flow through the coronary arteries, which feed blood and oxygen to the heart. It is why you'll also sometimes hear the term *ischemic heart disease* (*ischemic* is Latin for "insufficient blood and oxygen flow to the body's tissues"). When the heart can't receive enough oxygen-rich blood, coronary artery disease can lead to angina (chest pain) or even a heart attack. In this book I focus on strategies to help prevent coronary artery disease, which I refer to throughout as heart disease.

Your heart and circulatory system

For its small size, the heart is a pretty powerful organ. Only a little larger in size than a clenched fist, this strong muscular pump pushes blood continuously throughout the blood vessels.

Each day, your heart beats about 100,000 times. Over a lifetime, that's about 2.5 billion heartbeats, each one sending blood throughout your circulatory system, including your heart, lungs, arteries, arterioles (small arteries), capillaries (tiny blood vessels that connect arteries and veins), and veins. Arteries deliver oxygen-rich blood from the heart to all body tissues and organs, including the heart, whereas veins return deoxygenated blood from the body to the heart. That's a lot of territory to cover. If all your blood vessels were laid end to end, it's estimated they would extend roughly 60,000 miles!

ANATOMY OF YOUR HEART

Your heart has two sides connected by an inner wall called the *septum*. The right side pumps blood only to your lungs, to pick up oxygen. This life-giving blood then returns to the left side and is pumped to all parts of your body. Each side has two chambers. The upper, called the *atrium*, collects blood as it comes into the heart. The lower, called the *ventricle*, pushes blood out of the heart.

Four valves control blood flow from the atria to the ventricles and from the ventricles to arteries. The valves allow blood to flow in only one direction. When the valves between the atria and ventricles and those between the ventricles and arteries open and close, they make characteristic sounds that doctors can hear with a stethoscope.

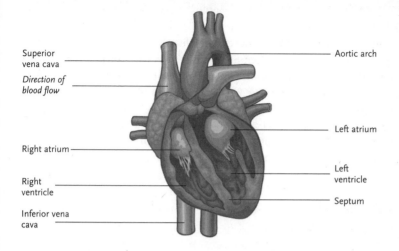

Superior vena cava

Direction of blood flow

Right atrium

Right ventricle

Inferior vena cava

Aortic arch

Left atrium

Left ventricle

Septum

By listening to these sounds, your doctor is able to measure your blood pressure. A small, portable instrument called a blood pressure cuff is usually used. It consists of an air pump, a pressure gauge, and a rubber cuff and measures your blood pressure in units called millimetres of mercury (mmHg).

The cuff is placed around your upper arm and inflated with an air pump to a pressure that blocks the flow of blood in the brachial artery, the main artery that travels through your arm. Your arm is then extended at the side of your body, at heart level, and the pressure of the cuff on the arm and artery is gradually released. As the pressure in the cuff decreases, your doctor listens with a stethoscope. The pressure at which your doctor first hears a pulse from the artery is your *systolic pressure* (the top number of your blood pressure measurement). As the cuff pressure decreases further, the pressure at which the pulse finally stops is your *diastolic pressure* (the bottom number). (You'll learn more about blood pressure and how it contributes to heart disease in Chapter 2, page 41.)

Blood travels to and from the heart through major blood vessels called arteries. The *aorta*, the main artery, sends oxygen-rich blood from the left side of your heart to your tissues and organs. The *coronary arteries* deliver oxygen- and nutrient-rich blood from the aorta to your heart, which like other organs needs oxygen to function properly. The *pulmonary artery* carries blood pumped from the right side of your heart to the lungs so it can pick up fresh oxygen. Think of these arteries as a fuel line to your heart muscle.

The pumping, or beating, of your heart is regulated by the *cardiac conduction system*, which sends signals that create an electrical current and contract the muscles. The signal starts in the right atrium—the *sinoatrial node* (SA node)—then moves across the heart's chambers causing sequential contractions. The SA node is also known as your body's pacemaker. If you've ever had an electrocardiogram (ECG) test and seen the printout of your results, you've witnessed your heart's electrical system at work. (Electrocardiograms and other heart tests are described later in this chapter, page 23.) Normally, electrical impulses are generated at a set rate, but emotions, stress, and hormones can affect the rate at which the SA node sends out electrical signals.

The process of heart disease

As you can see, the ability of your heart to pump blood efficiently depends on an intricate system of parts working together in a highly organized fashion. When heart disease disrupts your heart's electrical system and pumping action, it must work harder than normal to send oxygen-rich blood throughout your body. If the heart pumps too fast (tachycardia) or too slow (bradycardia), blood can't reach the body's vital organs efficiently, which in some cases can be life-threatening.

ATHEROSCLEROSIS

So what causes heart disease? By far, the most common cause of blocked coronary arteries is a disorder called *atherosclerosis*. Simply put, atherosclerosis is the buildup of fatty *plaques* (collections) on the inner lining of the arteries, like the accumulation of rust in a water pipe. These cholesterol-rich plaques cause hardening of the arteries and narrowing of the inner channel (*lumen*) of the artery. Narrowed arteries can't deliver enough blood and oxygen to maintain normal function. In the case of coronary arteries that deliver blood to the heart, reduced blood flow can cause angina, heart attack, sudden death, abnormal heart rhythms, and heart failure.

Atherosclerosis can also damage arteries in other parts of the body. For example, buildup of plaques in arteries leading to the legs can cause pain while walking or exercising as well as ulcers or delayed wound healing in the legs. When blood vessels outside the heart are affected, the condition is known as *peripheral vascular disease.*

In the case of atherosclerosis narrowing the arteries that feed the brain, the result may be *stroke* and *vascular dementia* (this mental deterioration occurs when the brain becomes damaged and blood cannot reach the brain cells so they eventually die).

Atherosclerosis is a progressive disease that can begin in childhood. (That's why it's so important to encourage your children to eat healthfully and be physically active from an early age.) As we get older, cholesterol and triglycerides (blood fats) are deposited on the lining of artery walls as fatty streaks. Being only slightly raised, these streaks don't cause any blockages or symptoms, but they are precursors to big obstructions that can occur later on.

Unhealthy lifestyle choices or genetics—or both—make some people susceptible to further buildup of fatty deposits, called *atheroma.* As atherosclerosis progresses, the atheroma begins to harden and turn into plaque, a substance made of fat, cholesterol, calcium, connective tissue, and other substances in the blood. The enlarging plaque obstructs blood flow through the arteries.

Atherosclerosis can remain silent, our bodies symptom-free, for years and even decades. Indications of a problem don't usually surface until blockage of the coronary arteries becomes severe. But heart disease is not related only to the narrowing of blood vessels. Researchers are now finding that many people who have heart attacks don't have arteries that are severely narrowed by fatty plaque. In fact, it's thought that these types of blockages cause only about 3 out of 10 heart attacks. Some people have what's called *vulnerable plaque*, which is buried inside the artery wall and may not always block blood flow through the artery. This type of plaque is filled with different types of cells that cause blood clots, making people more prone to suffering a heart attack.

Conditions such as high blood pressure, high cholesterol, and diabetes can speed up the process of atherosclerosis and cause earlier onset of symptoms.

ANGINA PECTORIS

When the coronary arteries become narrowed by more than 50%, they can't increase the flow of oxygen-rich blood to the heart. When the heart becomes starved for oxygen, chest pain occurs. The medical term for chest pain caused by coronary artery disease is *angina pectoris*, which means "squeezing of the chest" in Latin. Stable angina, the most common type, occurs when the heart is working harder than usual and requires more oxygen. Climbing a flight of stairs, physical exercise, emotional stress, or eating a heavy meal can trigger stable angina or exertional chest pain.

Angina pain feels like a pressure, heaviness, aching, or squeezing across the chest, behind the breastbone. The pain can also radiate to the neck, jaw, arms, and back. People who experience angina may also feel indigestion, heartburn, fatigue, nausea, cramping, and shortness of breath. Women are more likely to feel discomfort in their back, shoulders, and abdomen. In most cases, symptoms last less than 5 minutes and are relieved by rest or medication such as nitroglycerine placed under the tongue.

Unstable angina is less common and more serious. The symptoms are more severe, last longer (up to 30 minutes), and have a less predictable pattern than stable angina. Chest pain often comes as a surprise while at rest or sleeping at night, or upon mild physical exertion. Unlike stable angina, the pain of unstable angina is not relieved with rest or medication and may mean that a heart attack will happen soon.

Treatments for angina include lifestyle changes, medications, medical procedures such as angioplasty and stents, coronary artery bypass, and cardiac rehabilitation. (You'll learn more about angioplasty, stents, and coronary artery bypass procedures later in this chapter.)

HEART ATTACK

The medical term for heart attack is *myocardial infarction*. (And again, Latin provides an accurate description: *myo* means muscle, *cardio* refers to heart, and *infarct* means the death of cells from lack of oxygen.) Narrowed coronary arteries don't cause a heart attack on their own. Rather, a heart attack happens when a blood clot blocks the flow of blood through a coronary artery.

You might be wondering how a blood clot can occur in an artery that feeds the heart. Atherosclerosis is actually responsible. As heart disease advances, plaques within the inner lining of a coronary artery may develop a crack or rupture. The body treats this rupture as an injury and attempts to heal it in the usual way—by sealing the "wound" with a blood clot. However, the clot further obstructs blood flow through the artery and can cause angina. If the clot continues to grow, it can completely block the artery, cutting off blood flow to the heart. The end result: a heart attack.

A heart attack may also occur when a coronary artery temporarily contracts or goes into a severe spasm, preventing the flow of blood to the heart. Without oxygen, heart cells are injured, causing pain and pressure. The length of time the blood supply is cut off will determine the amount of damage to the heart. If blood flow isn't restored within 20 to 40 minutes, irreversible damage can occur: heart tissue dies and is replaced by scar tissue. Heart muscle continues to die for up to 8 hours, which is when the heart attack is over.

Heart attacks can occur at any time but more happen between 4:00 and 10:00 A.M. because of the higher amounts of adrenaline released by the adrenal glands in the morning. Adrenaline is a stress hormone that increases heart rate and dilates the blood vessels and airway passages. It's also thought that adrenaline may contribute to the rupture of plaques in artery walls.

Warning signs of a heart attack. Not all victims experience heart attacks to the same degree. In fact, some people, especially the elderly and those with diabetes, can have a "silent" heart attack, one with no symptoms. Women are more likely than men to suffer these. But silent heart attacks, or those with few symptoms, can be just as life threatening as attacks that cause severe pain.

Thousands of Canadians die each year from heart attacks because they don't get medical attention quickly enough. Too often, people pass off their symptoms as "indigestion," "stress," or "fatigue," or they fear the embarrassment of a false alarm. Of the people who don't survive a heart attack, most die within the first hour of signs and symptoms appearing.

Although chest pain is the most common indication of heart attack, people may suffer other symptoms. Knowing these common signs of heart attack can result in prompt medical attention and saved lives:

- increasing episodes of chest pain (angina)
- pressure, squeezing, tightness, or burning sensation in the centre of your chest that lasts for more than a few minutes
- pain that may extend to your shoulder, arm, neck, back, jaw, even teeth
- difficulty breathing
- sweating
- fainting

- indigestion, nausea, vomiting
- anxiety, impending sense of doom

Warning signals of a heart attack are less noticeable in women than in men. In addition to the above, women may experience the following symptoms:

- heartburn or abdominal pain
- cold, clammy skin
- dizziness, lightheadedness
- unexplained fatigue
- vague feeling of illness

Because of the indistinct nature of symptoms and the occasional difficulties doctors have in diagnosing heart attacks in women, women are less likely to receive aggressive treatment, and more likely to receive it later than men.

If you, or a loved one, are experiencing any of these symptoms, the Heart and Stroke Foundation of Canada advises the following[1]:

- Call 911 or your local emergency number immediately, or have someone call for you.
- Stop all activity and sit or lie down in whatever position is most comfortable.
- If you take nitroglycerine, take your normal dosage.
- If you are experiencing chest pain, chew and swallow one adult 325 milligram ASA tablet (acetylsalicylic acid or Aspirin) or two 80 milligram tablets. Pain medicines such as acetaminophen (e.g., Tylenol) or ibuprofen (e.g., Advil) do not work the same way as ASA and therefore will not help.
- Rest comfortably and wait for emergency medical services (EMS) (e.g., ambulance) to arrive.

Treatment for heart attack

Heart attack patients are treated with medications and, sometimes, surgical procedures. The following medications may be used:

- *Aspirin (ASA)* to decrease blood clotting and maintain blood flow through narrowed arteries by preventing blood cells called platelets from sticking together
- *Plavix* to help prevent new blood clots from forming
- *Heparin* to inhibit blood clotting
- *Thrombolytics* such as streptokinase or tPA (tissue plasminogen activator) to help dissolve a blood clot that's blocking blood flow to the heart. The sooner these drugs are administered after a heart attack, the greater the chance of survival and the less damage to the heart.
- *Statins* to lower levels of unwanted cholesterol and prevent a blockage from getting worse
- *Beta blockers* to relax the heart, slow the heart beat, and lower blood pressure
- *Nitroglycerine* to dilate the coronary arteries, improve blood flow, and reduce chest pain

Sometimes medications alone are unable to improve blood flow to the heart muscle. If not given soon enough after a heart attack, surgery may be required later.

CORONARY ANGIOPLASTY AND STENTING After a heart attack, doctors may perform emergency angioplasty, a procedure that opens blocked coronary arteries thereby greatly increasing blood flow, decreasing chest pain, and reducing the risk of a subsequent heart attack.

A deflated balloon is attached to special tubing that is threaded up to the coronary arteries. The procedure is commonly performed through an artery in the groin (the femoral artery), but it can also be done using an artery in the arm or wrist. The balloon is then inflated to widen blocked areas where blood flow to the heart muscle has been reduced or cut off.

Angioplasty is often combined with the implantation of a permanent stent, a metal wire mesh tube that's left in the artery to keep it open. This procedure, called stenting, improves blood flow and relieves angina pain. Within 3 weeks of the procedure, the inside lining of the artery grows over the surface of the stent.

Doctors often recommend angioplasty, and possibly stenting, for people who have angina that isn't helped by medication.

CORONARY ARTERY BYPASS GRAFT In some instances, doctors may perform this operation at the time of a heart attack, but most often it is scheduled for a later time. This procedure is advised for patients with multiple occurrences of narrowing in more than one of the four coronary arteries (this is often the case in people with diabetes). It's also recommended for patients who have not responded to medical therapy and who are not good candidates for angioplasty.

A healthy artery or vein from another part of the body (usually the leg) is grafted, or connected, to the blocked coronary artery. It bypasses, or goes around, the blocked portion of the coronary artery, creating a new route for oxygen-rich blood around the blockage to the heart.

Complications of heart attack

Depending on the amount of damage sustained by the heart muscle during a heart attack, complications can occur, including heart failure, arrhythmias (abnormal heart rhythms), and heart valve problems.

HEART FAILURE If a heart attack destroys a lot of tissue, the heart can't do an adequate job of pumping blood to meet the body's needs. Heart failure (also known as *congestive heart failure*) results in decreased blood flow to tissues and organs, and can cause shortness of breath, fatigue, and buildup of fluid (called edema) in the lungs, ankles, and feet. Treatment aims to relieve the symptoms and prevent the progressive decline in heart function. Lifestyle changes, medications, and, in some cases, medical devices that help the heart beat properly are used to manage heart failure.

ARRHYTHMIAS Injury to the heart can also disrupt the heart's electrical system causing irregular heartbeats, or arrhythmias, some of which can be fatal. Healed scar tissue in the heart can lead to arrhythmias days, weeks, even years after a heart attack.

Ventricular tachycardia, or rapid heart rate in the ventricles, may prevent the heart from pumping blood throughout the body. Tachycardia refers to a rate of more than 100 beats per minute.

The most serious type of arrhythmia is ventricular fibrillation, when the heart's lower chambers quiver or flutter, and the heart pumps little or no blood. Collapse and sudden death occurs unless medical help is provided immediately.

Heart rhythm disturbances can be treated with medications and an electronic device called an implantable cardioverter defibrillator (ICD). The ICD sends an electrical impulse to shock the heart back into a regular rhythm if it starts to beat irregularly.

HEART VALVE PROBLEMS If heart valves are damaged during a heart attack, they can develop serious and life-threatening leakage problems. In some cases surgery may be required to repair or replace a valve.

Blood tests

The chemistry of your blood offers a doctor many clues about the health of your heart. The most common blood screening tests to predict risk of heart disease are for cholesterol and triglycerides. However, there are an increasing number of other blood tests available that give doctors even more information. Keep in mind, though, that one abnormal blood test result does not determine your risk for heart disease. Likewise, a normal result from a blood test doesn't mean that you *don't* have atherosclerosis. Your doctor will evaluate all of your results, along with other important risk factors, to determine the need for further testing and preventative measures.

The interpretation of many blood test results involves comparing your results to the test's *reference range*, also commonly called the *normal range*. A reference range is established by testing a large number of healthy people and observing what appears to be "normal" for them. For some blood tests, like cholesterol, rather than worry about the "normal" range, you need to be concerned if your result falls above or below an applicable cut-off value. To determine your risk for developing heart disease, doctors look at your LDL (bad) cholesterol value and the ratio of your total cholesterol and HDL (good) cholesterol numbers.

The following blood tests help determine your risk of developing heart disease and also assist doctors in the treatment and management of heart disease.

LIPID PROFILE

The lipid profile, a group of blood tests often ordered together, measures the amount of lipids (fats) in your bloodstream. The profile includes LDL cholesterol ("bad" cholesterol), HDL cholesterol ("good" cholesterol), total cholesterol, and triglycerides. It can also include a calculated value for the total cholesterol:HDL ratio or a risk score based on lipid profile results, age, sex, and other risk factors.

Men, age 40 and older, and women who are post-menopausal or age 50 or older should have a lipid profile every 1 to 3 years. If you have other risk factors for heart disease, such as high blood pressure or diabetes, your doctor will routinely measure your lipid profile at a younger age. Younger adults should have a lipid profile at least once every 5 years. The test should be done when you are fasting (only water is allowed 12 hours before the test). Alcohol should not be consumed in the 24 hours prior to the test.

LDL cholesterol

Cholesterol is a waxy substance that can't dissolve in your blood. To circulate in your bloodstream, it piggybacks on carriers called lipoproteins. Low-density lipoprotein (LDL) cholesterol is referred to as "bad" cholesterol because too much of it in your bloodstream causes the buildup of fatty plaques on artery walls. The higher your LDL cholesterol, the greater your risk for heart disease.

What's a desirable LDL cholesterol level? That depends on your risk for developing heart disease—whether it be angina, heart attack, or even death from heart disease—during the next 10 years. Your doctor adds up points related to your age, LDL cholesterol, HDL cholesterol, blood pressure, and whether or not you smoke to calculate what's called the Framingham Risk Score. The Framingham Risk Score was developed from the Framingham Heart Study, an ongoing study that began in 1948 with 5209 healthy men and women from the town of Framingham, Massachusetts. The purpose of the study was to identify common factors that contribute to heart disease by following its development over a long period of time in men and women who had not yet developed symptoms of heart disease or suffered heart attack or stroke. Over the years, the Framingham Heart Study has identified major risk factors for heart disease such as high blood pressure, high cholesterol, smoking, obesity, diabetes, and physical inactivity. At the time of writing, this study continues to make important scientific findings that contribute to the treatment and prevention of coronary heart disease.

The Framingham Risk Score helps predict when a person may suffer angina, heart attack, or die from heart disease. The risk points are weighted differently for men and women. Your risk is stated as a percentage.

Framingham Risk Score

	Risk factors	10-year risk of heart disease
High	Those who have had a cardiac event or have been diagnosed with heart disease or diabetes	≥20%
Moderate	2 or more risk factors	10–19%
Low	Zero to one risk factor	<10%

Your Framingham Risk Score determines the target value for your LDL cholesterol. As you'll see in the chart below, if you are at low risk for developing heart disease, your target LDL cholesterol should be less than 5.0 millimoles per litre (mmol/L). If you are at high risk for heart disease (e.g., you have diabetes), your doctor will want your LDL cholesterol level to be less than 1.8 mmol/L. If your LDL value is higher than the desirable level, your doctor will recommend treatment with lifestyle changes such as diet and exercise, and possibly medication.

Risk ratio

Dividing your total cholesterol value by your HDL cholesterol value gives a risk ratio, a number that's helpful in predicting your likelihood of developing atherosclerosis. A high ratio indicates a higher risk of heart attack, whereas a low ratio denotes a lower risk. Having a high total cholesterol and low HDL cholesterol increases the ratio and is undesirable. Conversely, low total cholesterol and high HDL cholesterol lowers the ratio, and is desirable.

The following chart outlines LDL cholesterol and risk ratio targets based on the Framingham Risk Scores.

Framingham Risk Scores and Risk Ratio Targets

Framingham Risk	10-year risk of heart disease	LDL cholesterol target	Risk ratio target (total cholesterol/ HDL)
High	≥20%	<1.8 mmol/L	<4.0
Moderate	10–19%	<3.5 mmol/L	<5.0
Low	<10%	<5.0 mmol/L	<6.0

If you're considered low risk for developing heart disease, you might think that having an LDL cholesterol value of 4.5 mmol/L seems high even though it's considered acceptable. I tend to share this sentiment. I encourage all of my clients who are in the low risk category—and have an LDL cholesterol result between 3.5 and 5.0 mmol/L—to implement dietary strategies that will help lower their LDL value. In fact, the physicians I work with at the Medcan Clinic in Toronto encourage their low risk patients to do the same. If you're considered low risk and your LDL cholesterol is greater than 5.0 mmol/L, your doctor may advise medication, along with dietary and lifestyle modifications. (You'll learn more about nutrition strategies to lower LDL cholesterol in Chapters 4 and 5.)

HDL cholesterol

High-density lipoproteins (HDL) carry cholesterol away from the arteries towards the liver for degradation. HDL cholesterol keeps the arteries open and blood flowing through them. The higher your HDL level, the lower the risk for heart disease, which is why this one is called the "good" cholesterol.

Reference Ranges for HDL Cholesterol

	Desired	Increased risk
Males to age 19	0.90–1.60 mmol/L	<0.90 mmol/L
Males, 20+ years	≥1.0 mmol/L	<1.0 mmol/L
Females to age 19	0.90–2.40 mmol/L	<0.90 mmol/L
Females, 20+ years	≥1.30 mmol/L	<1.30 mmol/L

Total cholesterol

This is the sum of your LDL and HDL cholesterol values. If your blood's cholesterol content is high, you are at increased risk of heart disease.

Keep in mind that your total cholesterol value is not always relevant. Your LDL cholesterol and risk ratio values are more important in determining your risk for heart disease.

Desired total cholesterol: <5.2 mmol/L

Triglycerides

Triglycerides are fat that is made in the liver from the food you eat. They are transported in your blood on very low-density lipoproteins (VLDL). High triglyceride levels usually mean you eat more calories than you burn or you drink too much alcohol. Elevated blood triglycerides can also be associated with certain diseases such as diabetes and metabolic syndrome as well as some thyroid disorders. High triglyceride levels increase your risk of heart disease.

Desired triglycerides: <1.7 mmol/L

LIPOPROTEIN(a)

Lipoprotein(a), or Lp(a), is a type of LDL cholesterol. Some research has shown that high levels of Lp(a) may be a sign of increased risk of heart disease, though it's not clear how much risk. It's thought that high levels of Lp(a) inhibit the body's ability to dissolve blood clots, thereby increasing the likelihood of a heart attack.

Your doctor might order an Lp(a) test if you have a family history of early-onset heart disease or if you already have heart disease but appear to have otherwise normal total and LDL cholesterol levels. Lp(a) is also tested if your LDL cholesterol doesn't respond well to drug treatment.

Your Lp(a) level is determined by your genes and is not generally affected by diet or lifestyle.

Desired Lp(a): <0.30 grams per litre (g/L)

APOLIPOPROTEIN B (APO B)

Apo B is a protein that is an essential part of the VLDL and LDL carriers that piggyback cholesterol and fat through the bloodstream. Receptors on the surface of your body's cells recognize Apo B and bind to the protein, promoting the uptake of cholesterol into cells.

While the Apo B level tends to mirror the LDL cholesterol level, some experts think that it may prove to be the better indicator of heart disease risk. Apo B reveals the number of LDL particles in your bloodstream and whether you have more of the small, dense LDL cholesterol—the type that is thought to contribute to atherosclerosis. Others disagree but feel that Apo B may offer valuable additional information that can be used to evaluate cardiac risk. (For more information on LDL cholesterol size and risk of heart disease, see Chapter 2, page 38.)

Reference Ranges for Apo B

Males	0.55–1.4 grams per litre (g/L)
Females	0.55–1.25 g/L

The reference range for Apo B may vary among labs.

HIGH SENSITIVITY C-REACTIVE PROTEIN (HS-CRP)

CRP is produced as part of the body's inflammatory process, which responds to injury or infection. Studies suggest that inflammation plays an integral role in atherosclerosis. Think of the normal healing process after a scrape or cut. Immune cells rush to the injury site to fight off harmful bacteria and, in the process, often cause redness and swelling. Scientists now think that heart disease can start when inflammation overstays its welcome, causing a chronic, low-grade inflammatory state.

The amount of CRP in the blood indicates whether there is inflammation in the body; a heightened CRP level indicates inflammation and a higher risk of developing heart disease.

Large studies have found that high CRP levels correlate with a greater risk of heart disease. One such study of 18,000 healthy male physicians linked elevated CRP levels with a 3-fold increase in the risk of heart attack.[2] In the Harvard Women's Health Study, researchers found that CRP was a better predictor of heart attack or stroke than cholesterol levels. Compared to women with the lowest CRP levels, those with the highest level in their blood were seven times more likely to suffer a heart attack or stroke.[3]

What's more, studies show that high CRP levels consistently predict a recurrent cardiac event in patients who have unstable angina or have suffered a heart attack. An elevated CRP is associated with a lower survival rate in these patients.

Reference Ranges for High Sensitivity C-Reactive Protein

Low risk	<1.0 milligrams per litre (mg/L)
Average risk	1.0–3.0 mg/L
High risk	>3.0 mg/L

HOMOCYSTEINE

Homocysteine is an amino acid normally produced by the body to help build and maintain tissues. However, while the body needs homocysteine to function properly, too much is not a good thing. An elevated level in the bloodstream is linked with a greater risk of atherosclerosis, heart attack, stroke, and possibly even Alzheimer's disease. High homocysteine damages artery walls and promotes the buildup of fatty plaques.

Homocysteine is transformed into harmless compounds with the help of folic acid (a B vitamin also called folate), vitamin B12, and vitamin B6. A lack of these vitamins in the body can hamper the natural breakdown of homocysteine, causing it to accumulate in the bloodstream. Studies show that higher intakes of folic acid and higher blood levels of the B vitamin are associated with lower blood homocysteine levels. (You'll learn which foods help lower homocysteine in Chapter 5, page 140.)

Although it's well established that B vitamins, especially folic acid, can lower elevated homocysteine, it's not clear if doing so can actually ward off a heart attack. Even so, your doctor may order this blood test if you've had heart problems or if a family member developed heart disease at a young age.

Normal range for homocysteine: 5–15 micromoles per litre (μmol/L)

FIBRINOGEN

Fibrinogen is a protein made by the liver that helps your blood clot. The level of fibrinogen in your bloodstream then is a reflection of your body's blood-clotting ability. If your fibrinogen level is elevated, you might be at increased risk for developing a blood clot that could lead to a heart attack. Fibrinogen may also be an indicator of inflammation caused by atherosclerosis.

Fibrinogen level as a screening test for heart disease has not gained widespread acceptance because there are no direct treatments for an elevated presence. Nevertheless, many doctors feel that a fibrinogen result gives them additional information that may lead them to be more aggressive in treating risk factors such as high cholesterol and high blood pressure.

Normal range for fibrinogen: 2.0–4.0 grams per litre (g/L)

BRAIN NATRIURETIC PEPTIDE (BNP)

BNP is a protein produced by your heart and blood vessels, and indicates how well your heart is working. Normally, only a small amount of BNP is found in your bloodstream. However, if your heart is damaged and has to work harder than usual, it secretes more BNP into the blood. BNP levels can rise with new or worsening chest pain.

An elevated BNP presence may also be an indicator of heart failure or strain on the heart muscle. And doctors use BNP levels to assess the progress of heart failure treatment over time (the level should get lower if treatment is working). People with arrhythmias may also have a high BNP.

Some research suggests that BNP testing isn't much better at predicting your risk of heart disease than is assessing traditional risk factors, such as high cholesterol, obesity, and smoking. BNP is used more as a marker of the heart's pumping ability.

Reference Ranges for BNP

Range	Interpretation
0–125 picograms per millilitre (pg/mL)	No heart failure present
126–350 pg/mL	Heart failure may be present If repeat test still elevated, your doctor will refer you for further cardiac investigation.
351–900 pg/mL	Moderate heart failure; further cardiac tests required
>900 pg/mL	Severe heart failure

Normal values for BNP: vary among labs and depend on the method used for measurement.

HEMOGLOBIN A1c (HbA1c)

This test measures how well a person's diabetes is being controlled. Hemoglobin is a pigment within red blood cells that carries oxygen throughout the body. When diabetes is not controlled, sugar (glucose) builds up in your blood and combines with your hemoglobin, making it *glycated*, or sticky with sugar.

The HbA1c test provides an average of your blood glucose measurements over the previous 6 to 12 weeks. If levels have been high during those weeks, the HbA1c result will be higher.

You're probably wondering what blood sugar has to do with heart disease risk. The fact is, having diabetes substantially boosts your risk of angina, heart attack, and sudden cardiac death. What's more, research clearly shows that having elevated HbA1c is strongly linked with both the risk of developing and dying from heart disease.

The relationship between HbA1c and heart disease is even seen in people without known diabetes. In a study of 10,232 men and women, researchers found that those with an HbA1c reading of less than 5% had the lowest risk of heart disease. A rise of 1% in HbA1c increased the risk of dying from any cause by 24%.[4]

Reference Ranges for Hemoglobin A1c

0.040–0.060 (4–6%)	Non-diabetic
<0.070 (<7%)	Optimal diabetic control*
0.070–0.084 (7–8.4%)	Suboptimal diabetic control
>0.084 (>8.4%)	Inadequate diabetic control

*If you have diabetes, your doctor may prefer your HbA1c to be less than 0.060 if this can be achieved without the risk of low blood sugar reactions.

Screening procedures

Sadly, for many people, the first symptom of coronary artery disease is a heart attack or sudden death, with no chest pain to warn them that they have heart disease. For this reason, doctors use screening tests to detect signs of heart disease before a serious medical event occurs. The tests described below are especially important for people with heart disease risk factors such as diabetes, cigarette smoking, high blood pressure, high cholesterol, and family history. (For information about risk factors for heart disease, see Chapter 2.)

It's important to discuss your particular heart disease risks with your doctor in order to decide if screening tests are necessary. The choice of which and how many tests to perform will depend on your risk factors, history of heart problems, and presence of current symptoms such as chest pain.

CORONARY ANGIOGRAPHY

An angiogram is an X-ray that uses a special dye and camera to take pictures of the blood flow in a coronary artery. During an angiogram, which is performed in a clinic or hospital, a long, thin, flexible tube called a catheter is placed into either the femoral blood vessel in the groin or a vessel just above the elbow. The catheter is guided to the area to be studied, then an iodine dye is injected into the blood vessel to make the area show clearly on an X-ray. An angiogram tells doctors if atherosclerosis is present and how severe it is. Angiography may be recommended for people with angina or those with suspected heart disease. It may also be used if the doctor is considering surgery because it shows a clear picture of the blood vessels.

While an angiogram was once commonly used to check the condition of blood vessels, today other non-invasive tests provide the same information with less discomfort and risk to the patient.

CORONARY CATHETERIZATION

This gold-standard test is the one most commonly used to diagnose or confirm heart disease. Doctors will recommend this test for patients who have chest pain or an abnormal result on the exercise stress test or nuclear stress test (e.g., Cardiolite test). Done in a hospital, this test involves inserting a thin tube called a catheter into a blood vessel in your arm, groin, or neck. The catheter is then threaded to your heart. Through the catheter, cardiologists can evaluate heart valves, heart function, and blood supply. It may also be performed to determine if someone needs heart surgery. Cardiac catheterization is often used in conjunction with other tests, such as angiography.

COMPUTED TOMOGRAPHY ANGIOGRAM (CTA)

Like coronary catheterization, this test evaluates whether either fatty deposits or calcium deposits have built up in the coronary arteries, but it's less invasive, using only an IV in your arm. Patients undergoing a coronary CTA scan receive an intravenous contrast dye to ensure the best-possible images. The same IV may be used to give a medication to slow or stabilize heart rate in order to get a better image of the heart. During the test, beams of X-rays pass through the body and are picked up by special detectors in the scanner to create three-dimensional computerized images of the walls of the heart and coronary arteries.

The coronary CTA is controversial because it carries some risk from X-ray exposure (potential for stimulating cancer) and contrast dye exposure (allergic reactions and kidney damage).

In Canada, the coronary CTA is used for those considered high-risk patients and not good candidates for other screening tests. However, some doctors speculate there may be a role for CTA in screening patients who fall into the "intermediate" Framingham risk category. In the United States, the test has become more commercial despite its controversy.

DOPPLER ULTRASOUND

This non-invasive test, usually performed in a clinic, evaluates blood flow and pressure in blood vessels by bouncing high-frequency sound waves off red blood cells. Doctors use the test to diagnose narrowed or blocked arteries, the presence of blood clots, and heart valve defects.

Just prior to the test, a technician applies a special gel on your chest to improve sound quality. A hand-held transducer placed on your skin transmits sound waves that are picked up and converted into images of your blood vessels. The test is painless and takes about 30 minutes.

ECHOCARDIOGRAM

Like the Doppler test, an echocardiogram, or echo test, uses sound waves to take a moving picture of your heart. The recorded sound waves show the shape and size of your heart and its valves, how well they are working, and whether you have a blood clot. Your doctor may recommend this test if you have unexplained chest pain, shortness of breath, palpitations (sensation of rapid heartbeats), or a history of stroke.

An echocardiogram takes 15 to 45 minutes and involves no discomfort whatsoever.

ELECTROCARDIOGRAM (ECG OR EKG)

This test detects problems by recording the electrical activity that causes your heart to contract and pump blood. An electrocardiogram measures whether it takes a normal, fast, or irregular length of time for the electrical impulse to travel through your heart.

ECG readings can reveal evidence of a heart attack, lack of blood flow to the heart, an irregular heartbeat, and a heart that does not pump blood strongly enough. An ECG test may be advised if you are experiencing abnormal heart rhythms, palpitations, chest pain, unexplained fatigue, or dizziness.

The test is painless, takes about 10 minutes, and you just have to lie there. A technician attaches 12 sticky patches (electrodes) about the size of a quarter to the skin of the chest, arms, and legs. The electrodes detect the electrical signals of your heart, and a machine records them on graph paper or displays them on a screen.

EXERCISE ELECTROCARDIOGRAM (TREADMILL STRESS TEST)

An exercise electrocardiogram test checks for changes in your heart's electrical activity, heart rate, and blood pressure while you're exercising. Sometimes abnormal ECG readings can be seen only during exertion or while symptoms are present. An exercise ECG is performed while walking on a treadmill or pedalling a stationary bicycle.

Like the resting ECG described above, an exercise ECG translates the heart's electrical activity into line tracings on paper, which are then interpreted by your doctor. This test is performed in a clinic or hospital and takes between 15 and 30 minutes.

An exercise ECG is usually done to evaluate chest pain, especially if heart disease is suspected. If heart disease is already confirmed, an exercise ECG may be done to determine how far the disease has progressed and how much exercise can be done safely.

In general, the accuracy of the standard exercise electrocardiogram to diagnose heart disease is about 68% and, as a result, it may provide limited information. American television journalist Tim Russert's sudden cardiac death at age 58 in June 2008 highlighted the fact that Treadmill Stress Tests aren't foolproof and don't always reveal that heart problems are brewing. Two months prior to his death, Russert had performed well on an exercise stress test (as had former U.S. president Bill Clinton prior to complaints of chest pain and shortness of breath that prompted coronary bypass surgery). Plaque that's on the walls of a coronary artery but that's not yet thick enough to block blood flow to the heart won't affect a stress test. And there's no way to predict when plaque might rupture and obstruct blood flow to the heart.

The Treadmill Stress Test can also yield false positive results—as much as 30% of the time in women. For this reason, some doctors prefer a nuclear scan (e.g., thallium or Cardiolite test), which is more sensitive because it assesses blood flow.

THALLIUM AND CARDIOLITE SCANS

These scans determine the blood flow to the heart muscle when the heart is under stress (that is, during exercise) and at rest. The presence or absence of a significant problem can usually be documented with this test.

As with the electrocardiogram (ECG), electrodes are placed on your chest. Your blood pressure, heart rate, and ECG are recorded. The scan uses a radioactive tracer, thallium or Cardiolite, to see how much blood is reaching various parts of your heart.

This scan requires you to perform a "graded" exercise test on a treadmill. It begins with the treadmill at a slow speed and a little uphill inclination. Every 3 minutes, the treadmill increases in speed and incline. The technician may stop the test at any time for medical reasons, or you may stop the test because of significant fatigue or discomfort.

Just before you need to stop exercising, a small amount of the radioactive tracer is injected into a vein in your arm and circulates during the final minute of exercise. The heart muscle, in proportion to the blood flow through the coronary arteries, takes up the radioactive marker. Heart muscle receiving normal blood flow accumulates a larger amount of thallium/Cardiolite than cardiac muscle that is supplied by diseased coronary arteries.

After exercise, a special camera takes X-ray-like pictures of blood flow to the heart. Areas of the heart with poor blood supply show up as dark spots on the scan.

To prepare for the test, you will be advised not to eat or drink at least 3 hours prior and to avoid alcohol, cigarette smoking, caffeinated beverages, and over-the-counter medications for 24 hours before the test.

These nuclear scans are recommended for people with unexplained chest pain or to learn more about abnormal ECG readings. As well, your doctor may propose this screening test if you have multiple risk factors and previous testing is inconclusive for the presence of heart disease. A thallium or Cardiolite scan is also used to determine the size and location of damaged heart tissue after a heart attack.

HOLTER MONITORING

A Holter monitor is a portable ECG device that records your heart rhythm continuously for 24 hours while you're away from the hospital or clinic. Whereas a regular ECG examines your heart's electrical activity for a few minutes, the Holter monitor allows your doctor to examine changes over a sustained period as you carry on daily activities and as you sleep. Your heart's electrical impulses are transmitted to the Holter monitor recorder via sticky electrodes placed on your chest. The data is then played back on a computer and analyzed by your doctor.

Holter monitoring is usually used to evaluate symptoms such as dizziness and palpitations that might be related to heart rhythm disturbances.

EVENT MONITORING

An event monitor also records the electrical activity of your heart when you're away from the doctor's office. The monitor consists of two devices you wear while doing normal activities: one, the size of a beeper; the other, worn like a wristwatch. Sensors are attached to your chest with sticky patches. Wires connect the sensors to the monitor. You usually can clip the monitor to your belt or carry it in your pocket.

Unlike the Holter monitor, an event monitor does not record your heart's activity continuously over a 24-hour period. It's worn for a longer time—weeks to a month—and doesn't start recording until you feel symptoms and trigger the monitor. Event monitors tend to be smaller than Holter monitors because they don't need to store as much data.

After an event, you can transmit the recording over the phone to the monitoring station where the data will be saved. Or you can store the information in the monitor's memory and send it later to the monitoring station.

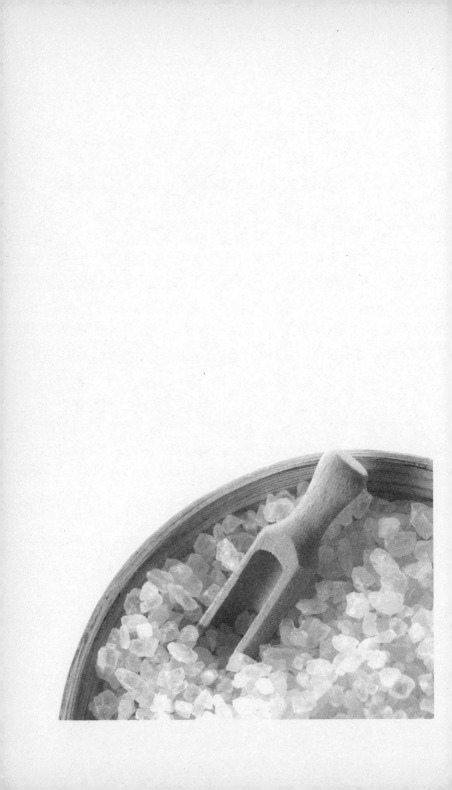

2

Are you at risk for heart disease?

By now you're probably wondering if you're at risk for heart disease. Or perhaps you've survived a heart attack and you're wondering how you got heart disease in the first place. There are many circumstances, called risk factors, that increase the likelihood of developing coronary artery disease and having a heart attack. The more risk factors you have, or the more severe their condition, the higher your risk for succumbing to heart disease. You may be born with some of these risk factors while others, like high blood pressure, overweight, and smoking, may develop over the years.

Researchers have learned that an overwhelmingly high proportion—90%!—of first heart attacks can be attributed to nine risk factors: cigarette smoking, high blood pressure, diabetes, abnormal blood lipid profile (high cholesterol), abdominal obesity, stress, physical inactivity, moderate alcohol drinking, and a lack of daily fruits and vegetables. The Canadian-led global study called INTERHEART involved 15,152 patients who had a first heart attack and 14,820 symptom-free control participants from 52 countries. Data about lifestyle and health status were collected from questionnaires, physical exams, and blood tests.

The INTERHEART findings should serve as a wake-up call to people who are not taking charge of risk factors that can be controlled. In the study, individuals who smoked more than one pack of cigarettes each day were nine times more likely than non-smokers to suffer a heart attack. People who had high blood pressure and diabetes and who smoked cigarettes boosted their risk of heart attack 13-fold compared to individuals who didn't have these risk factors. Even more alarming, having all nine risk factors mentioned above elevated the risk of heart attack more than 100-fold compared with not having any of these risk factors.[1]

The INTERHEART study investigators also discovered that certain risk factors affect men and women differently. High blood pressure, diabetes, physical activity, and moderate alcohol use were more strongly linked with heart attack in women than in men. On the other hand, the connection between heart attack and abnormal blood cholesterol, smoking, abdominal obesity, poor eating habits, and stress was similar in men and women.[2]

Major risk factors

Extensive scientific studies have identified a number of factors that increase the risk of developing heart disease, as well as major factors that significantly boost heart disease risk. Some of these risk factors, such as age, gender, and heredity, are beyond your control to change. Fortunately, though, there are other risk factors that you do have some—even a lot—of influence over. The major risk factors you can control include high blood pressure, high cholesterol, diabetes, overweight, physical inactivity, and cigarette smoking.

It's important to know your own constellation of risk factors in order to minimize their effect and reduce your risk of heart disease. Keep in mind that having one or more major risk factors doesn't mean that heart disease is unavoidable—but the reality is, the more risk factors you have, the higher your odds of developing heart disease at some point. According to the Heart and Stroke Foundation of Canada, 8 out of 10 Canadians have at least one risk factor for heart disease (e.g., smoking, overweight, physical inactivity, high blood pressure, diabetes) and 1 in 10 has three or more.[3]

AGING

As you grow older, your risk of heart disease increases. In fact, about 80% of people over the age of 65 have some form of heart disease. As we age, the heart's function tends to weaken, our arteries get stiffer, and the artery walls become thicker. What's more, other risk factors for heart disease—high blood pressure, elevated cholesterol, and diabetes—become more prevalent with aging.

Youth and heart disease

Adults aren't the only ones at risk for heart disease. Children are susceptible to atherosclerosis too. High blood pressure and high cholesterol are increasingly showing up in children and teenagers. Type 2 diabetes—previously considered an adult disease—has also escalated dramatically in kids. In fact, experts predict that today's children will be the first generation for some time to have poorer health and a shorter life expectancy than their parents.

The epidemic of childhood obesity is blamed for heart disease risk factors developing at an uncharacteristically young age. Today, it's estimated that 26% of kids aged 2 to 17 years are considered overweight or obese, and the number of children considered obese has tripled since 1978.[4]

In July 2008, in an effort to reduce a child's future risk of heart disease, the American Academy of Pediatrics (AAP) released recommendations to measure blood cholesterol in kids and teenagers who have a family history of high cholesterol or early-onset heart disease ($\leq$55 years of age for men and $\leq$65 years for women). It further advised that children whose family history is unknown, those who are overweight, and those who have high blood pressure or diabetes be screened after age 2, but no later than age 10. The report recommends that total cholesterol, LDL cholesterol, HDL cholesterol, and triglycerides be measured, and if results fall within the desirable range, retesting be done every 3 to 5 years. (See Chapter 1, page 13, for more information about these blood tests.)

Such screening might sound aggressive, but it's well established that heart disease begins in childhood and that it's progressive. One study conducted in youth who died of accidental causes found fatty streaks in the coronary arteries of 50% of children and 69% of young adults. What's more, the extent of fatty buildup in the arteries was shown to increase with age.

The AAP guidelines also recommend that doctors consider statin therapy in children 8 years and older who have high LDL cholesterol; in children with a family history of early heart disease; or those who have at least two risk factors for heart disease, such as obesity and high blood pressure. In addition, it's also recommended that doctors consider using statins for kids who have diabetes and elevated LDL cholesterol. At the time of writing, the Canadian Paediatric Society did not have a position on the use of statins in children, but Canadian doctors will undoubtedly take note of U.S. guidelines and treat kids on an individual basis.

The recommendation to prescribe cholesterol-lowering statin drugs to kids as young as 8 was met with harsh criticism from many health professionals. With no long-term safety data to back up the recommendations, critics can't fathom putting children on statins for decades. And some argue that prescribing these drugs is tantamount to giving up on dietary avenues to lower cholesterol. As a parent, you also might be reluctant for your child to pop a pill to lower cholesterol.

Most kids don't need statins to ward off a future heart attack—they need a healthy diet. The AAP's new guidelines should alert parents that their children could be building up fatty deposits in their arteries and should reinforce the need for a healthy lifestyle. The take-home message: It's imperative for both parents and children to take stock of personal risk factors and adopt heart healthy lifestyle behaviours early in life.

GENDER

Men are more likely than women to have heart attacks, and to have them at a younger age. The reasons are unclear but, on average, men develop heart disease 10 years earlier than women. The average age for a first heart attack is 56 in men versus 65 in women. Although heart disease was once seen as a male disease, the gap between men and women has narrowed. In fact, in Canada today, women are more likely to die of a heart attack or stroke than men.

Women and heart disease

A woman's risk of heart disease increases as she ages and rises significantly after menopause. During a woman's reproductive lifecycle, the naturally occurring hormone estrogen provides built-in protection from heart disease. Estrogen reduces the body's total cholesterol level by regulating the amount of cholesterol produced by the liver and by helping cells clear LDL (bad) cholesterol from the bloodstream. This helps raise a woman's HDL (good) cholesterol and lower her LDL cholesterol. Estrogen may also aid in keeping blood vessels more flexible.

It's important to note that estrogen does not protect all women from heart disease. Pre-menopausal women with diabetes are as likely to have a heart attack as men of the same age. (You'll learn more about why diabetes increases the risk of heart disease later in this chapter.)

During menopause, which usually occurs around the age of 51, a woman's ovaries start producing less and less estrogen. As a result, a woman's LDL cholesterol level rises as her HDL cholesterol level falls. By age 65, a woman's risk of heart attack equals a man's because she no longer produces estrogen.

If you're a female reading this book, it's important to understand that heart disease affects men and women differently. According to the Heart and Stroke Foundation of Canada, women are at higher risk of dying following a heart attack. They are less likely to be treated by a specialist, are less likely to be transferred to another facility for treatment, and are less likely to undergo certain cardiac medical procedures.

This gender gap may be due, in part, to the fact that men and women may experience different symptoms and respond differently to treatments. Compared to men, women who have heart attacks tend to be older, are more likely to have high blood pressure and diabetes, and often have other diseases such as arthritis or osteoporosis that can mask heart attack symptoms.

As well, if you recall from Chapter 1, the symptoms of heart attack are slightly different in women. Women, more than men, are prone to non-typical symptoms such as neck and shoulder pain, nausea, sweating, fatigue, and shortness of breath in addition to chest pain. Silent heart attacks are also more common in women. Whether out of denial or lack of awareness of both typical and non-typical symptoms, women tend to delay seeking treatment for signs of heart disease.

Hormone replacement therapy (HRT) and heart disease

You might be wondering if post-menopausal women should take estrogen therapy to regain the hormone's heart-protective benefits. In the 1980s and 1990s, several studies suggested that estrogen was an important strategy not only for preventing heart disease in healthy women, but also for reducing the risk of a recurrent heart attack in women with the disease. Many researchers believed this was due to estrogen's ability to maintain healthier, pre-menopausal HDL and LDL levels. Because of these study findings, there was a shift from prescribing hormone replacement therapy for short-term relief of menopausal symptoms such as hot flashes to prescribing it for the prevention of heart disease (and osteoporosis).

This prescribing pattern came to an end in 2002 when the long-term use of HRT fell out of favour in the medical community. That's when the Women's Health Initiative (WHI) Study investigating combined HRT (estrogen plus progestin) in 27,000 women aged 50 to 79 was abruptly halted after 5 years. The goal of the study was to determine whether HRT protected from heart disease and osteoporosis, and whether it increased the risk of cancer and blood clots.[5]

The results revealed that women taking HRT were at increased risk for heart disease, blood clots, stroke, and breast cancer. (The hormone regimen was found to safeguard against hip fracture and colon cancer, but more women suffered a serious health problem than a positive one.)

In 2004, a second group of WHI researchers investigating the effect of estrogen-only replacement therapy (i.e., no progestin) reported their results. Again, the women were told to stop taking their estrogen pills after the study concluded that estrogen alone did not appear to affect (neither increase nor decrease) heart disease risk. At the same time, estrogen appeared to increase the risk of stroke.[6]

As a result of these findings, the Heart and Stroke Foundation of Canada recommends that women do not begin to use or continue to use HRT, either estrogen alone or combined estrogen-progestin, for the sole purpose of preventing heart disease. If you are taking HRT and are concerned about your heart health, discuss the risks and benefits of HRT and the goals of your treatment with your doctor.

FAMILY HISTORY

Heart disease runs in families, so you are more likely to develop it if you have a parent or sibling with coronary heart disease. The link between family history and increased risk is limited to early-onset heart disease. If a male member of your immediate family developed heart disease before age 55 or a female relative was diagnosed before age 65, then you have a higher risk of developing the disease.

ETHNIC BACKGROUND

Your ethnicity, also tied to heredity, may also increase your risk. First Nations people and those of African or South Asian descent are at greater risk of heart disease and stroke than the general population because they are more likely to develop high blood pressure and diabetes.

CIGARETTE SMOKING

Without a doubt, smoking is one of the major avoidable causes of heart disease. Studies show that smokers are two to four times more likely to develop heart disease than non-smokers. Smoking also boosts the risk of sudden cardiac death among people with heart disease.

Smoking damages the heart in a number of ways. It speeds up heart rate, damages the cells that line your blood vessels, lowers HDL (good) cholesterol, and can cause irregular heartbeats. Smoking also increases the tendency for the formation of blood clots, which can cause heart attack and stroke.

The INTERHEART study involving 27,089 participants in 52 countries determined that the risk of having a non-fatal heart attack was nearly three times greater for smokers than for people who never smoked. Exposure to second-hand smoke also increased the risk of heart attack, with the amount of exposure making a difference. Compared to people who were not exposed to second-hand smoke, those with the least exposure (1 to 7 hours per week) were 24% more likely and those with the most exposure (more than 21 hours per week) were 62% more likely to suffer a heart attack.[7]

The good news is that quitting smoking immediately reduces your risk of heart disease—and the longer you're a former smoker, the greater the risk reduction. If you already have heart disease, you can lower your risk of dying from the condition if you stop smoking. A review of 20 studies in patients with a diagnosis of heart disease concluded that the risk of dying fell by 36% for those who quit smoking compared to those who continued.[8]

While smoking rates have declined among men and women of all age groups, it's estimated that 19% of the population aged 15 and older (slightly less than 5 million Canadians) still smoke an average of 15 cigarettes per day.[9]

HIGH BLOOD CHOLESTEROL

When you think about risk factors for heart attack, undoubtedly blood cholesterol comes to mind. We've known for years that excess cholesterol in your bloodstream directly increases your heart disease risk. This message has been kept top of mind through media reports of the latest scientific study or the constant commercial pitches for heart healthy foods like oat bran, psyllium-enriched breakfast cereals, and certain brands of margarine. The fact is, managing your blood cholesterol is a very important strategy to guard against atherosclerosis and heart attack.

Cholesterol is a wax-like fatty substance in your bloodstream. The majority of it—80% to 85%—is made by your liver. The rest comes from the foods you eat, like meat, poultry, fish, seafood, and dairy products. (Plant foods such as fruits, vegetables, whole grains, legumes, nuts, and seeds contain no cholesterol.)

Despite its bad reputation, we actually do need cholesterol. It is vital for maintaining cell membranes and nerve sheaths, forming sex hormones (estrogen, progesterone, and testosterone), and producing bile acids that aid digestion. Cholesterol also plays an important role in the skin's ability to make vitamin D when exposed to sunlight.

Your body produces all the cholesterol it needs to maintain health. When you eat foods rich in cholesterol and saturated (animal) fat, it triggers your liver to churn out more cholesterol. (You'll learn more about foods that raise—and lower—blood cholesterol in Chapter 4.) And if there's too much cholesterol in your bloodstream, it can accumulate on artery walls. Over time, this fatty buildup causes the arteries to become stiff and narrowed (what's called "hardening" of the arteries), which can slow or block blood flow to the heart. As you learned in Chapter 1, plaques on narrowed arteries can break off and obstruct blood flow to the heart and other parts of the body.

It's estimated than 40% of Canadians—as many as 10 million—have a cholesterol level higher than the recommended target.[10] Since high blood cholesterol causes no symptoms, the only way to know is to have your doctor measure your lipid profile—your total blood cholesterol, LDL (bad) cholesterol, HDL (good) cholesterol, and triglycerides—during your regular physical exams.

Your total cholesterol is the combined measure of your LDL and HDL cholesterol, and a healthy total is less than 5.2 mmol/L. While this number is important to know, your individual LDL and HDL levels are more important than your total cholesterol level. Each type of cholesterol has a distinct role in the body and impacts your risk for heart disease differently. Here's a quick overview of the "bad" versus "good" cholesterol.

LDL cholesterol

Most of the cholesterol in your blood is the LDL or "bad" type, which deposits on artery walls and increases the risk of heart disease. Normally, the cells in your body clear LDL cholesterol from your bloodstream for use in essential functions. LDL cholesterol particles attach to LDL receptors on the surface of the cell, and then enter. But if a cell has all the cholesterol it needs, it reduces its number of LDL receptors. LDL cholesterol then accumulates in the bloodstream and—you guessed it—slowly builds up on artery walls.

LDL cholesterol comes in all shapes and sizes, and some particles may carry a greater risk of heart disease than others. Scientists view LDL cholesterol particles under a powerful microscope to determine their size. It turns out that large, fluffy-looking particles are relatively harmless because they don't damage artery walls. On the other hand, small, dense particles do more damage because they are able to slip through the lining of artery walls. They are also more easily oxidized, or damaged by harmful free radicals that roam the body. These oxidized LDL cholesterol particles are more likely to form cholesterol-rich plaques. Research indicates that people with small LDL cholesterol particles have a 3-fold higher risk of heart disease than people with large-particle LDL cholesterol.

Experts now think that the lower your LDL cholesterol, the better. Your target number depends on your risk for developing or dying from heart disease over the next 10 years. Lowering elevated total and LDL cholesterol is important for everyone: children and adults, men and women, and people with and without heart disease.

Both genetics and diet have a significant influence on a person's cholesterol level. For instance, 1 in 500 people have the disorder familial hypercholesterolemia (inherited high cholesterol), caused by a genetic defect that results in few or no LDL receptors in the body. As a result, LDL cholesterol can't be removed from the body and builds up to very high levels in the bloodstream. People with familial hypercholesterolemia tend to develop heart disease during early adulthood. Medications are required to bring LDL cholesterol down to a safe level.

Most people with high cholesterol don't have familial hypercholesterolemia. Proper diet, exercise, and sometimes medications are necessary to lower cholesterol. You'll learn which foods to eat and which ones to limit to lower your cholesterol in Chapter 4.

Apo B cholesterol

The level of small, dense LDL cholesterol tends to rise with increasing blood triglyceride (fat) levels. High levels also tend to run in families. While some experts feel that determining the number of small, dense LDL particles is more predictive of heart attack than knowing the level of LDL cholesterol, it's not usually necessary for your doctor to measure the size of your LDL cholesterol. Knowing the results of your lipid profile, along with other risk factors for heart disease, is enough to determine appropriate treatment in most cases.

However, because about half of all heart attacks occur in people with normal levels of LDL cholesterol, there are circumstances in which your doctor may want to determine LDL particle size. If your LDL cholesterol number is healthy, and you have other risk factors for heart disease, your doctor may measure the apolipoprotein B (apo B) in your blood. This test reveals the number of LDL particles and indicates whether you have more of the small, dense LDL cholesterol.

HDL cholesterol

This type of cholesterol is considered good because it picks up excess cholesterol from different organs in your body and disposes of it through the liver, which helps prevent LDL cholesterol from damaging your arteries. Some experts also think that HDL removes cholesterol from plaques on artery walls, thereby slowing their growth.

The higher your HDL cholesterol, the lower your risk for heart disease. Studies indicate that even small increases in HDL cholesterol can reduce the odds of having a heart attack. Regular aerobic exercise, weight loss, and quitting smoking help to boost HDL cholesterol. As you'll read later on in this book, a daily intake of one to two alcoholic beverages and the B vitamin niacin can also raise HDL. But because of other health risks associated with moderate alcohol intake, I don't advise that you drink alcohol to increase your HDL level.

See Chapter 1, pages 13–17, for more information about the lipid profile and target values for total, LDL, and HDL cholesterol levels.

Triglycerides

There is controversy around whether high levels of this fat in the bloodstream increase the risk of heart disease. However, it is known that having elevated blood triglycerides and a high LDL cholesterol level creates more risk of heart attack than having elevated triglycerides alone. As well, it's recognized that people with high triglycerides also have other risk factors for heart disease, such as obesity, low levels of HDL, poorly controlled blood sugar, and small, dense LDL particles.

Triglycerides come from the liver and diet. In some instances, high triglyceride levels are the result of an inherited disorder. Elevated triglycerides can also be caused by diabetes, kidney disease, and estrogen-containing medications such as birth control pills. In most cases, however, high blood triglycerides arise from overweight, excessive alcohol consumption, and high sugar intakes. You'll learn more about lowering triglycerides through lifestyle modifications in Chapter 4.

See Chapter 1, page 17, for the desired level for blood triglycerides.

Medications to lower blood lipids

The first defence against high cholesterol and triglycerides is lifestyle changes such as diet, exercise, and weight loss if you're overweight. But sometimes lifestyle modifications aren't enough. Your doctor may prescribe medication if you've made these changes and your lipids are still high, if you're high risk and need to get your LDL cholesterol number very low, or if you have high LDL cholesterol in addition to other risk factors for heart disease. Several classes of medications are available in Canada to lower blood lipids.

Statins are the most commonly prescribed to lower cholesterol. They work by blocking the liver enzyme, HMG-CoA reductase, which promotes cholesterol production. Depletion of cholesterol in your liver cells causes your liver to remove cholesterol from your bloodstream. Studies show these drugs can lower LDL cholesterol by as much as 50%. Clinical trials have also demonstrated that statins prevent heart attacks in men who have elevated cholesterol and in members of both sexes who already have heart disease.

Drugs known as *resins*, or bile acid sequestrants, lower cholesterol but work differently than statins. Resins bind bile acids in the intestinal tract, causing them to be excreted in your stool. If you'll recall from earlier in this chapter, bile acids are made from cholesterol and help the body digest fat. The body reabsorbs a certain amount of these bile acids, but when resins remove more, they prompt your liver to use excess cholesterol to make more of these digestive aids.

Fibrates lower elevated blood lipids by reducing the liver's production of VLDL particles, the lipoprotein carriers that transport triglycerides in the blood, and by speeding up the removal of triglycerides from the bloodstream.

Drugs Used in Canada to Treat Elevated Blood Lipids

Medication	Used to lower	Possible side effects
Statins Lescol (fluvastatin) Mevacor (lovastatin) Zocor (simvastatin) Lipitor (atorvastatin) Pravachol (pravastatin) Crestor (rosuvastatin)	Total cholesterol LDL cholesterol Triglycerides And increase HDL cholesterol	Fever, muscle aches, cramps Unusual fatigue, weakness Headache Constipation, heartburn, stomach pain
Resins Questran (cholestyramine) Colestid (colestipol)	LDL cholesterol And increase HDL cholesterol	Muscle aches or pains Diarrhea Stomach pain, nausea, vomiting
Fibrates Lopid (gemfibrozil) Bezalip (bezafibrate) Lipidil (fenofibrate)	Triglycerides And increase HDL cholesterol	Fever, chills, sore throat Muscle pain Unusual fatigue, weakness Gas, upset stomach
Nicotinic acid Niacin	Total cholesterol LDL cholesterol Triglycerides And increase HDL cholesterol	Skin rash Flushing, itching Headache

Niacin, also known as nicotinic acid, may be prescribed in high doses to inhibit your liver's ability to make cholesterol and triglycerides. Niacin is more effective in raising HDL cholesterol and lowering triglycerides than it is in lowering LDL cholesterol. Nutrition supplements containing niacin, or vitamin B3, are not recommended for cholesterol lowering. Not only are they ineffective but high doses can damage your liver. Niacin should only be taken as a cholesterol-lowering medication if prescribed by your doctor. Side effects of high dose niacin include flushing, headache, and stomach upset. However, the greatest risk is liver damage. If you're prescribed this medication, your doctor will regularly monitor your liver function by measuring the liver enzymes in your blood stream.

The chart on page 40 outlines drugs used in Canada to lower elevated blood lipids.

In some cases, doctors will prescribe a combination of drugs to treat elevated blood lipids. Like any drug, cholesterol-lowering medications are not without side effects. Some disappear after a few days or weeks of taking the drug while others can be more serious. Always report any side effects to your doctor. Upon starting any new medication, your doctor will monitor your blood work, with particular attention to liver function. (Cholesterol-lowering statin drugs and niacin may cause abnormal liver enzyme levels.)

One rare but potentially serious side effect of statin drugs is *rhabdomyolysis*, a severe muscle deterioration that releases muscle proteins into the blood. Muscle pain usually starts in the larger muscles of the legs or shoulders. If this happens, see your physician immediately.

HIGH BLOOD PRESSURE (HYPERTENSION)

Anyone can have high blood pressure, but it's more common as we get older and become overweight. One in five Canadians has high blood pressure, a major risk factor for heart disease. Because as many as 43% of Canadians don't even know they have high blood pressure, the prevalence of hypertension may be much higher than estimated. One thing is certain: Thanks to our rising rates of obesity, the number of Canadians with high blood pressure is increasing. From 1995 to 2005, the number of adults in Ontario with hypertension more than doubled. What's more, the prevalence of high blood pressure was slightly higher among younger adults than older adults.[11]

Hypertension usually does not cause symptoms. But the effects of this silent condition on your health are not so subtle. Not only does hypertension cause heart attack, it can lead to stroke, congestive heart failure, dementia, and, over time, kidney disease. Having high blood pressure damages your arteries and increases your heart's workload, causing the heart to thicken and become stiffer.

Blood pressure is the force generated by your heart and exerted on your artery walls as your blood circulates. When your heart beats, blood pressure in your arteries rises. Between beats, when your heart relaxes, blood pressure falls. If the pressure remains elevated over time, it's called high blood pressure, or hypertension.

Blood pressure is measured in millimetres of mercury (mmHg). Your blood pressure is really two measurements: your *systolic blood pressure* and your *diastolic blood pressure*. You may have heard someone say his or her blood pressure is 115 over 75 (115/75). The first (or top) number is systolic pressure, the pressure created when your heart is pumping out blood. The second (or bottom) number is the diastolic pressure, the pressure when your heart muscle is relaxing and filling with blood.

Adults generally should have a blood pressure of less than 130/80. Hypertension is defined as a systolic pressure of ≥140 mmHg or a diastolic pressure of ≥90 mmHg. One in five Canadians fall into the category called prehypertension: 130–139/85–89 mmHg (high normal blood pressure). Unless lifestyle changes are made to bring blood pressure down, 60% of people with prehypertension will develop hypertension in 4 years.

Do You Have High Blood Pressure?

	Millimetres of mercury (mmHg)
Normal blood pressure	<120/<80
Prehypertension	130–139/85–89
Hypertension	≥140/≥90

Because prehypertension and hypertension usually don't cause symptoms, it's important to have your blood pressure checked annually as an adult. You should ensure annual monitoring if you have prehypertension and even more frequent checks if your blood pressure is high. Even children should have their blood pressure measured, beginning at the age of 2. A blood pressure reading is taken by putting a cuff around your arm when you are relaxed and at rest, inflating the cuff, and listening to the flow of blood. If you are under emotional or physical stress, your blood pressure may be elevated.

One high blood pressure reading does not mean you have hypertension. Your doctor will measure your blood pressure at more than one visit to determine if you have hypertension. However, if your blood pressure is extremely high, your doctor may diagnose hypertension after one reading.

White coat hypertension

Sometimes blood pressure numbers are high when people are in the doctor's office because the setting makes them feel anxious. When they leave the doctor's office and return to their normal activities, their blood pressure is normal. This is called *white coat hypertension*. People with this condition may still be at increased risk for some health problems, although the risk is lower than those diagnosed with hypertension. Since many who experience white coat hypertension go on to develop hypertension, it's important to monitor blood pressure on a regular basis.

Masked hypertension

Masked hypertension is the opposite of white coat hypertension: people have normal blood pressure at the doctor's office but high blood pressure elsewhere. People with masked hypertension have a greater likelihood of developing heart disease and stroke. If your doctor suspects you may have this condition, you may be asked to take your blood pressure reading at home using a monitor and then review these readings with him or her.

Risk factors for hypertension

Most people who are diagnosed with high blood pressure have a type that's called *primary* or *essential hypertension*. This means that the exact cause is unknown. That said, there are several known factors that increase your chances of developing hypertension—some of these risk factors are within your control, others are not.

AGE The risk of hypertension increases as we get older. Through middle age, men are more likely to develop high blood pressure, but after menopause, women are at greater risk.

GENETICS If you have a family member with hypertension, you are at increased risk for developing the condition. High blood pressure is more common in people of South Asian and African American descent and it develops at a younger age than in Caucasians.

OVERWEIGHT AND OBESITY Quite simply, as your body weight increases your blood pressure rises. A larger body mass requires more blood to supply oxygen and nutrients to your tissues. And as more blood circulates through your blood vessels, the pressure on your artery walls increases.

LACK OF EXERCISE People who are sedentary tend to have higher heart rates, causing the heart to work harder with each contraction. That extra exertion puts extra pressure on your artery walls. Being inactive also increases the risk of being overweight.

DIET Excess sodium in your diet can cause fluid retention and increased blood pressure, especially if you're sodium-sensitive. A lack of potassium-rich fruits and vegetables can also contribute to hypertension since potassium helps balance the amount of sodium in your cells. Too little potassium can cause too much sodium to build up in your blood.

EXCESS ALCOHOL Consuming more than 2 drinks per day can increase blood pressure and, over time, damage your heart.

SMOKING Cigarette smoking damages the lining of your artery walls, causing them to narrow. As a result, blood pressure rises.

If you have hypertension

If your blood pressure is elevated, it's imperative to have it checked regularly by your doctor. He or she will also want to measure your lipid profile and blood sugar level to see if you have other risk factors for heart disease. Blood tests and urine tests will assess your kidney function. If you have been diagnosed with hypertension, make sure to tell your family members since they may also be at risk and should have their blood pressure checked.

The health problems associated with high blood pressure—heart attack, stroke, kidney disease—can be prevented by controlling your blood pressure. Lowering your blood pressure can cut your risk of stroke by up to 40% and of heart attack by as much as 25%. Treating hypertension involves lifestyle changes such as diet, exercise, and weight loss, and usually two or more medications. (You'll learn more about dietary modifications that lower blood pressure in Chapters 5 and 6.)

Your doctor may also advise you to monitor your blood pressure at home. With a device that has either memory storage or a printout function, your doctor can review all the readings you take. Home blood pressure monitoring devices recommended by the Canadian Hypertension Society include models by A&D, LifeSource, Omron, Microlife, and Thermor. When purchasing a device, make sure the retail staff helps you choose the right cuff size and features for you. You should also be instructed on the proper technique for taking your own blood pressure reading.

Medications for hypertension

There's no argument that taking medication to lower blood pressure prevents heart attacks and strokes. In general, blood pressure should be lowered to less than 140/90 mmHg and to less than 130/80 mmHg in people with diabetes or kidney disease. With many medications, it can take up to 6 weeks for your blood pressure to respond. Some people get better results from one medication versus another, but all of the following may be used to treat high blood pressure.

DIURETICS Also known as water pills, diuretics cause the kidneys to remove more sodium and water from the body, which helps to relax the blood vessel walls, thereby lowering blood pressure. These drugs are often combined with other medications to lower blood pressure. Some diuretics cause your body to lose potassium and your doctor may advise you to increase your intake of potassium-rich foods or to take a potassium supplement. Commonly prescribed diuretics include Aldactone (spironolactone) and Apo-Hydro (hydrochlorothiazide).

BETA BLOCKERS These medications reduce the nerve impulses to the heart and blood vessels, which causes the heart to beat slower and with less force. As a result, blood pressure drops and the heart doesn't work as hard. People with heart disease often take these. Commonly prescribed beta blockers include Lopresor (metoprolol), Tenormin (atenolol), and Inderal (propranolol hydrochloride).

ACE INHIBITORS Angiotensin converting enzyme (ACE) inhibitors help the blood vessels relax by blocking the formation of a hormone called angiotensin II. Normally, angiotensin II causes blood vessels to narrow. Commonly prescribed ACE inhibitors include Altace (ramipril), Vasotec (enalapril maleate), Accupril (quinapril hydrochloride), and Monopril (fosinopril sodium).

ANGIOTENSIN RECEPTOR BLOCKERS These medications shield blood vessels from the action of angiotensin II by preventing the hormone from binding to its cell receptor. The receptor blocking action of these drugs widens blood vessels and lowers blood pressure. Commonly prescribed angiotensin receptor blockers include Cozaar (losartan potassium), Diovan (valsartan), and Avapro (irbesartan).

CALCIUM CHANNEL BLOCKERS This class of drugs relaxes the muscles of the blood vessel walls by preventing calcium from entering the cells of the heart and blood vessels. Some calcium channel blockers slow heart rate. Commonly prescribed calcium channel blockers include Adalat (nifedipine), Cardiazem (diltiazem hydrochloride), and Norvasc (amlodipine besylate).

A word of advice if you are taking a calcium channel blocker: Avoid grapefruit juice and grapefruit products. Flavonoids—natural compounds present in the pulp and peel of grapefruit as well as the juice—inhibit the body's ability to break down these drugs, thereby increasing the amount of drug that gets into the bloodstream and causing potential toxic effects. Talk to your doctor or pharmacist if you're concerned about interactions.

RENIN INHIBITORS This new medication targets a kidney enzyme called renin. By inhibiting the action of renin, these drugs can decrease the production of angiotensin and aldosterone, which are both potent hormones that raise blood pressure. Currently there is only one renin inhibitor available in Canada called Tekturna (aliskiren).

PHYSICAL INACTIVITY

Like smoking, high blood cholesterol, and hypertension, lack of physical activity is considered a major risk factor for heart disease. In fact, leading a sedentary lifestyle doubles your chances of having a heart attack. According to the Heart and Stroke Foundation of Canada, nearly half (48%) of Canadians aged 12 and older report being physically inactive. Among women, 50% are inactive, and 45% of men don't get enough exercise.[12] Furthermore, only 2 out of 10 Canadian teenagers are active enough to meet international guidelines for optimal growth and development.[13]

We all know that exercise is good for us, but its protective effect on our cardiovascular system is considerable. For starters, regular aerobic exercise (e.g., brisk walking, jogging, cycling, swimming, cross-country skiing) strengthens your heart and makes it pump blood more efficiently. Physical activity also lowers triglycerides and increases the level of HDL (good) cholesterol in your bloodstream. If you have diabetes, exercise helps to lower blood pressure and blood sugar. Burning calories through regular physical activity helps prevent weight gain and promotes weight loss if you're overweight. And of course, there's nothing like a brisk walk or workout at the gym to help reduce the stress of daily life.

Evidence indicates that all it takes is 30 minutes of moderate exercise most days of the week to have a significant protective effect on your heart and blood vessels. You'll learn more about which types of exercise are best for preventing heart disease and how much is enough in Chapter 10.

OBESITY AND OVERWEIGHT

It's no surprise that being overweight or obese increases your risk for atherosclerosis and heart attack. Excess weight puts added pressure on your heart muscle to pump blood throughout your body. In fact, research has revealed that being overweight or obese causes the heart to pump blood less efficiently, even in the absence of heart disease. Being overweight is also linked with higher levels of LDL cholesterol, triglycerides, and blood glucose; lower levels of HDL cholesterol; and elevated blood pressure—all risk factors for heart attack.

Where you carry your extra weight also has a significant effect on your risk for heart disease. Excess fat around the middle, called abdominal obesity, creates even greater risk. The size of your waist is a good measure of visceral fat. That's the deep fat that packs itself around the organs and secretes chemicals that increase the body's resistance to insulin and cause inflammation throughout the body. (Recent research suggests that hip and thigh fat may actually offer some unique protection against heart disease.)

It's estimated that 6 out of 10 Canadians are overweight or obese and 15% are obese. Statistics for overweight among Canadian kids are equally dismal: One-quarter (26%) of children aged 2 to 17 are either overweight or obese. What's more alarming, the number of kids considered obese has tripled over the past 25 years, soaring from 3% in 1984 to 8% in 2004.[14]

Most people who are overweight or obese simply consume more calories than they burn off. It's the combination of eating foods high in calories, fat, and sugar and being sedentary that leads to weight gain. In Chapter 9, pages 206–210, you'll find tools to determine if you're overweight along with plenty of strategies to help you control your weight.

DIABETES

Having diabetes and pre-diabetes (also called *impaired fasting glucose*) puts you at risk for developing heart disease and stroke, often at an earlier age. Roughly 21% of people with diabetes, compared to 4% without diabetes, have heart disease or are suffering the effects of a stroke. In the 35 to 64 age group, people with diabetes are six times more likely to have heart disease or a stroke than those without the condition. Sadly, 80% of people living with diabetes will die as a result of cardiovascular disease.[15]

Diabetes is a condition in which your blood sugar (glucose) is higher than it should be. This occurs because your pancreas does not secrete enough insulin, the hormone that removes sugar from the bloodstream, and/or the cells in the body do not use insulin properly. Over time, excess sugar in the blood damages blood vessels by causing increased fat deposits on vessel walls, which can lead to atherosclerosis and blocked arteries.

There are two types of diabetes. *Type 1 diabetes*, formerly called insulin-dependent diabetes, typically occurs in childhood or the teen years and requires daily insulin injections. Most often, type 1 diabetes is caused by the body's immune system destroying the insulin-producing cells of the pancreas. Type 1 diabetes accounts for 10% of all diabetes cases in Canada.

The majority of people with diabetes (90%) have *type 2 diabetes*, previously known as non-insulin dependent diabetes. Type 2 diabetes usually develops after the age of 40, but it's increasingly being diagnosed in children and adolescents. The underlying cause of type 2 diabetes is thought to be insulin resistance—your cells are unable to use insulin properly. In the early stages, your body responds by telling the pancreas to produce more insulin to clear sugar from the bloodstream. But over time, the pancreas can't keep up with demand, blood sugar rises, and diabetes results.

Pre-diabetes (impaired fasting glucose)

As the name implies, impaired fasting glucose is a condition that precedes type 2 diabetes. Perhaps your doctor has said you have "borderline" diabetes or that you're blood sugar levels are "borderline" high. This means that your fasting glucose is higher than normal but not high enough to be diagnosed as diabetes. (Your fasting glucose is the amount of sugar in your bloodstream when you have not eaten for 12 hours.) If you fall into this category, waste no time in taking charge of your blood sugar: Type 2 diabetes is not inevitable. Regular exercise and loss of excess body weight can lower your fasting blood sugar to the normal range and prevent full-blown diabetes.

The Diabetes Prevention Program, a major clinical trial involving 3234 adults with impaired fasting glucose, found that diet and exercise dramatically reduced the risk of developing diabetes. In the three-year study, participants were assigned to one of three groups on different regimens: lifestyle intervention, the drug metformin taken twice daily (it helps the body use insulin more efficiently thereby reducing the risk of diabetes), or a twice-daily placebo pill. The lifestyle intervention involved losing 7% of body weight (e.g., 14-pound weight loss for a 200-pound person) and exercising for a total of 150 minutes per week. The results: Participants who exercised and lost weight lowered their risk of developing diabetes by an impressive 58% relative to those taking placebo pills. Those in the metformin group were also less likely to develop diabetes, although less dramatically. Compared to the placebo group, these individuals lowered their risk by 31%.[16]

Risk factors for type 2 diabetes

Researchers don't fully understand why some people develop type 2 diabetes and others don't. Genetic makeup as well as numerous environmental factors play a role. The following are thought to increase the risk of type 2 diabetes. As you'll see, many are the same risk factors that contribute to heart disease.

AGING Becoming older increases the odds of developing type 2 diabetes, largely because people tend to exercise less and gain weight as they age. However, type 2 diabetes is increasing in children, too, because of these lifestyle factors.

GENETICS If you have a parent, brother, or sister with diabetes, you're at increased risk for developing diabetes. Being of Aboriginal, Hispanic, Asian, South Asian, or African descent also increases the likelihood of developing diabetes since these are considered high-risk populations. Unfortunately, you can't change your genes but there are other important risk factors you can control.

OVERWEIGHT Carrying excess body weight, especially around the middle, is the main risk factor for type 2 diabetes. The more body fat you have, the more resistant your cells become to the action of insulin. The good news: Losing weight can reverse insulin resistance.

SEDENTARY LIFESTYLE Physical inactivity boosts the risk of diabetes by making you more likely to gain weight. Regular exercise also uses glucose in your body for energy, thereby making your cells more sensitive to insulin.

IMPAIRED FASTING GLUCOSE Having an elevated fasting blood sugar, slightly higher than normal, often progresses to type 2 diabetes if it's not managed through healthy lifestyle behaviours and, in some cases, medication.

GESTATIONAL DIABETES This type of diabetes occurs during pregnancy, usually during the second trimester. While gestational diabetes usually disappears after childbirth, it increases a woman's future risk for type 2 diabetes. As well, giving birth to a baby weighing 9 pounds (4.1 kilograms) or more, increases the chances of developing diabetes.

Today it's estimated that more than 2 million Canadians have diabetes, and the number is expected to hit 3 million by the end of this decade. Unlike type 1 diabetes, which cannot be prevented, it is possible to prevent or delay the onset of type 2 diabetes through healthy lifestyle choices such as physical activity, healthy eating, weight control, and not smoking. In the chapters that follow, you'll learn plenty of strategies to lower your risk of impaired fasting glucose and type 2 diabetes.

METABOLIC SYNDROME

Chances are you haven't heard the term *metabolic syndrome*. It is characterized by a cluster of risk factors and is gaining attention among researchers and medical professionals as a potent predictor of heart attack and type 2 diabetes. While you won't find metabolic syndrome listed among traditional risk factors for heart disease—at least not yet—it's important to understand how this constellation of conditions impacts your risk. What's more, an increasing number of Canadians have metabolic syndrome. It's estimated that 25% of the population has this disorder, with a greater prevalence in Aboriginal and South Asian populations.[17]

A person is thought to have metabolic syndrome if he or she has a large waist circumference plus two or more of the following conditions: high blood triglycerides, high blood pressure, elevated fasting glucose, and low HDL (good) cholesterol. Having metabolic syndrome is thought to double the risk of heart attack and increase by 5-fold the likelihood of developing type 2 diabetes.

The principal underlying risk factors for metabolic syndrome are abdominal obesity and insulin resistance. Other risk factors linked with metabolic syndrome include genetics, physical inactivity, aging, and cigarette smoking.

There are no well-accepted criteria for diagnosing metabolic syndrome. Over the past decade, experts have proposed various, slightly different criteria for identifying the syndrome. The most recent criteria were proposed by the International Diabetes Federation in 2005 and are widely used in research and medical settings.

Criteria for Metabolic Syndrome[18]

To be diagnosed as having metabolic syndrome, a person must have:

An elevated waist circumference:

Men:	≥94 cm (37 inches)
Women:	≥80 cm (31.5 inches)

Plus any two of the following four risk factors:

Elevated blood triglycerides	≥1.7 mmol/L
Reduced HDL cholesterol Men: Women: Or on medication for low HDL	 <1.03 mmol/L <1.29 mmol/L
Elevated blood pressure Or on medication for high blood pressure	≥130 mmHg systolic pressure (upper number) or ≥85 mmHg diastolic pressure (lower number)

Elevated fasting blood sugar Or previously diagnosed with type 2 diabetes	≥5.6 mmol/L

Source: The IDF consensus worldwide definition of the metabolic syndrome, International Diabetes Federation, 2006. Table 1: the International Diabetes Federation definition (of the Metabolic Syndrome).

The waist circumference cut-offs given are for Caucasians of European origin. Ethnic-specific values exist for other populations. For instance, lower thresholds for waist circumference are recommended for Asian populations because studies suggest that health risk increases among many Asian populations at lower levels of body weight than in Caucasian populations.

The primary goal of treatment is to reduce the risk for cardiovascular disease and type 2 diabetes by losing excess weight, lowering cholesterol and blood pressure, and reducing blood sugar to the recommended levels. In the chapters that follow you'll be given plenty of tips to help you do these very things.

Contributing risk factors

Other risk factors are linked to heart disease, but their significance hasn't yet been precisely determined. These are called *contributing risk factors*.

DIET AND NUTRITION

By now it's probably obvious how unhealthy eating habits can contribute to a greater risk of heart disease. A diet laden in saturated (animal) and trans fats can lead to high LDL cholesterol. Eating too much sodium and not enough fruits and vegetables can cause your blood pressure to climb above what's considered healthy. Consumption of too many calories coupled with inactivity can cause weight gain and boost your risk of impaired fasting glucose and type 2 diabetes, not to mention elevated blood triglycerides and low HDL cholesterol. Poor eating habits can also increase inflammation in your body, a factor thought to contribute to atherosclerosis.

The following chapters deal specifically with dietary modifications that can lower your future risk for coronary heart disease. You'll learn which foods to eat, which ones to limit, and which nutritional supplements might guard against heart disease. I'll give you tips to use at the grocery store and when dining out in restaurants. And you'll learn proven strategies to help you achieve and maintain a healthy weight.

ALCOHOLIC BEVERAGES

You might be wondering why I include alcoholic beverages among factors that increase the risk of heart disease. After all, you've probably heard that a moderate intake of alcohol reduces, rather than increases, the likelihood of heart attack. It's true that numerous studies have found that people who consume one or two drinks per day are less likely to develop heart disease than non-drinkers. But consuming more than this can boost both your blood pressure and blood triglycerides, two factors that increase the chances of developing heart disease.

You'll learn more about the effects of alcohol on your heart in the next chapter, but suffice to say, it's recommended that women limit intake to one drink per day and men to no more than two. And if you're a non-drinker, it is not advised that you starting consuming alcohol.

STRESS

We all need some stress in our life to perform well. But depending on how you respond to it, too much stress may increase the risk of heart attack. The link between stress and heart disease isn't completely clear, but scientists have uncovered a few ways in which stress might make you more prone to atherosclerosis and heart attack. For starters, when you're under stress, your body releases so-called *stress hormones* that increase blood pressure. Over time, that elevated pressure can damage the lining of your artery walls, promoting the accumulation of fatty plaques. Stress also increases clotting factors in the blood, which could lead to a blood clot forming and blocking an artery. In people who already have coronary heart disease, stress speeds up the heart rate and increases the heart's demand for oxygen. If the heart and coronary arteries aren't in good enough shape to deliver this oxygen, chest pain (angina) can occur.

As well, how you cope with stress can influence other risk factors for heart disease. If you turn to food, alcohol, or cigarettes to deal with stress, you're further increasing your risk.

It's impossible to escape life's stresses. What matters most is how you deal with stress. Learning to manage stress through communicating with family and friends, exercise, relaxation techniques, or professional counselling can help reduce its harmful impact. Managing stress, or preventing it if possible, is especially important for people who already have heart disease.

PART 2

PREVENTING HEART DISEASE WITH DIET AND NUTRITION

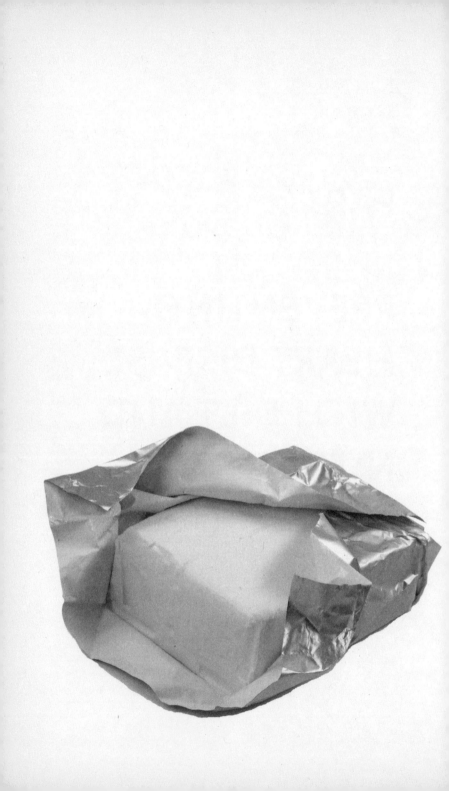

3
Foods and nutrients to limit or avoid

Scientists have been busy studying the link between diet and heart disease since the 1950s, when it was proposed that the differences in the rates of heart attack between populations were due to some aspect of lifestyle, especially fat in the diet. At that time, observational studies in countries revealed that as fat intake increased so did rates of heart disease. (An observational study examines populations, rather than individuals, to observe and compare characteristics of groups of people living in different countries.)

The famous Seven Countries Study was the first to explore the association between diet, health risk, and disease in contrasting populations living in Greece, Italy, Yugoslavia, Finland, the Netherlands, Japan, and the United States. The study's principal investigator was physiology professor Ancel Keys, Ph.D., who hypothesized that a type of fat—saturated fat—increased blood cholesterol, which in turn boosted the risk of heart disease. The Seven Countries Study lasted from 1958 to 1970 and successfully demonstrated the degree to which makeup of the diet—in particular, levels of saturated fat—predicted present and future rates of coronary heart disease in population groups.

Then, almost two decades later, researchers began demonstrating the cholesterol-lowering properties of oat bran and, in so doing, fuelled the demand for everything oat bran, from cereals, breads, muffins, and cookies to even potato chips. In recent years, foods such as fish, soy, nuts, and chocolate have all made headlines as foods to help ward off heart attack.

The truth is, no one "magical" food will lower your risk for developing heart disease. There are many foods, which when eaten regularly as part of a healthy diet, work together to protect your heart and blood vessels. Food is directly involved in many of the risk factors for heart disease—high cholesterol, hypertension, diabetes, inflammation, obesity, and so on. That's why paying attention to what you eat—and don't eat—is one of the most important preventative measures you can take.

In this chapter and the next you'll learn how certain foods and food components work to guard against or contribute to atherosclerosis and heart attack. I'll give you plenty of tips to help you limit your intake of foods that can harm your heart. And I'll tell you easy ways to add heart healthy foods to your daily diet. In Part III, *Recipes to Prevent Heart Disease*, you'll find delicious ways to turn many of these powerful foods into heart healthy meals.

I'll start with the "bad news" first by telling you what types of foods you need to cut back on. It's very clear that eating certain foods on a regular basis can increase the likelihood of developing risk factors that lead to heart disease. Certain fats boost LDL cholesterol, while others increase LDL and lower HDL cholesterol. Too much salt contributes to high blood pressure, as does excess alcohol. And a steady intake of refined sugars can lead to weight gain, high triglycerides, and elevated blood sugar. In the following sections, you'll learn which foods may increase your future risk of heart disease and how to reduce your intake of them.

Saturated fat

When it comes to heart health, the evidence is pretty strong that what's most important is the type of fat you eat, rather than the total amount. Studies have failed to find a link between one's total fat intake and the onset of heart disease. But that's not to say it's okay to follow a high-fat diet. Too much of any kind of fat can lead to weight gain since dietary fat is a concentrated source of calories.

Dietary fat, be it in ice cream, potato chips, steak, or vegetable oil, is actually a mixture of different types of *fatty acids*, the individual building blocks that make up the fat in food. Fatty acids are either *saturated* or *unsaturated*, terms that reflect their chemical structure. (You'll learn more about unsaturated fats, the so-called "good fats," later in this chapter.) We refer to a fat as being either saturated or unsaturated based on the main type of fatty acid present. For instance, butter is called a saturated fat because most of its total fat—63%—is comprised of saturated fatty acids.

Fats are simple molecules built around a series of carbon atoms linked to each other on a chain. In saturated fatty acids, the carbon atoms are completely full, or saturated, with hydrogen atoms; in unsaturated fatty acids, some of the hydrogen atoms are missing. It's the chemical structure of fatty acids that determines how they behave in the body and, ultimately, how they impact your health.

Saturated fats are typically solid at room temperature. In general, they're found in animal foods such as meat (beef, pork, lamb), milk, yogurt, cheese, butter, and ice cream. (Non-fat dairy products contain virtually no saturated fat.) However, saturated fat also occurs in some plant foods, including coconut oil, coconut milk, palm kernel oil, cocoa butter, and palm oil. Three of these—coconut oil, palm kernel oil, and palm oil, which are also called tropical oils—are not sold on grocery store shelves; instead, they're used as ingredients in packaged foods such as crackers, cookies, ice cream, and non-dairy creamers.

There are actually four different saturated fatty acids, with varying numbers of carbon atoms, and they are not all created equal when it comes to heart health.

Saturated Fats in Food

Saturated fatty acid	Food sources
Lauric acid	Coconut oil, palm oil
Myristic acid	Milk, dairy products
Palmitic acid	Palm oil, meat
Stearic acid	Meat, cocoa butter (e.g., chocolate)

A high intake of saturated fat is widely believed to contribute to the development and progression of coronary heart disease. The ongoing Nurses' Health Study, which followed 80,082 healthy women aged 34 to 59, found that consuming 5% of daily calories from saturated fat, compared to getting those same calories from carbohydrate, was associated with a 17% greater risk of developing heart disease over 14 years.[1] (For a 2000-calorie diet, 5% of calories from saturated fat is equivalent to 100 calories or 11 grams of saturated fat.)

Studies have consistently demonstrated that excess saturated fat in the diet raises total and LDL cholesterol levels, a major risk factor for heart disease. What's more, there is clear evidence that reducing your intake of these so-called bad fats can lower blood cholesterol, which helps to guard against heart attack. In a 2003 review of 60 clinical trials, researchers from the Netherlands concluded that reducing saturated fats and replacing them with unsaturated fats significantly improved the ratio of total cholesterol to HDL (good) cholesterol. In other words, eating less saturated fat and more of the good fats lowered total cholesterol and increased HDL cholesterol levels.[2] (See Chapter 1, page 15, for more information about the risk ratio.)

But it turns out that not all classes of saturated fatty acids raise your blood cholesterol to the same degree. Studies have revealed that lauric (coconut and palm oil), myristic (dairy products), and palmitic (palm oil) acids elevate blood cholesterol, whereas stearic acid (meat, chocolate) does not. Among the cholesterol-raising saturated fats, myristic acid is the most potent. And although lauric acid in coconut and palm oil boosts total blood cholesterol, this effect is mostly due to its ability to increase HDL cholesterol.

For those of you who love chocolate cake or a juicy steak, it probably comes as good news that the saturated fatty acid in these foods, stearic acid, appears to have a neutral effect on blood cholesterol. Some experts have even suggested that stearic acid not be included with saturated fat on food labels. The bad news: Scientists have learned that this fatty acid impacts your blood chemistry in other ways. It lowers HDL cholesterol and increases lipoprotein (a), a type of LDL cholesterol that, when elevated, is thought to increase your risk for heart disease. Consuming too much stearic acid may also activate clotting factors in the bloodstream and impair your body's ability to dissolve blood clots.[3]

RECOMMENDATIONS FOR SATURATED FAT

Rather than worrying about different types of saturated fat, it's much easier to focus on reducing your overall intake of these fats. That will help keep your LDL cholesterol in check, or lower it to the desired level if you have high cholesterol. The Heart and Stroke Foundation of Canada does not give a recommended daily intake limit for saturated fat. Instead, it advises keeping your total fat intake between 20% and 35% of your day's calories and choosing unsaturated rather than saturated fats. For the average woman following a 2000-calorie diet, this works out to 45 to 75 grams of fat a day, and for men consuming 2700 calories, 60 to 105 grams of fat a day. Of course, if you're trying to lose weight you'll need to consume less fat.

The American Heart Association gives a specific limit for saturated fat to help people reduce their intake. In its most recent dietary guidelines, released in 2006, the association recommends keeping saturated fat to less than 7% of daily calories. That means, if you need about 2000 calories per day, no more than 140 of them should come from saturated fat. Since 1 gram of fat delivers 9 calories, that means no more than 15 grams of saturated fat per day. If you're following a 1400-calorie weight-loss diet, you should limit your intake to 10 grams of saturated fat per day.

I don't want you to get bogged down with numbers and percentages. All you really have to do is make a habit of choosing animal foods that are lower in fat. High-fat dairy products and fatty cuts of meat such as lamb chops, rib eye steak, and spareribs are high in saturated fat. Lean cuts of meat (sirloin, tenderloin, flank steak, eye of round), skinless poultry breast, 1% or skim milk, 1% or non-fat yogurt, and part-skim or skim-milk cheese are examples of animal foods lower in saturated fat. If you use butter, do so sparingly since it packs 7 grams of saturated fat per 2 teaspoon (10 ml) serving. In addition, many baked goods contain high levels of saturated fat if they're made with butter, palm oil, or palm kernel oil.

Use the following chart to help you choose foods lower in saturated fat.

Saturated Fat Content of Selected Foods

	Total fat (grams)	Saturated fat (grams)
Dairy products		
Cheese, cheddar, low-fat, 7% milk fat (MF), 1 ounce (30 g)	2.0	1.2
Cheese, cottage, 1% MF, 1/2 cup (125 ml)	1.1	0.8
Cheese, cottage, fat-free, 1/2 cup (125 ml)	0.5	0.3
Cheese, mozzarella, part-skim, 16.5% MF, 1 ounce (30 g)	4.6	2.9
Milk, 1% MF, 1 cup (250 ml)	2.5	1.7
Milk, skim, 0.1% MF, 1 cup (250 ml)	0.5	0.3
Yogurt, frozen, vanilla, 5.6% MF, 1/2 cup (125 ml)	4.0	2.5
Meat and Poultry		
Beef, steak, eye of round, grilled, 3 ounces (90 g)	7.7	2.7
Beef, steak, inside round, grilled, 3 ounces (90 g)	3.9	1.4
Beef, steak, strip loin, broiled, 3 ounces (90 g)	9.2	3.5
Beef, steak, top sirloin, grilled, 3 ounces (90 g)	6.8	2.6
Beef, tenderloin, roasted, 3 ounces (90 g)	7.3	2.3
Beef patty, ground, extra lean, broiled, 3 ounces (90 g)	7.8	2.1
Pork, back (peameal) bacon, grilled, 3 ounces (90 g)	7.5	2.5
Pork, ham, lean (5% fat), 3 ounces, (90 g)	4.8	1.6
Pork, tenderloin, roasted, 3 ounces (90 g)	3.2	1.0
Veal, cutlets, grain-fed, pan-fried, 3 ounces (90 g)	2.5	0.8
Veal, ground, broiled, 3 ounces (90 g)	6.8	2.7
Veal, loin chop, grain-fed, lean, broiled, 3 ounces (90 g)	5.7	2.4
Veal, sirloin, roasted, 3 ounces (90 g)	5.6	2.2
Chicken, breast, roasted, skinless, 3 ounces (90 g)	1.9	0.6
Chicken, dark meat, roasted, skinless, 3 ounces (90 g)	8.7	2.4
Chicken, white meat, roasted, skinless, 3 ounces (90 g)	4.0	1.1
Turkey, dark meat, roasted, skinless, 3 ounces (90 g)	2.7	0.9
Turkey, white meat, roasted, skinless, 3 ounces (90 g)	0.9	0.2
Eggs		
Egg whites, 2 large	0	0
Egg, whole, 1 large	5.3	1.6

Source: Canadian Nutrient File, 2007b, Health Canada. Retrieved June 2008 from: http://205.193.93.51/cnfonline/newSearch.do?applanguage=en_CA. Adapted and Reproduced with the permission of the Minister of Public Works and Government Services Canada, 2008

USING NUTRITION LABELS TO REDUCE SATURATED FAT INTAKE

It's easy to cut saturated fat when buying packaged foods. The introduction of mandatory nutrition labelling on food packages in December 2005 resulted in manufacturers having to disclose the grams of saturated fat—along with many other nutrients—per one serving of the food product. In the Nutrition Facts box, you'll find the grams of saturated fat listed after the grams of total fat. You can use this information to compare different brands of similar products, such as cookies, crackers, and frozen desserts, and to choose one that's lower in saturated fat. Just be sure to check the serving size! Nutrient numbers are given for *one* serving of the food. If you usually eat more than the specified serving size, you'll need to adjust the saturated fat number accordingly.

In the next section, on trans fats, I'll tell you how to use the Daily Value for saturated plus trans fats to seek out healthier foods.

QUICK TIPS TO REDUCE SATURATED FAT

- Choose leaner cuts of poultry and meat such as skinless chicken; extra lean ground chicken or turkey; extra lean ground beef, sirloin, tenderloin, top round, and flank steak.
- Before cooking meat and poultry, trim away any visible fat and remove the skin from poultry.
- Use cooking methods that drain fat from meat such as grilling, broiling, baking, poaching, and steaming.
- Substitute meat or poultry with beans. Add kidney beans, chickpeas, or lentils to soups, salads, chilis, pasta sauces, and tacos.
- Replace ground beef with ground soy or soy-based veggie burgers more often.
- Choose lower fat luncheon meats, such as sliced turkey or chicken breast, lean ham, or lean roast beef.
- Switch to 1% or skim milk and other non-fat or lower fat dairy products such as fat-reduced sour cream.
- Save desserts high in saturated fat, such as ice cream, for special occasions and, when you do enjoy them, have a small portion. As a rule, choose sorbet or low-fat frozen yogurt over ice cream.

- Use 1% or non-fat cottage cheese or part-skim hard cheese (both less than 20% milk fat, or MF), or skim-milk cheese (7% MF or less) instead of regular full-fat cheese (31% MF).
- Use spreads that have very little or no saturated fat, such as jam, fruit spread, apple butter, reduced-fat mayonnaise, hummus, or mustard, instead of butter.
- Read the Nutrition Facts box on packaged foods to seek out foods that are lower in saturated fat.

Trans fats

With all the media attention around the evils of trans fats, you're no doubt aware of these man-made fats that lurk primarily in commercial baked goods and fried foods. Over the past 50 years, industry-produced trans fat has become a common ingredient in hundreds of popular foods: You'll see it listed as partially hydrogenated vegetable oil and/or vegetable short-ening. Roughly 90% of the trans fat in our food supply is found in cookies, cakes, pastries, doughnuts, snack foods, fried fast foods, and some brands of margarines. In fact, in some of these foods, trans fats make up 45% of the total fat content!

Trans fats are formed during partial hydrogenation, a food industry process that hardens and stabilizes liquid vegetable oils. This maintains the taste and smell characteristics of oils, giving them a longer shelf life—a boon to food manufacturers.

Why are trans fats so harmful? Ever since the 1990s, scientists have raised concerns about the detrimental effects of trans fats. Growing evidence indicates that trans fats are more harmful than saturated fats and, when the two are compared, trans fats are linked with a 2.5- to 10-fold higher risk of heart disease. That's because trans fats increase LDL choles-terol and decrease levels of good, HDL cholesterol. Studies also show that a steady intake of trans fats can trigger inflammation in the body, disrupt the normal functioning of blood vessel walls, and impair the body's use of insulin. As well, researchers have found that higher intakes of trans fat are linked with a greater risk of developing coronary heart disease.[4]

Low levels of trans fats also occur naturally in foods from ruminant animals, such as beef, lamb, goat, and dairy products. A 1 ounce (30 gram) serving of cheddar cheese, for example, has roughly 0.3 grams of naturally occurring trans fat, and a similar serving of part-skim cheese contains

0.1 grams. Bacteria in the stomach of these animals convert small amounts of polyunsaturated fats to trans fatty acids. Unlike industry-produced trans fats, naturally occurring trans fats are not considered harmful. Moreover, it would take an amount well above what we consume in our typical diet to raise blood cholesterol.[5]

RECOMMENDATIONS FOR TRANS FAT

In 2002, the Institute of Medicine of the National Academy of Sciences in the U.S. recommended that our intake of trans fat be as low as possible. This panel of experts did not set a safe upper limit because any increase in trans fat boosts the risk of heart disease. A year later, the World Health Organization advised that our trans fat intake be restricted to a mere 1% of daily calories. Health Canada advises that we keep trans fat *plus* saturated fat to a maximum of 10% of our daily calorie intake. If you consume 2000 calories per day, this means keeping your daily intake of trans plus saturated fat combined to 20 grams at most.

Limiting or avoiding trans fat is getting easier to do in Canada. Mandatory nutrition labelling has forced food manufacturers to list the grams of trans fat on the Nutrition Facts box. Heightened consumer aware-ness has prompted many—but not all—food manufacturers and restaurant chains to reduce or eliminate trans fat from foods. Today, you'd be hard pressed to find trans fat in french fries served in fast food restaurants. As well, most brands of potato chips and many brands of store-bought cookies are also trans fat–free.

Despite the progress, you nonetheless need to read labels on many foods to determine if trans fat is present. Some baked goods, instant noodles, puddings, baby foods, pastries, microwave popcorn, hard margarines, and shortening still harbour this cholesterol-raising fat. That's why Health Canada and the Heart and Stroke Foundation of Canada have proposed regulations for reducing trans fat in our food supply. In June 2006, the Trans Fat Task Force submitted its report, *Transforming the Food Supply*, to Canada's Minister of Health. It recommends that over the next few years, trans fat be limited to 2% of total fat in all vegetable oils and soft, spreadable margarines sold to consumers or used in restaurants, and that other foods contain no more than 5% of total fat as trans fat.[6]

In June 2007, the Canadian government accepted these recommen-dations and called on the food industry to achieve these limits by June 2009. If significant progress has not been made by that time, Health

Canada is expected to develop regulations to ensure that the recommended levels are met.

USING NUTRITION LABELS TO LIMIT OR AVOID TRANS FAT INTAKE

Scanning the Nutrition Facts box will help you choose food products with little or no trans fat. You'll find the grams of trans fat listed per one serving of the food. More useful, however, is the Daily Value (DV) for saturated plus trans fat combined, which is written as a percentage. This value tells you whether there is a little or a lot of these cholesterol-raising fats in a food. I told you earlier that the Daily Value for saturated plus trans fat is set at 20 grams, 10% of the calories in a standard 2000-calorie diet. If you notice that one serving of your favourite brand of cookies has 50% of the DV for saturated plus trans fat, it means there's a fair bit of artery-clogging fat present—half your daily limit. If you really want to eat those cookies, you'll have to curb your intake of saturated and trans fats for the rest of the day.

As food companies make the switch to trans fat–free oils, you'll notice many packaged foods boldly stamped with the claim "trans fat–free." To make this assertion, foods must contain less than 0.2 grams of trans fat and no more than 2 grams of saturated fat per serving. While such a claim helps you spot foods that contain zero trans fats, it doesn't always help you identify heart healthy food products. Keep in mind that many trans fat–free foods can contain undesirable amounts of sodium and refined sugars. Bottom line: You need to read the Nutrition Facts box to get the complete picture.

QUICK TIPS TO REDUCE TRANS FAT

- Read the Nutrition Facts box on foods you buy at the store and choose foods with little or no trans fat. Foods with a Daily Value for saturated plus trans fat combined of 5% or less are low in these fats.
- Read the ingredient list if a packaged food does not have a Nutrition Facts box, as may be the case for foods prepared in-store. Avoid buying food that lists partially hydrogenated vegetable oil, hydrogenated vegetable oil, and shortening.
- If you plan on eating at a fast food or family-style restaurant, check the company's website in advance. Most fast food outlets and some chain restaurants post the nutrient content of their menu items. If you're uncertain, ask what kind of oil is used in cooking before you order.

- Eat meals that are mostly prepared at home so you can control ingredients and know precisely what you're eating.
- Cut down on your consumption of processed foods such as crackers, cookies, snack foods, and toaster pastries since these foods supply most of the trans fat we consume.
- Choose margarine that is made from non-hydrogenated vegetable oil, since it will be trans fat–free.

Dietary cholesterol

For much of the past 40 years, we've been warned away from eggs because of their link with heart disease risk. The concern has to do with high cholesterol content—190 milligrams per egg yolk. Consuming too much cholesterol from food was thought to increase LDL cholesterol in the bloodstream, a major risk factor for coronary heart disease. As a result, nutrition guidelines to keep LDL blood cholesterol in the desirable range have long emphasized limiting dietary cholesterol, which is abundant in egg yolks, shrimp, liver, and duck.

It seems that such alarm over dietary cholesterol has been exaggerated. While there's compelling evidence that high cholesterol intakes can cause hardening of the arteries in rabbits, pigs, and mice, there's little evidence of this occurring in humans. For most people, only a small amount of the cholesterol in food passes into the bloodstream. A number of short-term studies have demonstrated that feeding healthy people as many as 3 whole eggs per day does not raise LDL cholesterol. In fact, some research has even found that an egg-rich diet increases HDL cholesterol.[7] (Despite this finding, I wouldn't recommend eating 3 eggs per day to boost your level of HDL cholesterol. You're much better off adding aerobic exercise to your daily routine.)

Furthermore, 30 years of research has not yet turned up a connection between eating eggs and heart disease risk. Studies have determined that healthy people who eat 1 egg per day do not have an increased risk of coronary heart disease or stroke.[8]

However, if you have diabetes, you might want to limit your egg consumption. The Physicians' Health Study, from Harvard Medical School, followed 21,327 male physicians for 20 years and found that egg consumption—up to 6 per week—was not linked with a greater risk of heart attack, stroke, or dying from all causes overall. But among men with diabetes, those who ate 7 or more eggs each week—versus less than 1 egg per week—were twice as likely to die from any cause. Interestingly, this study also reported a relationship between egg consumption and risk of heart disease in people with diabetes. Among those with diabetes, egg-a-day eaters were slightly more likely to develop heart disease than those who rarely ate eggs.

Scientists speculate that individuals with diabetes absorb higher amounts of cholesterol from foods. Consuming too much dietary cholesterol might also lead to the formation of smaller and denser LDL cholesterol particles in people with diabetes. (If you'll recall, small, dense LDL particles are more often associated with hardening of the arteries than large, "fluffy" LDL particles.)

Another report from the Physicians' Health Study found that men who ate at least 2 eggs per day were 64% more likely to be diagnosed with heart failure than those who ate less than 1 egg per week.[9]

RECOMMENDATIONS FOR DIETARY CHOLESTEROL

By now you're probably wondering, how much cholesterol is too much? How many eggs can you safely eat each week? Nutrition guidelines aimed at preventing heart disease generally recommend consuming less than 300 milligrams of cholesterol per day. If you already have high blood cholesterol, the American Heart Association advises consuming less than 200 milligrams of cholesterol each day. The Heart and Stroke Foundation of Canada, on the other hand, does not recommend a specific cholesterol intake for healthy people but, rather, stresses the importance of limiting saturated and trans fat to help control blood cholesterol. That's because, as you read earlier, higher intakes of these fats raise LDL cholesterol to a much greater degree than do higher amounts of dietary cholesterol.

Cholesterol is found in meat, poultry, eggs, dairy products, fish, and seafood. It's particularly plentiful in shrimp, duck, liver, and egg yolks. I tell my clients not to worry about eating shrimp. A 3 ounce (90 g) serving is a great source of protein that's very low in fat and calories, and contains virtually no saturated fat. Instead, to limit dietary cholesterol, pay attention to your intake of animal foods. As you'll see from the chart below, choosing animal foods low in saturated fat will also help you reduce your cholesterol intake.

Cholesterol Content of Selected Foods

	Cholesterol (milligrams)
1 egg, white only	0
1 egg, whole	190
Beef sirloin, lean only, 3 ounces (90 g)	64
Calf liver, fried, 3 ounces (90 g)	416
Chicken breast, skinless, 3 ounces (90 g)	73
Pork loin, lean only, 3 ounces (90 g)	71
Salmon, 3 ounces (90 g)	54
Shrimp, 3 ounces (90 g)	135
Butter, 1 teaspoon (5 ml)	10
Cheese, cheddar, 31% MF, 1 ounce (30 g)	31
Cheese, mozzarella, part-skim, 1 ounce (30 g)	18
Cream, half and half, 12% MF, 2 tablespoons (25 ml)	12
Milk, skim, 1 cup (250 ml)	5
Milk, 2% MF, 1 cup (250 ml)	19
Yogurt, 1.5% MF, 3/4 cup (175 ml)	11

Source: Canadian Nutrient File, 2007b, Health Canada. Retrieved June 2008 from: http://205.193.93.51/cnfonline/newSearch.do?applanguage=en_CA. Adapted and Reproduced with the permission of the Minister of Public Works and Government Services Canada, 2008

How many eggs can you eat? If you're healthy, 1 whole egg a day seems perfectly safe. If you're a male with diabetes, it's prudent to limit egg yolks to 4 per week. Instead of a 3-egg omelet packed with 570 milligrams of cholesterol, try a whites-only omelet for a good source of protein, riboflavin (a B vitamin), and selenium. Some eggs might actually offer protection from heart disease. Research has demonstrated that eating eggs enriched with the omega-3 fatty acid DHA (docosahexaenoic acid) found in fish oil helps lower triglycerides, a blood fat linked to heart disease.

Some whole eggs are enriched with another omega-3 fatty acid called ALA (alpha-linolenic acid), which is abundant in flaxseed. As you'll learn in Chapter 4, page 88, consuming more of this omega-3 fatty acid may help guard against heart disease. My recommendation: When buying whole eggs, choose ones that are enriched with omega-3 fatty acids.

A Guide to Buying Eggs

Brown eggs
Produced by Rhode Island Red breed hens, which are slightly larger and require more food than Leghorn hens (white-shell eggs). Eggshell colour does not affect the quality, flavour, or nutrients of an egg.

Free-run eggs
Produced by hens that are free to roam in wide open-concept barns equipped with nests and perches. Their nutrient content is the same as regular eggs.

Free-range eggs
Produced by hens that have outdoor access as well as space for nesting and perching. Due to the cold Canadian winter, hens get outdoors only seasonally. Nutrient content is the same as for regular eggs.

Liquid eggs
Contain pasteurized egg whites, a small amount of pasteurized egg yolk, beta carotene, and natural flavour. They're convenient for omelets and baking. Four tablespoons (60 ml) is equivalent to 1 large egg. One carton (250 ml) is the equivalent of 5 large eggs. Burnbrae Farms Naturegg Break-Free liquid eggs contain 80% less cholesterol than 1 regular egg.

Liquid egg whites
Pasteurized egg whites that contain no fat or cholesterol. One carton (250 ml) is equivalent to 8 large egg whites (4 tbsp/60 ml equal 1 large egg).

Omega-3 eggs
Laid by hens fed a diet enriched with flaxseed or fish oil, sources of the omega-3 fatty acids ALA (alpha-linolenic acid) and DHA (docosahexaenoic acid) respectively. As a result, these eggs are good sources of either ALA or DHA, both linked with protection from heart disease.

Organic eggs
Laid by hens fed certified organic grains grown without the use of synthetic chemicals or genetically modified crops. Organic eggs have the same nutritional content as regular eggs.

Egg substitutes
Found in the freezer section, these products contain egg whites, corn oil, colouring, and additives and preservatives.

QUICK TIPS TO REDUCE DIETARY CHOLESTEROL

- Choose lean cuts of meat, skinless poultry, and low-fat dairy products. Remove visible fat from meat and poultry before cooking.
- Use spreads that contain little or no cholesterol, such as non-hydrogenated margarine, olive oil, nut butters, and hummus.
- Substitute canola oil in recipes that call for butter when sautéing.
- Use 1 whole egg per person when making egg dishes such as scrambled eggs and omelets, then add egg whites or a cholesterol-reduced liquid egg product to make up the difference.
- Replace 1 whole egg with 2 egg whites in baking and other recipes.
- Read the Nutrition Facts box on packaged foods. Foods with a Daily Value (DV) for cholesterol of 5% or less will be low in cholesterol.
- Don't worry if you eat one food that's high in cholesterol. Balance your day by including others that are low in cholesterol.

Added sugars

Prior to the advent of modern food processing, we didn't consume much sugar in our diet. Today, however, it's estimated that Canadians consume, on average, 16 teaspoons (80 ml) of sugar each day. And it's not just from the usual culprits like soft drinks, cookies, and candy. Sugar also lurks in salad dressings, frozen dinners, pasta sauces, soy milk, and even peanut butter and bread.

By added sugars, I am referring to those added to foods during processing and preparation. On food packages, you'll see them listed as a number of different ingredients, including brown sugar, corn syrup, dextrose, fructose, high fructose corn syrup, fruit juice concentrate, glucose-fructose, honey, invert sugar, liquid sugar, malt, maltose, molasses, rice syrup, table sugar, and sucrose. Manufacturers add sugars to foods to enhance flavour, contribute bulk and texture, and aid in the browning of foods. Added sugars are not to be confused with naturally occurring sugars, such as lactose in milk and yogurt and fructose in fruit and sweet vegetables.

No studies have linked higher intakes of added sugars with a greater risk of heart disease. That said, there are still several reasons why you should limit your intake of added, or refined, sugars. Eating too much sugar can negatively affect your lipid profile. A number of studies have found that a high sugar intake lowers the level of protective HDL cholesterol. A 7-year study of over 3000 young men and women found a consistent link between increased sugar intakes and low HDL cholesterol levels.[10] Findings from animal research and a few small studies in humans also suggest that high intakes of sugar raise blood pressure.

It's well known that excess sugar can cause your blood triglycerides to rise to an undesirable level. Getting more than 20% of your day's calories from sugar can boost your triglycerides by as much as 60%. A high sugar intake triggers your liver to produce more triglycerides and impairs the ability of your body to clear triglycerides from the bloodstream. Reducing your intake of sugar and sugar-laden foods is a key strategy to lowering elevated triglycerides.

Of course, a steady intake of sugary foods can also lead to overweight and obesity by adding a surplus of calories to your diet. Recent research has shown our increased use of sweeteners, especially high-fructose corn syrup, over the past 20 years correlates with rising obesity rates. This correlation doesn't prove that high-fructose corn syrup causes weight gain, but some experts contend that fructose in corn syrup is processed differently than glucose in cane or beet sugar. Fructose doesn't trigger hormone responses that regulate appetite and satiety, which could trick you into overeating.

High intakes of sugary foods, which have a high glycemic index, can also increase your risk for insulin resistance, a condition in which the body cannot effectively remove sugar (glucose) from the bloodstream. Insulin resistance, in turn, ups your risk for developing type 2 diabetes and metabolic syndrome, two potent predictors of heart disease. (Foods with a high glycemic index are quickly digested and cause high spikes in blood sugar and an outpouring of insulin from the pancreas. Over time, the overworked pancreas can't keep up and blood sugar remains elevated. You'll learn more about the glycemic index in the next chapter.)

A 2008 review of 37 studies concluded that low-glycemic diets are associated with significant protection from diabetes and coronary heart disease. In fact, compared to a low-glycemic diet, an eating plan based on carbohydrates that spike blood sugar increased the risk of developing heart disease by 25%.[11]

RECOMMENDATIONS FOR ADDED SUGARS

The World Health Organization recommends we limit added sugars to no more than 10% of daily calories. If you follow a 2000-calorie diet, this translates to a daily maximum of 12 teaspoons (48 g) of added sugars. To me, that still sounds like a lot. But it's shocking how quickly those sugars add up if you eat processed foods.

Breakfast cereals can hide as many as 15 grams of sugar per serving (almost 4 teaspoons' worth). If you pour 1 cup (250 ml) of light vanilla soy milk over that cereal, you could be adding another 3 teaspoons (13 g) of sugar. A can of maple-style beans in sauce harbours 24 grams of sugar per 1 cup (250 ml) serving. A low-fat frozen dinner can weigh in with up to 10 grams of sugar. Even 2 slices of whole-grain bread can add 6 grams of sugar to your diet. And if you drizzle your salad with 1 tablespoon (15 ml) of low-fat dressing, you could very well be tossing your greens with a teaspoon's worth of sugar.

You need to read labels to sleuth out hidden sugars. The Nutrition Facts box on prepackaged foods discloses the grams of sugars contained in one serving of the food, and you can easily do the math to convert grams of sugar to teaspoons of sugar (4 grams equals 1 teaspoon). But keep in mind that the sugar numbers on nutrition labels include both naturally occurring sugars (e.g., fruit or milk sugars) and refined sugars added during food processing (e.g., sucrose, honey, corn syrup).

To find added sugars, you need to read the ingredient list. You might be surprised to see how many different types of refined sugars can go into one product!

QUICK TIPS FOR REDUCING ADDED SUGARS

- Limit sugary drinks. Replace soft drinks and fruit drinks with water, low-fat milk, unflavoured soy beverages, vegetable juice, or tea.
- Satisfy your sweet tooth with natural sugars. Choose fruit, yogurt, or homemade smoothies over candy, cakes, cookies, and pastries.
- Reduce portion size. Avoid the temptation to order king-sized desserts, pastries, and candy bars when eating away from home. When eating sweets at home, take a small serving.

- Choose breakfast cereals that have no more than 8 grams of sugar per serving. An exception includes cereals with dried fruit (natural sugars in the fruit will bump up the sugar numbers).
- Sweeten foods with spices instead of sugar. Add cinnamon and nutmeg to hot cereals, a dash of vanilla to coffee and lattes, and grated fresh ginger to fruit and vegetables.
- Reduce sugar in recipes. As a rule, you can cut the sugar in most baked goods by a third.
- Read the Nutrition Facts box when buying packaged baked goods. Compare products and choose a brand that has fewer grams of sugar per serving. (Be sure to look for products that are low in saturated and trans fats too!)

Sodium

It probably comes as no surprise that sodium is on my list of nutrients to limit. Study after study has linked excess sodium with elevated blood pressure. And as you're well aware, high blood pressure can lead to heart attack, stroke, and eventually, kidney disease. The problem: Canadians of all ages are consuming too much sodium. The latest survey estimates daily sodium intakes at somewhere between 2300 and 2800 milligrams in women and between 2882 and 4066 milligrams in men—amounts in excess of what our bodies need. (One teaspoon of table salt—sodium chloride—contains 2300 milligrams of sodium.)

Having said that, we do require some sodium for good health. It is an essential mineral that regulates fluid balance and blood pressure and keeps muscles and nerves working properly. The following table shows how much sodium we're consuming relative to what we actually need each day.

Sodium Intakes Versus Daily Requirements

Age (years)	Gender	We're consuming (milligrams/day)	We need (milligrams/day)	Upper safe intake (milligrams/day)
1–3	Both	1918	1000	1500
4–8	Both	2677	1200	1900
9–13	Males	3515	1500	2200

Age (years)	Gender	We're consuming (milligrams/day)	We need (milligrams/day)	Upper safe intake (milligrams/day)
	Females	2959	1500	2200
14–18	Males	4130	1500	2300
	Females	2938	1500	2300
19–30	Males	4066	1500	2300
	Females	2793	1500	2300
31–50	Males	3607	1500	2300
	Females	2806	1500	2300
51–70	Males	3334	1300	2300
	Females	2573	1300	2300
>70	Males	2882	1200	2300
	Females	2300	1200	2300

The vast majority of sodium we consume each day (77%) is hidden away in processed and restaurant foods. Only 11% of our daily sodium comes from salt that's added during cooking and while eating. The remainder occurs naturally in foods, including milk, shellfish, and tap water. Some of the worst sodium culprits are soups, canned vegetables, frozen dinners, processed meats, and snack foods. Many restaurant meals also deliver a hefty dose of salt, especially breakfasts, Chinese entrees, and deli sandwiches. Consider these facts: Denny's Country Scramble packs 3995 milligrams of sodium, a typical order of chow mein serves up roughly 3600 milligrams, and a Rueben sandwich has about 3200 milligrams!

Sodium is added to food as sodium chloride (table salt), monosodium glutamate (MSG), sodium nitrite, sodium bicarbonate, and sodium benzoate. However, sodium from sources other than sodium chloride may have a lesser effect on blood pressure. Besides enhancing flavour, sodium helps control the growth of bacteria and moulds, preserves texture, and extends shelf life.

The major risk of a high-salt diet is elevated blood pressure. Studies show that, on average, blood pressure rises progressively with increasing sodium intakes. People with high blood pressure, diabetes, and chronic kidney disease as well as older adults and African Americans are more sensitive than others to the blood pressure–raising effects of sodium.

What's Your Blood Pressure?

	Millimetres of mercury (mmHg)
Normal blood pressure	<120/<80
Prehypertension	130–139/85–89
Hypertension	≥140/≥90

To learn more about blood pressure, see Chapter 2, page 41.

Well-controlled trials have clearly demonstrated that cutting back on sodium can lower blood pressure in people with hypertension. The DASH-Sodium Trial (DASH stands for Dietary Approaches to Stop Hypertension) was a landmark study that assigned 412 people with prehypertension and hypertension to either a typical American diet or a diet high in fruits, vegetables, and low-fat dairy products (the DASH diet). Participants following each diet ate foods with low (1150 milligrams), medium (2300 milligrams), and high (3450 milligrams) daily levels of sodium for 1 month. (You'll learn more about how the DASH diet works to lower blood pressure in Chapter 6, page 159.)

Reducing sodium intake substantially lowered blood pressure in both diets in a linear fashion: the greater the sodium reduction, the greater the effect. However, at every sodium level, the DASH diet group had lower blood pressure than the American diet group. The combination of the DASH diet and a low-sodium intake reduced blood pressure the most in people with hypertension, and more in women than in men.[12]

Evidence shows that controlling your sodium intake over the long term translates into less risk of heart disease. British researchers followed 3126 adults with prehypertension, aged 30 to 54, over time to determine if a lower sodium intake reduced the risk of heart attack and stroke. Those assigned to a low-sodium diet were counselled on how to identify sodium in the diet, how to monitor their intake, and how to select and prepare low-sodium foods.

Follow-up done for 10 and, in some cases, up to 15 years, showed that people who had lowered their daily sodium intake by 760 to 1000 milligrams were 25% less likely to suffer a cardiovascular event, including heart attack, stroke, coronary artery bypass surgery, angioplasty, or cardiac death.[13]

If you don't have prehypertension or hypertension now, consuming less sodium can reduce your future risk for developing the condition.

SODIUM AND POTASSIUM IN BALANCE

If the majority of Canadians over-consume sodium, you might be wondering why we all don't experience high blood pressure. Heredity is one explanation: Some people's genetic makeup predisposes them to developing hypertension. Potassium, a mineral involved in nerve function, muscle control, and blood pressure, is another reason why many people don't succumb to hypertension. Studies show that people with a low daily intake of potassium (less than 1560 milligrams) are more likely to develop high blood pressure and suffer a stroke.

Scientists aren't certain how potassium works to keep blood pressure in check. Some think that the mineral somehow makes blood vessels less sensitive to hormones that normally trigger constriction. Other experts feel that potassium acts directly on blood vessels causing them to relax. A higher potassium intake also causes the kidneys to excrete more sodium, thereby preventing blood pressure from rising.

Adults need 4.7 grams (4700 milligrams) of potassium each day. It's found in many foods, especially meat, milk, fruits, and vegetables. The best way to increase your potassium intake is to eat more fruits and vegetables. While you can get the mineral in a supplement, research has shown that potassium in foods is far superior for keeping blood pressure within the normal range. (Check with your doctor before increasing your intake of potassium. Some people, for example those with kidney disease, may need to avoid potassium-rich foods.)

Potassium-rich Foods

	Potassium (milligrams)
Buttermilk, 1%, 1 cup (250 ml)	391
Milk, skim, 1 cup (250 ml)	404
Yogurt, plain, 1%, 3/4 cup (175 ml)	410
Apricots, 4	362
Avocado, 1/2	345
Banana, 1 medium	422

	Potassium (milligrams)
Cantaloupe, cubed, 1 cup (250 ml)	440
Dates, 4	217
Honeydew, diced, 1 cup (250 ml)	426
Nectarine, 1 medium	273
Orange, 1 medium	237
Orange juice, 1/2 cup (125 ml)	262
Prunes, dried, 4	245
Prune juice, 1/2 cup (125 ml)	373
Raisins, 1/4 cup (50 ml)	275
Spinach, cooked, 1/2 cup (125 ml)	443
Sweet potato, baked, 1 small	285
Swiss chard, cooked, 1/2 cup (125 ml)	508
Tomato juice, 1/2 cup (125 ml)	294
Winter squash, 1/2 cup (125 ml)	214
Black beans, cooked, 3/4 cup (175 ml)	452
Chickpeas, cooked, 3/4 cup (175 ml)	353
Kidney beans, cooked, 3/4 cup (175 ml)	528
Lentils, cooked, 3/4 cup (175 ml)	540
Molasses, blackstrap, 1 tablespoon (15 ml)	518
Nuts, mixed, 1/4 cup (50 ml)	207

Source: Canadian Nutrient File, 2007b, Health Canada. Retrieved June 2008 from: http://205.193.93.51/cnfonline/newSearch.do?applanguage=en_CA. Adapted and Reproduced with the permission of the Minister of Public Works and Government Services Canada, 2008

QUICK TIPS TO REDUCE SODIUM INTAKE

- Read the Nutrition Facts box on packaged foods. Sodium levels vary widely across different brands of like products. Compare brands of similar foods and choose one with a lower % Daily Value (DV) of sodium. Foods with a 5% or less DV of sodium are low in sodium. (The DV for sodium on nutrition labels is set at 2400 milligrams.)

- Pay attention to portion size. Sodium numbers on a nutrition label will underestimate your intake if you consume more than the serving size indicated.

- Limit your intake of processed meats such as bologna, ham, sausage, hot dogs, bacon, and deli meats and of smoked salmon. (Many of these foods are high in saturated fat too.)
- Limit your use of bouillon cubes, soy sauce, Worcestershire sauce, or barbecue sauce.
- Rely less on convenience foods such as canned soups, frozen dinners, and packaged rice and pasta mixes.
- Choose pre-made entrees or frozen dinners that contain no more than 200 milligrams sodium per 100 calories.
- Choose lower sodium products when possible. Many sodium-reduced brands contain 25% less sodium than the original version and some, like V8 juice, contain 75% less. If you can't find low-salt products in your supermarket, ask your grocer to stock them.
- Read ingredient lists. Salt, sodium chloride, baking soda, baking powder, sodium nitrate, sodium benzoate, and monosodium glutamate are all ingredients that indicate sodium has been added to the food.
- Substitute herbs and spices for salt when cooking—try garlic, lemon juice, salsa, onion, and vinegar too.
- Remove the salt shaker from the table to break the habit of salting food when it's on your plate.

Alcoholic beverages

You've likely heard that one to two drinks per day can keep your heart healthy. Many studies have revealed that this level of moderate alcohol consumption is linked with 20% to 30% reductions in heart disease risk. Alcohol is thought to protect against heart disease in a few ways. It increases the level of HDL (good) cholesterol in the bloodstream. There's also evidence that alcohol reduces the ability of blood cells called platelets to clump together and form clots. But keep in mind that alcohol's protective effects are limited to middle-aged and older adults. We don't know if drinking moderately when you are younger benefits your heart when you're older.

RED WINE VERSUS OTHER ALCOHOLIC BEVERAGES

Despite popular belief, there's no evidence that drinking red wine offers greater protection than drinking any other type of alcoholic beverage. The beneficial effects on HDL cholesterol and platelets occur with wine, spirits, and beer. (The notion of red wine's protective merits may stem from the so-called "French Paradox"—the observation that death from coronary heart disease is relatively low in France despite high levels of saturated fat (e.g., cheese, paté) in the diet and of cigarette smoking.) While some studies have found that wine drinkers have a lower risk of heart disease than beer or liquor drinkers, most have found no difference. In fact, research suggests that people who prefer red wine tend to have higher incomes, more education, smoke less, consume less saturated fat, and eat more fruits and vegetables—factors that may explain part of the additional benefits observed in some studies.

It is true that red wine, made from the skins and seeds of grapes, contains antioxidants that may benefit blood vessels. Test-tube studies have demonstrated that one such antioxidant, resveratrol, reduces blood clot formation, relaxes blood vessel walls, and inhibits inflammation. But the amount used to effect these reactions was much greater than found in a glass or two of red wine. Animal studies also point to the cardio-protective effects of resveratrol. At this time, however, there is no convincing evidence that antioxidants in red wine offer additional benefits beyond the alcohol content itself. (Resveratrol is also found in red grapes, purple grape juice, peanuts, blueberries, and cranberries.)

HOW MUCH ALCOHOL?

If you're thinking it might be wise to add a glass of wine or pint of beer to your daily diet, think again. The Heart and Stroke Foundation of Canada does not recommend that you drink alcohol for the purpose of reducing your risk for heart attack and stroke: The harmful effects of alcohol outweigh any benefits.

Consuming more than 2 drinks per day boosts blood pressure and increases the long-term risk of developing hypertension.[14] Drinking alcoholic beverages can also increase blood triglycerides—even 1 drink a day can increase these blood fats in susceptible people. If you have elevated triglycerides, limiting or avoiding alcohol is strongly advised. Moderate alcohol intake also increases the risk for several cancers, including breast and colon cancers.

If you do drink alcohol, limit yourself to 1 drink per day for women and 2 for men. Keep in mind that for elderly people, 2 drinks may be too much to be considered a low-risk intake. And avoid binge drinking, which can elevate blood pressure.

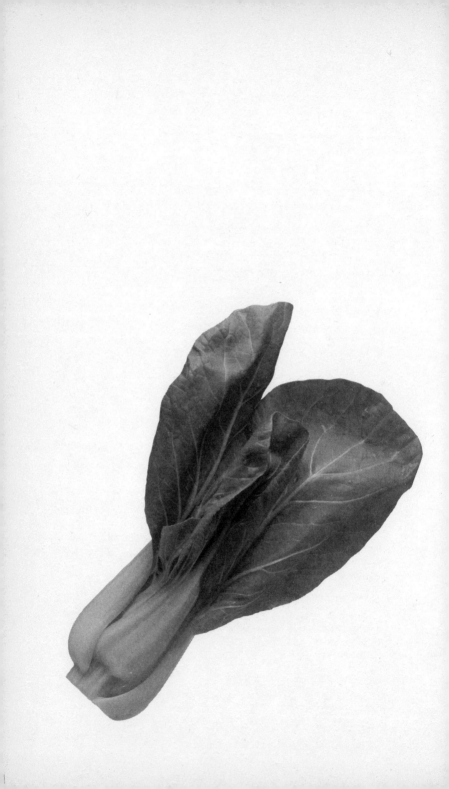

4

Heart healthy foods

In the previous chapter, I told you that there isn't one special food that will guard against heart disease. Rather, there are many foods that, when eaten regularly as part of a healthy diet, can help protect your heart. And by *healthy diet*, I mean one that's low in saturated and trans fats, refined sugars, and sodium. Adding a bowl of oat bran to a high-fat, high-salt diet won't do you much good. More and more, scientists are learning that certain *dietary patterns*, and not individual foods and food components, defend against many chronic disorders, including heart disease. Over the past decade, research certainly suggests that it's the cumulative effect of eating many heart healthy foods and nutrients that offers protection from heart disease.

A good example of a heart healthy dietary pattern is the Mediterranean diet, followed by people who live in countries that border the Mediterranean Sea. This eating pattern is characterized by plenty of fruits and vegetables, legumes and nuts, fish, and, of course, extra-virgin olive oil—a combination that includes several heart healthy foods. What's more, foods considered bad for your heart if eaten in excess form a very small part of the Mediterranean diet. Red meat is seldom eaten and wine is consumed in low to moderate quantities. You'll learn about other heart healthy dietary patterns in Chapter 6.

In order to put together an effective, heart healthy dietary plan, it's important to learn which foods and nutrients make up an eating pattern that reduces the risk of heart disease. Understanding how these foods work in your body to fight disease—and how to add them to your family's meals—is the first step in developing your own personal heart healthy diet.

Omega-3 fats

By now you know which fats contribute to heart disease: saturated and trans fats. However, some fats are well known for their ability to protect the heart—omega-3 fatty acids being the most famous. Omega-3 fats belong to the *polyunsaturated* family of fats. Chemically speaking, polyunsaturated fats are not saturated with hydrogen atoms (as are saturated fats), and they remain liquid both at room temperature and when refrigerated. (Vegetable oils such as corn, soybean, and safflower are also rich in polyunsaturated fat; however, they contain omega-6 fatty acids, the other main type of polyunsaturated fat.)

There are three types of omega-3 fatty acids in foods: DHA, EPA, and ALA. DHA and EPA are found in oily, cold water fish such as salmon, trout, sardines, tuna, mackerel, and herring. ALA is plentiful in flax, canola, and walnut oils as well as soybeans. DHA and ALA can also be found in a growing number of fortified food products such as eggs, yogurt, fruit juice, soy beverages, and breads. Numerous studies have shown that higher intakes of each type of omega-3 fat is linked with protection from heart disease.

FISH: DHA AND EPA

The cardiovascular benefits of eating fish have been documented in several prospective studies and randomized controlled trials. A 2006 report published in the *Journal of the American Medical Association* concluded that eating 1 to 2 servings of fish per week is enough to reduce the risk of dying from heart attack by 36%. Researchers from Harvard School of Public Health and Harvard Medical School based their conclusions on a review of hundreds of studies about fish and health.[1]

Omega-3 fats in fish protect the heart in several ways: They make the blood less likely to form clots, reduce inflammation, and guard against irregular heartbeats that cause sudden cardiac death. There's even evidence that fish oil helps blood vessels relax, preventing increases in blood pressure. When it comes to blood cholesterol, fish oil may help raise HDL levels as well as increase the size of LDL cholesterol particles, resulting in larger, fluffy LDLs that are less damaging to artery walls. One trial, which enrolled 11,323 subjects who survived their first heart attack, demonstrated that even a small amount of omega-3 fatty acids (1000 milligrams per day) was effective at reducing overall death and the risk of sudden cardiac death by 20% and 45% respectively. Another study, from Finland, conducted in post-menopausal women with heart disease, found that higher levels of DHA in the blood—consistent with their reported fish intake—was associated with less progression of the disease.[2]

It's well documented that omega-3 fish oils can reduce elevated blood triglycerides by 20% to 50%. It's thought that DHA and EPA reduce secretion of triglycerides from the liver and increase their clearance from the bloodstream. People who are overweight and who have poorly controlled diabetes often have high triglycerides in their bloodstream—one reason why having diabetes increases the risk of heart attack. A pooled analysis of 23 randomized trials, that included 1075 people with type 2 diabetes, concluded that fish oils can significantly lower blood triglycerides.[3]

How much fish should you eat?

The Heart and Stroke Foundation of Canada advises eating fish, especially fatty fish, twice per week to increase your intake of heart healthy omega-3 fatty acids. Many experts recommend an intake of 300 to 500 milligrams of DHA and EPA (combined) per day to help reduce the risk of heart disease—a target that most of us don't achieve. It's estimated that Canadian children, aged 2 to 3, consume 19 milligrams of DHA each day and that adults, on average, get 78 milligrams. There are no official recommended DHA and EPA intakes for Canadians because the ideal intake is unclear at this time.

As you'll see from the chart below, eating oily fish is an excellent way to boost your intake of omega-3 fats. (Keep in mind that since the body stores omega-3 fats, you don't need to eat fish every day to reap its health benefits.)

DHA and EPA Content of Fish and Other Foods

For fish, per 3 ounce (90 gram) cooked portion

	DHA + EPA combined (milligrams)
Fish	
Haddock	203
Halibut, Atlantic and Pacific	395
Herring, Atlantic	1712
Mackerel, Atlantic	1022
Salmon, Atlantic	1825
Salmon, Chinook	1476
Salmon, sockeye, canned	982
Salmon, Coho	900
Sardines, Atlantic	835
Shrimp	267
Tilapia	115
Trout, rainbow	981
Tuna, skipjack	733
Fish oil capsule, 1000 milligrams	300–600
Fortified foods	
Naturegg Omega Pro, 1/4 cup (50 ml)	293
Naturegg Omega 3 Pro Eggs, 1 whole egg	82
Black Diamond DHA Omega 3 Cheese, 1 ounce (30 g)	20
PC Blue Menu Oh Mega j Orange Juice, 1 cup (250 ml)	50
Tropicana Essentials Omega-3 Orange Juice, 1 cup (250 ml)	20
Neilson Dairy Oh! homogenized milk, 1 cup (250 ml)	20
Neilson Dairy Oh! 2% milk, 1 cup (250 ml)	10
Silk Plus Omega-3 DHA Soy Beverage, 1 cup (250 ml)	25

Source: Food manufacturers and USDA National Nutrient Database for Standard Reference, Release 17

Fish and mercury

Eating fish is not without risks. Some species contain high levels of mercury, which can accumulate in the body and affect the developing nervous system, especially the brain, of infants and young children. If women consume too much mercury before and during pregnancy, it may increase the risk of birth defects and learning disabilities in children. Some, but not all, studies have found associations between a women's mercury exposure during pregnancy and the baby's neurologic test scores during childhood.

Fortunately, the types of fish that provide the most omega-3 fatty acids are also low in mercury and can be safely enjoyed by women and young children. Women who are pregnant or breastfeeding, women who could become pregnant, and children aged 11 and younger should limit—or avoid, in my opinion—swordfish, shark, marlin, orange roughly, escolar, fresh and frozen tuna, king mackerel, and canned albacore (white) tuna. Canned light tuna (e.g., skipjack, yellowfin, tongol) is low in mercury and safe to eat regularly. Health Canada advises that women and children limit their intake of high-mercury fish to a small portion once per month.

Fish oil supplements

If you don't like the taste of fish or can't convince your family to enjoy it, you might consider getting your DHA and EPA in a fish oil capsule. The American Heart Association recommends that people who have coronary heart disease consume 1000 milligrams of DHA + EPA combined each day, which requires taking a supplement in addition to eating fish twice per week.

Most studies using fish oil supplements have been conducted in people with existing heart disease to determine if the supplements prevent arrhythmias, irregular heartbeats that can cause sudden death. Randomized controlled trials have found that fish oil reduces the risk of heart attack, stroke, sudden cardiac death, and dying from all causes. Findings from studies undertaken in people without documented heart disease also suggest that fish oil supplements benefit the heart. One study conducted in overweight men who had high blood pressure and high cholesterol or elevated triglycerides found that a daily fish oil supplement and regular exercise resulted in lower triglycerides, increased HDL cholesterol, and a loss of body fat.[4]

But fish oil capsules may not be safe for everyone. Researchers from St. Michael's Hospital (Toronto), the University of Toronto, and Cardiff University in Wales, U.K., analyzed the results of three randomized trials involving patients with implantable cardioverter defibrillators (ICDs) who were at risk for sudden cardiac death caused by abnormal heart rhythms. ICDs are very small devices that monitor heart rhythms and correct an irregular, life-threatening heartbeat with an electrical shock. They're used in patients whose lower heart chambers, or ventricles, beat too quickly (tachycardia) or flutter rather than beat (fibrillation). ICDs are also implanted in patients at risk for these conditions due to previous heart attack and heart failure.

When the results of the three studies were pooled, there was no overall effect of fish oil on the risk of an ICD discharge (e.g., arrhythmia) after 1 year of fish oil supplementation. But the results of each individual study varied considerably. After 1 year of fish oil supplementation, one study reported a significant anti-arrhythmic effect, another found no benefit, and the smallest study showed a tendency towards increasing irregular heart-beats.[5]

The variation in inconclusiveness of these findings suggests that people with implantable defibrillators should use fish oil with caution. If you have an ICD, consult with your doctor before taking a fish oil supplement.

Fish oil supplements are made from species of fish rich in omega-3 fatty acids: salmon, anchovies, sardines, herring, and mackerel. Most capsules (1 gram each) provide 300 milligrams of DHA + EPA combined, but some deliver as much as 600 milligrams (check the label to be sure).

For lowering triglycerides, studies have used 1 to 4 grams (1 to 4 capsules) per day. Because fish oil thins the blood, taking high doses may increase the risk of bleeding in people taking prescription anticoagulants such as heparin or warfarin (Coumadin). If you're on such medication, check with your doctor before taking a fish oil supplement.

When it comes to chemical contaminants, fish oil capsules are generally considered safe. Mercury accumulates in the flesh (protein) rather than the oil of fish, which explains the lack of detectable mercury in most supplements. Also, the deodorizing process seems to reduce levels of contaminants such as polychlorinated biphenyls (PCBs).

FLAX, CANOLA, AND WALNUTS: ALA

If you don't have access to fish, are allergic to it, or just don't like it, consuming foods rich in ALA is an alternative way to increase your intake of omega-3 fatty acids. While the evidence isn't nearly as abundant or compelling as that for DHA and EPA, numerous studies do suggest ALA may offer some cardio-protective benefits.

A decade ago, researchers from Harvard School of Public Health found that among 76,283 healthy women who were followed for 10 years, those with the highest intake of ALA were half as likely to die from heart disease as those who consumed the least. A higher intake of oil and vinegar salad dressing, a major source of ALA, was also linked with a lower risk of death from heart disease.[6]

A more recent analysis of this large group of women revealed that after 18 years of follow-up, a greater ALA intake was linked with significant protection from sudden cardiac death. Women who consumed 1.16 grams of ALA per day were 40% less likely to die suddenly of cardiac arrest than women whose diets provided only 0.66 grams per day. However, a greater intake of ALA did not reduce the risk of non-fatal heart attacks.[7]

Sudden cardiac death is unexpected death resulting from an abrupt loss of heart function (cardiac arrest). Death can occur within minutes after symptoms appear. The majority of all cardiac arrests occur in homes and public places—not in the hospital. Sadly, less than 5% of people who have a cardiac arrest outside the home survive. People who suffer sudden cardiac death may or may not have diagnosed heart disease, but the most common underlying reason for individuals to die suddenly from cardiac arrest is coronary heart disease.

Research on the relationship between ALA intake from foods and death from heart disease has also been conducted in men. While one study found that ALA had no effect, two others reported protective effects from higher intakes of ALA. In a large study of healthy men, the findings hinted that a higher ALA intake reduced the overall risk of heart disease. Men with low intakes of omega-3 fats from fish appeared to benefit the most from consuming more ALA in their diet.[8]

Consuming more ALA might also help prevent atherosclerosis, the process that leads to heart attack. Researchers from the Boston School of Medicine examined the diets and coronary arteries (using high-resolution ultrasound) of 1575 men and women, and found that a diet high in ALA was associated with significantly less plaque buildup in the coronary arteries.[9]

It's thought that alpha-linolenic acid may benefit the heart in many of the same ways as fish-derived omega-3 fatty acids, by helping to prevent abnormal heart rhythms and fatal ventricular arrhythmias. As well, once consumed, small amounts of ALA are converted by the body to EPA and, to a lesser extent, DHA, both of which have anti-arrhythmic effects. ALA's cardio-protective abilities are believed to include inhibiting the body's production of inflammatory compounds such as C-reactive protein. Some evidence also suggests that ALA can reduce blood fibrinogen, a protein made by the liver that causes the blood to clot.

Recommendations for ALA

Alpha-linolenic acid is considered an essential fatty acid, which means your body can't produce it so it must be supplied by your diet. In order to meet the body's need for this omega-3 fatty acid, women require 1.1 grams(1100 milligrams) of ALA per day and men need 1.6 grams (1600 milligrams). During pregnancy and breastfeeding, women require 1.6 grams and 1.4 grams per day respectively.

Is the official recommended daily intake for ALA sufficient to guard against heart disease? For the most part, yes, although women may need to add a little more ALA to their diet. Research points to a daily ALA intake of 1.2 to 2 grams (1200 to 2000 milligrams) to prevent heart disease in healthy people. If you have existing heart disease, an intake of 1.6 grams (1600 milligrams) appears to help lower the risk of dying from heart disease and sudden cardiac death.

The richest sources of ALA are flaxseed oil, walnut oil, and canola oil. It's also found in soybean oil, tofu, and food products fortified with flaxseed oil. Flaxseed oil capsules sold in drug stores and health food stores are also an excellent source of ALA. Use the following chart to help you boost your intake of this essential fatty acid.

ALA Content of Selected Foods

	ALA (milligrams)
Walnuts, English, 14 halves (28 g)	2575
Salba, ground, 2 tablespoons (25 ml)	2500
Flaxseed oil, 1 teaspoon (5 ml)	2416
Flaxseed, ground, 2 tablespoons (25 ml)	2400
So Good Omega Soy Beverage, 1 cup (250 ml)	700
So Nice Plus Soy Beverage, 1 cup (250 ml)	700

	ALA (milligrams)
Country Harvest Whole Grain Breads, 2 slices	600 to 2000
Soybeans, 1/2 cup (125 ml)	514
Flaxseed oil capsule, 1 capsule (1000 mg)	500
Lactantia Healthy Attitude Omega 3 Margarine, 2 teaspoons (10 ml)	500
Walnut oil, 1 teaspoon (5 ml)	470
Canola oil, 1 teaspoon (5 ml)	419
Astro Biobest Omega 3 Yogurt, 1/2 cup (113 g)	300
Beatrice Omega 3 Milk Beverage, 1 cup (250 ml)	300
Natrel Omega 3 Milk Beverage, 1 cup (250 ml)	300
Naturegg Omega 3 Eggs, 1 whole egg	300

Source: Food manufacturers and USDA National Nutrient Database for Standard Reference, Release 17

ALA and prostate cancer risk

There is some concern that high intakes of ALA might increase the risk of prostate cancer. Lab studies have shown that ALA can stimulate prostate tumour growth, but the risk in humans remains unclear. One study reported higher levels of ALA in prostate tissue of men with prostate cancer that correlated with higher PSA (prostate specific antigen) levels. (PSA is a protein produced by the prostate gland. The higher a man's PSA level, the more likely it is that cancer is present; however, there are other possible reasons for elevated PSA.) Another study of 29,592 men aged 55 to 74 found no association between ALA intake and overall risk of developing prostate cancer, but did uncover a slightly higher risk of advanced prostate cancer with high ALA intakes. However, this increased risk was statistically insignificant, meaning it could have occurred by chance.[10]

ALA association with prostate cancer seems to depend on the source. Alpha-linolenic acid from dairy and meat has been positively associated with prostate cancer, whereas ALA from plant sources, such as flaxseed, doesn't seem to affect prostate cancer risk.

If you're a male who's at high risk for prostate cancer (e.g., you have a father or brother with the disease, especially if they were diagnosed at a young age), I advise that you play it safe and avoid high intakes of ALA from supplements and oils.

QUICK TIPS TO INCREASE OMEGA-3 FATTY ACID INTAKE

- Add fish to your menu twice per week. For more omega-3 fatty acids, try salmon, trout, Arctic char, sardines, herring, and mackerel.
- Consider taking a fish oil capsule if you don't like fish. (Speak to your doctor first if you have an implantable cardioverter defibrillator.)
- Look for foods fortified with DHA, such as orange juice, milk, cheese, and whole eggs. Read labels to determine if the source of omega-3 fat is DHA or ALA (from flaxseed oil).
- Use flaxseed oil in salad dressings or add it to foods at the end of cooking (you can't cook with flaxseed oil because high heat destroys the essential fatty acids and causes the oil to burn).
- Add a little walnut oil to your olive oil and vinegar salad dressing.
- Snack on walnuts and dried fruit for a mid-afternoon energy boost.
- Try yogurt fortified with ALA from flaxseed oil for breakfast or a snack.
- Add ground flaxseed to hot cereal, smoothies, yogurt, or applesauce.
- Use canola oil for high-heat cooking such as sautéing and stir-frying. (Canola oil has a higher smoke point than flaxseed oil, which means it does not burn or break down at high cooking temperatures.)
- Choose soy beverages that are fortified with ALA from flaxseed oil.

Recipes

Avocado Lime Dressing, page 266
Chickpea and Black Bean Salad with Flaxseed Dressing, page 256
Grilled Salmon with Sesame Cilantro Pesto, page 320
Honey Balsamic Dressing, page 268
Lemon Pepper Salmon Dip, page 321
Lemon Thyme Grilled Trout, page 322
Mussels Steamed in a White Wine Sauce, page 323
Pepper-Crusted Salmon, page 324
Seared Tuna Sandwich with Caramelized Onions, page 325
Smoked Salmon Sandwich with Capers and Red Onions, page 326

Monounsaturated fats

There's another family of fats that appears to offer significant protection from heart disease: monounsaturated fats. Like polyunsaturated fat, its carbon atoms are not completely full of hydrogen atoms and it's a liquid at room temperature; but monounsaturated fats turn semi-solid when refrigerated. The word *monounsaturated* undoubtedly brings to mind olive oil. Among cooking oils, olive oil is the richest source of monounsaturated fat, which makes up 77% of the oil's total fat content. Other good sources include canola oil, peanut oil, avocado, nuts, and nut butters.

WHAT MAKES MONOUNSATURATED FATS HEART HEALTHY?

Many studies have demonstrated that replacing saturated and trans fats with monounsaturated fats helps to lower the risk of heart disease. In studying populations, researchers have learned that higher intakes of monounsaturated fats are linked with lower death rates from heart disease. In particular, the death rate from heart disease is very low in Mediterranean populations that use olive oil as a primary fat source. A 1997 report from the Nurses' Health Study estimated that replacing as few as 5% of daily calories' worth of saturated and trans fats with an equivalent amount of unsaturated (mono- and polyunsaturated) fats would reduce the risk of coronary heart disease by 42%.[11]

During the past several decades, the main focus of dietary recommendations to prevent heart disease has been reducing total fat. Today, however, we've realized that message has unintended health consequences. Filling our shopping carts with low-fat cookies, baked potato chips, cereal bars, and sorbet has resulted in a low-fat, high-carbohydrate diet that tends to depress HDL (good) cholesterol and raise blood triglycerides.

More recently, researchers have investigated the cardiovascular effects of replacing a proportion of daily calories from carbohydrates with monounsaturated fats. Findings have demonstrated the ability of monounsaturated fat to raise HDL cholesterol without increasing LDL cholesterol. Among people with diabetes, monounsaturated fat may also improve how the body uses glucose.

Researchers from Johns Hopkins University School of Medicine have also validated the cardio-protective effects of monounsaturated fat. In the OmniHeart study (Optimal Macronutrient Intake Trial to Prevent Heart

Disease), 164 men and women with prehypertension or hypertension were assigned to one of three different diets for 6 weeks. The purpose of the study was to determine whether replacing calories from saturated fat with calories from protein or unsaturated fat (mainly monounsaturated fat from olive oil) lowered blood pressure and cholesterol more effectively than replacing those saturated fat calories with carbohydrate.

The OmniHeart Diets

Diet	Percentage of daily calories from ...		
	Carbohydrate	Protein	Fat
High carbohydrate	58%	15%	27%
High protein	48%	25%	27%
High unsaturated fat	48%	15%	37%

Compared to the study diet with more carbohydrate, the one with more protein lowered blood pressure, LDL cholesterol, and triglycerides. But this diet also lowered the level of protective HDL cholesterol. The diet high in monounsaturated fat had the best results: It lowered blood pressure and triglycerides, and raised HDL cholesterol. Although it didn't lower LDL cholesterol, the increase in HDL cholesterol improved the risk ratio. While following their diets, all participants lowered their risk of heart disease, but both the protein and monounsaturated fat diets resulted in a greater risk reduction than the high carbohydrate diet.[12]

Another benefit of foods plentiful in monounsaturated fats: most are high in vitamin E. When consumed in the diet rather than taken as a supplement, this nutrient is believed to guard against heart disease. Vitamin E is a potent antioxidant that protects LDL cholesterol particles from oxidation by harmful free radicals. (I mentioned earlier that oxidized LDL cholesterol is thought to stick more readily to artery walls.)

OLIVE OIL'S PROTECTIVE PROPERTIES

When it comes to preventing heart disease, olive oil has received the most attention among foods rich in monounsaturated fat—and for good reason. In addition to lowering blood pressure and LDL cholesterol and raising HDL cholesterol when part of a diet that's low in saturated and trans fats, olive oil also seems to help prevent oxidization of LDL cholesterol by free radicals. This heart healthy oil also contains phytochemicals, naturally occurring compounds that seem to help dilate blood vessels and inhibit blood clotting. Furthermore, thanks to a phytochemical (a naturally occurring plant chemical) called oleocanthal, olive oil has anti-inflammatory properties in the body.

Not all olive oils are created equal. Olive oils graded virgin and extra-virgin are not refined in any way—olives are pressed using minimal heat and no chemicals. They contain the highest amount of phytochemicals and nutrients. (*Pure olive oil* and *olive oil* are usually refined oils that have been treated with heat and/or chemicals. *Light olive oil*—light in colour, not calories—is a refined olive oil.)

RECOMMENDATIONS FOR MONOUNSATURATED FATS

There is no official recommended intake for monounsaturated fat. Instead, current dietary guidelines advise that you keep your *total fat* intake to no more than 25% to 35% of your daily calorie intake. What does this mean in practical terms? Well, how much fat you should consume in a day will depend on how many calories you consume. If you eat 2000 calories a day, the upper fat limit of 35% amounts to 77 grams of total fat. If your daily calorie intake is 1500 calories, 35% amounts to 58 grams of total fat. (The math: 1500 calories × 0.35 = 525 calories. Since 1 gram of fat contains 9 calories, 525 fat calories is equivalent to 58 grams of fat.)

Since you should limit your daily intake of saturated plus trans fat to 10% of calories, the majority of your fat should come from heart healthy monounsaturated and polyunsaturated oils. As a rough guide, one-third to two-thirds of your daily fat (10% to 20% of calories) should come from monounsaturated fats. The rest should come from polyunsaturated fats found in oily fish and vegetable oils.

Recommended Intake of Fats

Daily calories	Total fat grams (25% to 35%)	Saturated + trans fat grams (maximum 10%)	Monounsaturated fat grams (10% to 20%)
1600	44–62	18	18–35
1800	50–70	20	20–40
2000	56–78	22	22–44
2200	61–85	24	24–48
2400	67–93	27	27–54
2800	78–109	31	31–62

You needn't worry about counting grams of monounsaturated fat. You won't often find this information on labels anyway because it's not among the 13 nutrients required to be listed on the Nutrition Facts box. In some cases, however, food manufacturers will voluntarily disclose the grams of monounsaturated fat. For instance, you'll find these numbers on labels of soft tub margarines made from olive oil. Most brands supply 4.5 grams of monounsaturated fat per 2 teaspoon (10 ml) serving.

The easiest way to meet your fat recommendations is to replace saturated and trans fats and refined sugars with foods rich in monounsaturated fats. (If you've read Chapter 3, then I'm sure you're well on your way to cutting back on the so-called bad fats and sugars.) In fact, the most recent version of Canada's Food Guide (2007) advises consuming 2 to 3 tablespoons (25 to 45 ml) of unsaturated fat per day. But don't go overboard.

While monounsaturated fats are good for your heart, large portions can lead to weight gain because all dietary fats—olive oil, butter, margarine—deliver 120 calories per 1 tablespoon (15 ml). When it comes to weight control, your waistline doesn't know the difference between unsaturated and saturated fats. That's why the guidelines for dietary fat emphasize substituting heart healthy fats for the less healthy fats and refined carbohydrates.

Foods Rich in Monounsaturated Fat

	Monounsaturated fat content (as a percentage of total fat)
Hazelnut oil	82%
Olive oil	77%
Safflower oil	75%
Hazelnuts (filberts)	75%
Avocado	67%
Almond butter	65%
Almonds	62%
Canola oil	62%
Pistachios	52%
Peanuts	50%
Peanut oil	48%
Peanut butter	47%

QUICK TIPS TO INCREASE MONOUNSATURATED FAT INTAKE

- Use extra-virgin olive oil in salad dressings and marinade recipes.
- Use canola oil when sautéing and baking for a boost of monounsaturated fat and ALA.
- Add a drizzle of hazelnut oil to an oil and vinegar salad dressing.
- Add slices of avocado, instead of cheese, to a sandwich.
- Toss chunks of avocado in salads, burritos, and tacos.
- Snack on a small handful of almonds or peanuts instead of pretzels, potato chips, or crackers.
- Spread peanut or almond butter instead of butter on whole-grain toast.
- Add slivered or chopped nuts to salads, stir-fries, and baked good recipes.

- Try a margarine made from 100% olive oil. (Read the label to make sure it is non-hydrogenated.)

Recipes

Grilled Chicken and Mixed Vegetable Pasta, page 296
Honey Balsamic Dressing, page 268
Pasta Salad with Tuna, Capers, and Lemon, page 300
Roasted Vegetable Pasta, page 302
Roasted Vegetables, page 290
Sautéed Cherry Tomatoes with Garlic and Fresh Basil, page 291

Whole grains

There's little doubt that a steady intake of whole grains protects the heart. Many large studies have revealed that a higher intake of whole grains is associated with significant protection from coronary heart disease. In general, those with the highest intakes of whole grains (about 3 servings per day) had a risk of heart disease or stroke that was 20% to 40% lower than those whose diets contained little or no whole-grain foods. Whole-grain foods consumed in these studies included dark bread, whole-grain breakfast cereals, popcorn, cooked oatmeal, brown rice, bran, barley, and other grains such as bulgur and kasha. (One serving of whole grain is equivalent to 1 slice of whole-wheat bread, 1/2 cup (125 ml) cooked oatmeal, 1/2 cup (125 ml) of cooked brown rice, and 1/2 cup (125 ml) cooked whole-wheat pasta.)[13]

A steady intake of whole grains may also delay the progression of heart disease by slowing the buildup of plaque in the arteries. A study from Tufts University in Boston found that, among post-menopausal women with established heart disease, those who consumed more than 6 servings of whole grains each week had decreased narrowing of the coronary arteries compared to women whose diets contained fewer whole grains.[14]

WHAT ARE WHOLE-GRAIN FOODS?

All grain—be it wheat, rye, oats, or spelt—starts out as whole-grain kernels composed of three layers: the outer bran layer that has nearly all the fibre; the inner germ layer that's rich in nutrients, antioxidants, and unsaturated fats; and the endosperm that contains most of the starch. Whole-grain foods contain *all* parts of the grain kernel and, with that, all of the nutrients, phytochemicals, and fibre. Because they contain all components of the kernel, whole grains are darker and chewier than refined grains.

When whole grains are refined, milled, and heat-processed into flakes, puffs, or white flour, the bran and germ are removed, leaving only the starchy endosperm. Minus the bran and germ, grain loses about 25% of its protein—along with at least 17 nutrients. In addition to less protein, refined grains have less fibre, fewer vitamins and minerals, and 75% fewer phytochemicals. Refined grains are enriched with some, but not all, of the vitamins and minerals lost during processing. However, phytochemicals that benefit the heart are not added back to refined grains.

Whole grains can be eaten whole (e.g., wheat berries, oats), cracked, split, flaked, or ground. Often they're milled into flour and used to make whole-grain breads, cereals, pastas, and crackers. A whole grain can be a single food like oatmeal, brown rice, flaxseed, popcorn, or quinoa, or it can be an ingredient in another food such as bread, crackers, and ready-to-eat breakfast cereal.

Whole-Grain Foods

Barley, pot
Bulgur
Corn
Emmer
Farro
Flaxseed
Kamut
Kasha (buckwheat groats)
Millet
Oatmeal
Oat Bran
Popcorn
Pasta, whole-wheat
Quinoa
Rice, brown
Rice, wild
Rye: whole, rye berries, rye kernels
Spelt: whole, spelt berries
Wheat: whole, cracked, wheat berries

HOW DO WHOLE GRAINS PROTECT THE HEART?

There are many ways in which whole grains protect the heart. For starters, they're good sources of vitamins and minerals thought to prevent heart disease, including folate, vitamin E, magnesium, and potassium. Soluble fibre found in certain whole grains can also keep LDL cholesterol in the healthy range, thereby reducing heart disease risk. (You'll learn more about soluble fibre on page 101.) In a study of 3588 older adults, only fibre from cereal grains—not fibre from vegetables and fruit—was found to guard against heart attack and stroke. The most protective fibre came from dark breads such as wheat, rye, and pumpernickel.[15] Whole grains also contain natural compounds called phytosterols, which have been shown to lower elevated blood cholesterol levels.

A diet based on whole grains can also promote weight loss and improve heart disease risk factors in people with metabolic syndrome. (Metabolic syndrome is a strong risk factor for heart attack and type 2 diabetes. For more information about metabolic syndrome, see Chapter 2, page 50.) In a study from Pennsylvania State University, 50 obese men and women with metabolic syndrome were given a low-calorie diet with all of its grain servings being either whole grain or refined grain. After 12 weeks, the researchers found that, compared to those eating refined grains, the whole-grain eaters lost more abdominal body fat and reduced their blood level of C-reactive protein by 38%. C-reactive protein did not change among those on the calorie-reduced refined-grain diet.[16] (C-reactive protein is an inflammatory compound linked to heart disease; see Chapter 1, page 18, for more information.)

Compounds in whole grains seem to keep blood vessel walls healthy as well. One study found that among 1178 men and women, whole-grain eaters had carotid arteries that were less thick.[17] (The carotid arteries supply your head and neck with oxygen-rich blood. The thickness of carotid arteries is a marker of atherosclerosis or hardening of the arteries.)

Eating mainly whole grains can help prevent heart attack by reducing your risk for developing type 2 diabetes. The Iowa Women's Health Study, conducted among 35,988 healthy post-menopausal women, revealed that those with the highest intake of whole grains (4.7 servings per day) were 21% less likely to develop type 2 diabetes than those who consumed less than 2 daily servings. A 10-year study of 75,521 younger women also found whole-grain intake protective from diabetes while high intakes of refined grains increased the risk.[18]

Whole grains are good sources of magnesium, vitamin E, antioxidants, and soluble fibre, all of which play a role in lowering blood sugar. What's more, many whole-grain foods have what's called a low glycemic index, which means they are digested slowly and raise blood sugar gradually. Refined grains such as white bread and white rice have a higher glycemic index and raise blood sugar quickly. This causes your pancreas to produce excess insulin to lower blood sugar to normal. Over time, a steady intake of high-glycemic foods can overwhelm your pancreas such that it can't meet the body's demand for insulin. Blood sugar rises and type 2 diabetes can eventually develop.

Low-Glycemic Whole Grains
Barley
Bread, whole-grain pumpernickel
Bread, whole rye
Corn
Oatmeal, large flake and steel-cut
Oat bran
Pasta, whole-wheat
Popcorn
Rice, brown
Rice, wild
Quinoa

SOLUBLE FIBRE AND CHOLESTEROL-LOWERING

I mentioned earlier that one of the nutritional benefits of certain whole-grain foods is their soluble fibre content. Foods such as whole grains, fruits, vegetables, legumes, and nuts are made up of two types of fibre: soluble and insoluble. Both are always present in varying proportions in plant foods, but some foods will be rich in one or the other. For instance, dried peas, beans, lentils, oats, oat bran, barley, psyllium husks, apples, and citrus fruits are good sources of soluble fibre. Foods like wheat bran, whole grains, and certain vegetables contain mainly insoluble fibre. This fibre has a significant capacity for retaining water and acts to increase stool bulk and promote regularity.

When it comes to preventing heart disease, you want to increase your intake of soluble fibre. Ever since the early 1990s, studies have demonstrated the ability of soluble fibre–rich foods such as legumes, oats and oat bran, and psyllium to lower elevated LDL blood cholesterol in adults and children. Most of the research suggests that including a good source of soluble fibre in your daily diet can lower LDL cholesterol by 9%. A combined analysis of eight clinical trials involving people with high blood cholesterol concluded that, in conjunction with a low-fat diet, consuming 10.2 grams of psyllium per day lowered total cholesterol by 4% and LDL cholesterol by 7%. Another study involving men and women with elevated cholesterol found that eating a 1 ounce (28 g) serving of oat bran twice a day provided significant added cholesterol-lowering power to a low-fat diet, particularly for men and post-menopausal women.[19]

You'll sometimes hear soluble fibre referred to as *viscous* fibre. That's because it forms a viscous or sticky gel in your stomach and slows the rate of digestion and absorption. As soluble fibre passes through the digestive tract, its gel-like property can bind bile acids causing them to be excreted from the body rather than reabsorbed in the intestine. This forces the liver to remove cholesterol from the bloodstream to make more bile acids. Soluble fibre may also trap dietary cholesterol and fat in the digestive tract and speed their removal from the body.

Soluble fibre in your diet might do more than keep your cholesterol level in the desirable range. Adding 3 to 10 grams of soluble fibre to a low-fat diet can also help improve some of the abnormalities of metabolic syndrome and improve blood sugar control in people with diabetes.

How much soluble fibre?

You need to consume *at least* 3 grams of soluble fibre each day to lower your LDL cholesterol. If you have high blood cholesterol, be consistent! Include soluble fibre in your diet most days of the week—in addition to limiting saturated and trans fats. Eating a soluble fibre–rich breakfast cereal twice a week won't do the trick! The following chart shows you how much food it takes to get 3 grams of soluble fibre. You don't have to get all of it in one meal; you might prefer to add a little soluble fibre to several meals or snacks each day.

Best Food Sources of Soluble Fibre

	Total fibre (grams)	Soluble fibre (grams)
Barley, cooked, 1^1/2 cups (375 ml)	12	3
Flaxseed, ground, ^{1}/4 cup (50 ml)	8	2.6
Kellogg's All Bran Buds with Psyllium, ^{1}/3 cup (75 ml)	12	3
Kellogg's All Bran Guardian, 1 cup (250 ml)	6	4
Nature's Path Smart Bran, ^{2}/3 cup (150 ml)	13	3
Oat bran, cooked, 1 cup (250 ml)	6	3
Oatmeal, cooked, 1^1/2 cups (375 ml)	6	3
Oatmeal, instant, unflavoured, 3 packs	8.4	3
Baked beans, cooked, ^{1}/2 cup (125 ml)	6	3
Black beans, cooked, ^{3}/4 cup (175 ml)	8.2	3
Kidney beans, cooked, ^{1}/2 cup (125 ml)	6	3
Lentils, cooked, 1^1/2 cups (375 ml)	24	3

QUICK TIPS TO INCREASE WHOLE GRAINS AND SOLUBLE FIBRE INTAKE

- Read labels. Choose breads, cereals, and crackers made from 100% whole grain. If this information is not on the front of the package, check the ingredient list. Look for a whole grain to be listed first. This means that the product is predominately whole grain. If a whole grain is listed second, you might be getting only a little or nearly half whole grain.
- Try pasta made from whole wheat, brown rice, spelt, or kamut.
- Substitute cooked bulgur, quinoa, or wild or brown rice for potatoes and white rice.
- Sneak whole grains into recipes—add oatmeal to pancakes, ground flaxseed to muffins, bulgur and barley to soups and stews.

- Replace half the white flour with whole-wheat flour in recipes for baked goods.
- Start the day with a bowl of "stick to your ribs" oatmeal or hot oat bran cereal.
- Sprinkle ¼ cup (50 ml) of Kellogg's All Bran Buds over low-fat yogurt and fruit.
- Add 1 to 2 tablespoons (15 to 25 ml) of ground flaxseed to hot cereal, smoothies, yogurt, or applesauce.
- Add raw oats or oat bran to recipes for cookies, muffins, loaves, and pancake batters.
- Bake fish or chicken with an oat bran/ground flaxseed breading. Dip pieces in egg whites first, and then lightly dust with the breading. Add seasonings as desired.

Recipes: whole grains

Apple Raspberry Crisp with Maple Oat Topping, page 362
Chicken Barley Soup, page 271
Marbled Chocolate Banana Bread, page 356
Pumpkin Quinoa Muffins, page 358
Quinoa Tabbouleh, page 262
Wild Rice and Black Bean Salad with Cilantro Lime Dressing, page 265

Recipes: soluble fibre

Apple Blueberry Bran Muffins, page 342
Apple Cinnamon Hot Oats, page 246
Cinnamon Flax French Toast, page 251
Honey Garlic Soy Meatballs, page 313
Orange Fig Granola Bars, page 373
Strawberry Almond Oat Bran Cereal, page 255
Turkey Burgers, page 340

Legumes and soy

Unless you're a vegetarian, you probably don't eat legumes and soy on a regular basis. Many of my clients tell me that they seldom eat these heart healthy foods because they don't know how to prepare them, not because they don't like them! If that sounds familiar, you'll find plenty of tips and recipes in this book to help you incorporate legumes and soy foods into your menu.

Legumes are dried beans (e.g., kidney beans, black beans, lima beans, navy beans, garbanzo beans), peas, and lentils. You can buy them dried in packages or from bulk food bins or you can buy them canned. If you buy dried legumes, you'll have to cook them before you can eat them (see tip on page 107). To save time, I buy legumes in cans, already cooked. All I have to do is open the tin, drain the legumes in a colander, rinse them under cold running water to remove excess sodium, and then add them to soups, salads, and pasta sauces.

Researchers have learned that legumes are definitely an important part of a heart healthy diet. One large study from Tulane University School of Public Health followed 9632 healthy men and women for 19 years and found those who ate dried beans or peas, or peanuts at least four times per week had a 22% lower risk of coronary heart disease than people who ate them less than once a week.[20] Harvard University scientists found that, compared to following a typical Western diet (i.e., one high in red meat, processed meat, refined grains, and sweets), eating legumes as part of a healthy diet that included fruits, vegetables, whole grains, fish, and poultry was associated with a 30% lower risk of heart disease in men.[21]

HIGH CHOLESTEROL AND BLOOD PRESSURE Many studies have demonstrated the ability of legumes to modify risk factors for heart disease. A combined analysis of 11 studies that examined the impact of eating legumes (not including soybeans) on blood cholesterol, showed that legumes significantly lowered total cholesterol, LDL cholesterol, and blood triglyceride levels.[22]

Legumes also help lower blood pressure. The well-known randomized clinical trial, Dietary Approaches to Stop Hypertension (DASH), proved that a diet that includes legumes four times per week has a potent blood pressure–lowering effect. Individuals on the DASH diet who had mild hypertension achieved a reduction in blood pressure similar to that obtained by drug treatment. What's more, blood pressure reductions occurred within 2 weeks of starting the eating plan.[23] (The DASH diet is low in saturated fat and refined carbohydrates and includes fruit, vegetables, legumes, and low-fat dairy products. You'll learn more about the DASH diet in Chapter 6, page 159.)

TYPE 2 DIABETES Making legumes a regular part of your diet might also reduce the risk of developing type 2 diabetes. Numerous studies have linked diets rich in legumes, especially soybeans, to a lower diabetes risk. In a study of 64,227 Chinese women living in Shanghai, those who consumed the most legumes (peanuts, soybeans, and other legumes) were 38% less likely to develop type 2 diabetes than their peers whose diets contained the least.[24]

WHAT MAKES LEGUMES HEART HEALTHY?

There are many components in legumes that make them heart healthy. Legumes are an excellent source of magnesium, a mineral that helps keeps heart rhythm steady, promotes normal blood pressure, and helps regulate blood sugar. Legumes are among the top food sources of cholesterol-lowering soluble fibre. Researchers also attribute the cardio-protective effects of legumes to their vegetarian protein, folate, potassium, calcium, and phytochemical content. The B vitamin folate helps keep blood homocysteine levels in check, while potassium and calcium are needed to regulate blood pressure. It's the unique package of nutrients and phyto-chemicals in legumes that works synergistically to reduce the risk of heart disease.

Like whole grains, legumes are a good source of slow-released carbo-hydrate (i.e., they have a low glycemic index). As such, eating them regularly can improve blood sugar control and reduce insulin secretion, thereby lowering the risk of type 2 diabetes. And there's one more benefit of adding low glycemic legumes to your diet: Because they're digested slowly, they keep you feeling full longer and can help you eat less food at later meals. In other words, adding legumes to meals could help you lose a few pounds!

Heart Healthy Nutrients in Legumes

Per 3/4 cup (175 ml) serving, cooked

	Calories	Carbohydrates (g)	Protein (g)	Fibre (g)	Folate (mcg)	Magnesium (mg)
Black beans	170	30	11.4	11.2	192	90
Garbanzo beans	202	34	11.0	9.3	212	59
Kidney beans	169	30	11.5	8.5	173	56

	Calories	Carbohydrates (g)	Protein (g)	Fibre (g)	Folate (mcg)	Magnesium (mg)
Lentils	172	30	13.4	11.7	269	53
Lima beans	162	29	11.0	10.0	117	61
Navy beans	191	35.5	11.2	14.3	191	72
Pinto beans	183	33.6	11.6	11.5	221	64
Soybeans	223	12.8	21.5	7.7	70	111
Edamame	142	11.5	12.6	6.0	362	74

Source: Canadian Nutrient File, 2007b, Health Canada. Retrieved June 2008 from: http://205.193.93.51/cnfonline/newSearch.do?applanguage=en_CA. Adapted and Reproduced with the permission of the Minister of Public Works and Government Services Canada, 2008

To help put these nutrient numbers in perspective, adults require 400 micrograms of folate every day. With the exception of soybeans, 1 food guide serving of cooked legumes, 3/4 cup (175 ml), supplies at least half of your daily requirements. Women aged 19 to 50 need 25 grams of fibre per day and men require 38 grams. After age 50, daily fibre requirements decrease to 21 grams for women and 30 grams for men. When it comes to fibre, a serving of legumes ranks right up there with bran cereal! And legumes are one of the best sources of magnesium, providing at least 15% of your recommended daily intake. Women need 310 to 320 milligrams per day while men need 400 to 420 milligrams.

Cooking with dried legumes

If you prefer to buy dried legumes, you'll have to soak them before cooking. Soaking rehydrates the beans and reduces cooking time. During soaking, legumes can double in size, so be sure they're well covered in at least three times their volume of water. Once rehydrated, they'll cook in 30 minutes to 2 hours, depending on the type of legume.

• *Overnight-Soak Method.* This takes time and some advance planning, but requires very little effort. First, cover the beans with cool or room temperature water (hot water may cause the beans to sour; cold water slows rehydration and the beans will take longer to cook). Soak them overnight or for 8 to 10 hours. Drain and then cook.

- *Quick-Soak Method.* This convenient shortcut rehydrates dried legumes in little more than an hour. Cover the legumes with water for soaking. Bring legumes and water to a boil. Boil for 2 minutes. Remove the legumes from the heat and cover the pot. Let them stand in the soak water for 1 hour. Discard the soak water and cook the legumes.

- *Cooking.* Cooking times will vary depending on the type, size, and age of the legume. In general, beans triple in size after cooking. To cook, add 3 cups (750 ml) of unsalted water for every 1 cup (250 ml) of soaked and drained beans. The water should be 2 inches (5 cm) above the top of the beans. Add 1 to 2 tablespoons (15 to 25 ml) of vegetable oil to prevent boiling over. Bring the beans to a gentle boil, and then reduce to a simmer, partially covering the pot. Gently stir beans occasionally during cooking. Skim off any foam that develops during cooking.

   Small legumes (black beans, pinto beans, navy beans, lentils) may take 30 to 45 minutes to cook; medium-sized legumes (kidney beans, garbanzo beans, lima beans) can take 1 to 2 hours. When the beans are tender, remove the pot from the heat and let the beans cool in the cooking liquid (this prevents them from drying out). Once cooked, legumes are ready to use in salads, soups, tacos, burritos, and pasta dishes.

SOY AND BLOOD CHOLESTEROL

The soy and heart disease link became popular back in 1995 when researchers from Lexington, Kentucky published a report in the *New England Journal of Medicine* that analyzed 38 studies on soy and cholesterol. The review concluded that eating soy protein instead of animal protein significantly lowered high levels of LDL cholesterol and blood triglycerides. Subsequent studies continued to confirm soy's cholesterol-lowering properties. One study showed that 20 grams of soy protein significantly improved cholesterol levels in 53 women who had normal cholesterol levels to begin with. Another study found that a high-soy diet lowered LDL cholesterol by 4% in people with mildly elevated cholesterol. This same study found the effect of soy to be even more pronounced in individuals with higher cholesterol levels: LDL cholesterol dropped by 10%.[25]

   In October 1999, after reviewing research from 27 studies showing soy's ability to lower total and LDL cholesterol, the U.S. Food and Drug

Administration passed a regulation allowing manufacturers of soy foods to add a health claim on food labels. Most of the evidence showed that substituting at least 25 grams of soy protein for animal protein each day lowered LDL cholesterol by 10%. If you shop for soy milk, tofu, or veggie burgers in a U.S. supermarket, you're bound to read: "Diets low in saturated fat and cholesterol that include 25 grams of soy protein a day may reduce the risk of heart disease. One serving of (name of food) provides x grams of soy protein." Foods that carry the claim must provide 6.25 grams of soy protein per serving and be low in fat, saturated fat, and cholesterol.

In 2000, the American Heart Association recommended adding soy protein to a low–saturated fat diet to help lower cholesterol levels. But in January 2006, the association changed its tune after analyzing 22 studies published since the 2000 advisory. The analysis found that large amounts of soy protein in the diet didn't produce a significant cholesterol-lowering effect—it lowered LDL cholesterol by about 3%.

The reason for the inconsistent results isn't clear. It may have to do with different study designs, different types of products used (e.g., various soy foods and soy supplements), and the types of patients enrolled in the studies. As well, the studies included in the American Heart Association's 2006 review looked at the effect of adding soy protein to a low-fat diet. Researchers from the University of Toronto have demonstrated that soy has a significant cholesterol-lowering effect if it is added to your diet in combination with other known cholesterol-lowering foods. (You'll learn more about this diet, called the portfolio diet, in Chapter 6, page 168.)

Even if they lower your cholesterol only modestly, soy foods are a healthy addition to your diet. They're very low in saturated fat and an excellent source of vegetarian protein. And soy might protect your heart in other ways besides lowering LDL cholesterol. Studies suggest that a regular intake of soy raises HDL cholesterol, lowers blood pressure, and keeps blood vessels healthy. Soy also seems to prevent oxidation or damage to LDL cholesterol. When damaged by free radicals, it sticks to artery walls much more easily.[26]

The heart-protective effects of soybeans are attributed to their protein and isoflavone (a phytochemical) content. To lower cholesterol levels, you need both components, which is why studies using only isoflavone supplements don't show a cholesterol-lowering effect. If you want to keep your LDL cholesterol level in the healthy range, I recommend adding 10 grams of soy protein to your heart healthy diet each day. (Keep in mind that research does suggest greater cholesterol reduction with higher intakes of soy protein.)

Protein Content of Selected Soy Foods

	Soy protein (grams)
Soy beverage, 1 cup (250 ml)	9
Soy flour, defatted, 1/4 cup (50 ml)	13
Soy nuts, 1/4 cup (50 ml)	14
Soy protein powder, isolate, 1 scoop	25
Soybeans, canned, 1/2 cup (125 ml)	14
Tempeh, 1/2 cup (125 ml)	16
Tofu, firm, 1/2 cup (125 ml)	19
Tofu, regular, 1/2 cup (125 ml)	10
Veggie Burger, Yves Veggie Cuisine, 1	11
Veggie Dog, small, Yves Veggie Cuisine, 1	11

QUICK TIPS TO INCREASE LEGUMES AND SOY INTAKE

- Enjoy a mixed bean salad in a pita pocket for a high protein, vegetarian sandwich.
- Add black beans to tacos and burritos. Use half the amount of lean ground meat you usually would and make up the difference with beans.
- Make a vegetarian chili with kidney beans, black beans, and chickpeas.
- Sauté chickpeas with spinach and tomatoes and serve over pasta.
- Add white kidney beans to tomato-based pasta sauce.
- Toss chickpeas or lentils into your next salad or soup.
- Use beans as dips for vegetables or fillings for sandwiches.
- Try a soy-based veggie burger for a change from beef burgers. Most veggie burgers require only 3 minutes grilling per side. Overcooking causes them to dry out.

- Substitute soy ground round for ground beef or chicken in pasta sauce and chili recipes.
- Try an unflavoured soy beverage on cereal or in smoothies. You might need to try a few brands before you find one you like.
- Snack on roasted soy nuts with dried fruit for an afternoon energy boost.
- Replace up to half the all-purpose flour with soy flour in baked goods recipes.

Recipes

Chickpea and Black Bean Salad with Flaxseed Dressing, page 256
Chipotle Chili, page 312
Cinnamon Orange Loaf, page 348
Honey Garlic Soy Meatballs, page 313
Miso Soup, page 276
Slow Cooker Stewed Lentils, page 317
Spicy Black Bean Soup, page 278
Sweet and Sour Tofu Stir-Fry, page 303
Tempeh Stir-Fry with Orange Garlic Sauce, page 305
Thai Tofu Cutlets, page 319

Nuts

Here's a snack that won't be hard to add to your diet because it tastes so good! (Unless, of course, you have a nut allergy, in which case all types of nuts must be avoided.) Botanically speaking, nuts (tree nuts) include almonds, Brazil nuts, cashews, hazelnuts, macadamia nuts, pecans, pine nuts, pistachios, and walnuts. Peanuts are technically considered legumes rather than nuts, but their nutrient makeup and health benefits are similar to nuts so they're grouped with the heart healthy tree nuts.

There is compelling evidence that eating nuts on a regular basis can lower your risk of developing heart disease and dying from it. To date, four large studies involving 172,000 men and women have found that those who eat nuts at least four times per week are almost 40% less likely to succumb to heart disease than those who eat nuts less than once per week. In one study, Harvard researchers followed 21,454 healthy men for 17 years and found that, compared to men who rarely ate nuts, those who included nuts in their diet at least twice per week had a 47% lower risk of sudden cardiac death. (Sudden cardiac death results from an abrupt and unexpected loss of heart function, with the major cause being coronary heart disease.)[27]

HIGH CHOLESTEROL AND BLOOD PRESSURE Nuts can help control certain risk factors for heart attack such as high cholesterol and high blood pressure. Study after study has consistently demonstrated that adding almonds, peanuts, hazelnuts, walnuts, pistachios, macadamia nuts, or pecans to the diet lowers LDL cholesterol in the bloodstream. One study from St. Michael's Hospital in Toronto, Ontario, suggests that the larger the portion of nuts, the greater the cholesterol-lowering effect. The study, conducted among 27 adults with high cholesterol found that snacking on 1/4 cup (50 ml) of whole raw almonds each day lowered LDL cholesterol by 4.4%, while a 1/4 cup portion (50 ml) reduced LDL by 9.4%! The larger portion size of almonds also lowered lipoprotein(a) and oxidized LDL cholesterol.[28] (For more information about lipoprotein(a), see Chapter 1, page 17.) The scientifically tested DASH (Dietary Approaches to Stop Hypertension) diet demonstrated that eating nuts (and legumes) four times per week helps lower elevated blood pressure in people with mild hypertension.

TYPE 2 DIABETES Making nuts a regular part of your diet might also lower your odds of developing type 2 diabetes, a major risk factor for heart attack. The ongoing Nurses' Health Study found that among 83,818 healthy women who were followed for 16 years, those who ate 1 ounce of nuts (roughly 1/4 cup/50 ml) at least five times per week were 27% less likely to develop type 2 diabetes than women who rarely or never consumed nuts. Peanut butter also offered protection, but to a lesser degree. Women who used peanut butter five times per week had a 21% lower risk of type 2 diabetes than women who never or almost never ate it.[29]

The evidence on the cardiovascular benefits of nuts was compelling enough to prompt the U.S. FDA in 2003 to approve a health claim for seven types of nuts. Packages of almonds, hazelnuts, peanuts, pecans, some pine nuts, pistachios, and walnuts can state: "Scientific evidence suggests, but does not prove, that eating 1.5 ounces per day of most nuts as part of a diet low in saturated fat and cholesterol may reduce the risk of heart disease." (These nuts were approved because they contain less than 4 grams of saturated fat per 50 gram serving.)

WHAT MAKES NUTS HEART HEALTHY?

The unsaturated fat found in nuts plays a powerful role in guarding against heart disease since, as you read earlier in this chapter, these fats help lower LDL blood cholesterol. Nuts are high in protein and unusually rich in arginine, an amino acid thought to improve blood vessel function. They are a good source of magnesium, a mineral that helps maintain a healthy blood pressure and regulate blood sugar. As well, nuts deliver a fair amount of vitamin E, folate, B vitamins, potassium, and fibre, nutrients demonstrated to have cardio-protective properties.

Some nuts have unique ingredients that make them especially heart healthy. Walnuts, for example, are an excellent source of alpha-linolenic acid (ALA), the omega-3 fatty acid you read about earlier in this chapter. Studies suggest a steady intake of ALA plays a role in preventing athero-sclerosis and sudden cardiac death, and protecting against irregular heart rhythms. Peanuts contain resveratrol, an antioxidant also found in red grapes and red wine. Animal studies have shown that resveratrol greatly improves blood flow to the brain, and lab studies have demonstrated this antioxidant's ability to reduce blood clots, relax blood vessel walls, and inhibit inflammation.

Nutritional Content of Nuts

Per 1 ounce (30 g) serving

	How many?	Calories	Notable heart healthy nutrients
Almonds	24	160	Vitamin E, magnesium
Brazil nuts	6–8	190	Vitamin E, magnesium
Cashews	18	160	Magnesium
Hazelnuts	20	180	Vitamin E, B6, folate, magnesium
Macadamia nuts	10–12	200	Vitamin B6, magnesium
Peanuts	28	170	Vitamin E, folate, magnesium, resveratrol
Pecans	20 halves	200	Vitamin E

	How many?	Calories	Notable heart healthy nutrients
Pine nuts	157	190	Vitamin E, magnesium
Pistachios	49	160	Vitamin B6, magnesium, potassium
Walnuts	14 halves	190	Vitamin B6, folate, magnesium, ALA

Plant sterols in nuts

Nuts also contain natural compounds called plant sterols, which scientific studies have shown lower LDL cholesterol. Plant sterols are essential components of plant membranes; they're found naturally in nuts, vegetable oils, whole grains, fruits, and vegetables. The ability of plant sterols to lower cholesterol levels has prompted food manufacturers to develop a number of plant sterol–enriched foods such as margarine, milk beverages, yogurt, and yogurt drinks.

Ironically, plant sterols have a similar chemical structure to cholesterol in foods. But rather than boosting blood cholesterol, plant sterols compete with dietary cholesterol for absorption in the digestive tract—and have been shown to reduce the absorption of dietary cholesterol by 30% to 40%. The decrease in stored cholesterol, which is used to make hormones, bile acids, and vitamin D, causes the body to pull cholesterol from the bloodstream for these important functions. Scientists believe it's in this way that plant sterols lower LDL cholesterol levels.

Sounds good so far. The problem? To achieve a substantial cholesterol-lowering effect, you need to consume more plant sterols than you'll find in a handful or two of nuts. A review of 41 clinical trials on plant sterols and blood cholesterol concluded that an intake of 2 to 2.5 grams of plant sterols daily lowers LDL cholesterol, on average, by 10%—a reduction that's associated with a 20% lower risk of heart disease![30] The average North American diet provides 0.15 to 0.3 grams of plant sterols. If you're a vegetarian, you'll consume more—about 0.6 grams per day.

If you have high blood cholesterol, you'll need to increase your intake to 2 grams daily, an amount you can only get from foods enriched with plant sterols. You'll find these foods in the United States, Europe, Australia, Israel, and Japan. Unfortunately, our government has not yet approved plant sterol–enriched foods in Canada. If you happen to travel to the United States, consider stopping by a grocery store to pick up margarine with added plant sterols. Brands include Becel Pro-Activ, Take Control, and Benecol. For most products, you'll need to consume roughly 5 teaspoons (25 ml) of enriched margarine to get 2 grams of plant sterols.

Although the amount of plant sterols found in a serving of nuts won't offer a potent cholesterol-lowering effect, it will certainly help. What's more, emerging research suggests that plant sterols also have anti-inflammatory and antioxidant properties.

QUICK TIPS TO INCREASE NUT INTAKE

While nuts are nutritious and good for your heart, they're also high in calories, thanks to their high fat content. When adding nuts to your diet, especially in $1/4$ cup (50 ml) (~200 calories) or $1/2$ cup (125 ml) (~400 calories) portion sizes, you'll need to subtract a similar number of calories from your diet in order to prevent weight gain. Substitute nuts for less healthy foods like cookies, ice cream, candy, soft drinks, chips, and refined (white) starchy foods. In my opinion, the best way to eat nuts is portion-controlled: pre-measure 1 serving of nuts and store in a small Ziploc bag. Don't snack directly from a large package or jar of nuts! You'll end up eating more than you intended—and more than you need for heart health.

- Toss a handful of peanuts into an Asian-style stir-fry.
- Stir-fry Swiss chard or kale with cashews.
- Add walnuts or pine nuts to a green or spinach salad.
- Sprinkle slivered almonds over a bowl of oatmeal.
- Blend ground almonds into a breakfast smoothie.
- Add chopped pecans or walnuts to muffin, loaf, or pancake batters.
- Snack on a handful of almonds with dried apricots or mango.
- Sprinkle your casserole with a handful of mixed nuts or pine nuts.
- Use nut butter on toast in place of butter or cream cheese.

Recipes

Almond and Berry Yogurt Breakfast Parfait, page 245
Almond-Crusted Tofu, page 307
Blueberry Almond Smoothie, page 247
Carrot Walnut Bread, page 344
Cinnamon Pecan Baked Apples, page 368
Fig and Roasted Walnut Salad, page 259
Green Beans with Toasted Almonds, page 284
Strawberry Almond Oat Bran Cereal, page 255

Fruit and vegetables

We've long been told that eating more fruit and vegetables can help ward off disease, and heart disease is no exception. Studies consistently show that high intakes of these nutrient-packed foods significantly reduce the risk of heart disease and death from heart disease. In a 2007 review of 13 studies involving nearly 280,000 people, researchers concluded that compared to individuals whose diets had less than 3 servings of fruit and vegetables per day, those who ate more than 5 daily servings were 17% less likely to develop heart disease.

Adding more fruit and vegetables to your daily diet benefits both women and men. When researchers from Harvard Medical School followed 39,876 healthy women for 5 years, they learned that eating 7 to 10 servings of fruit and vegetables per day—versus 2 servings—lowered the risk of heart disease by 32%. Among women, a higher fruit and vegetable intake was also linked with protection from heart attack. When the same research group investigated the effect of vegetables on heart disease risk in healthy men, they found that eating at least 2.5 servings per day, compared to less than 1 serving, reduced the risk of heart disease by 23%. The protective effects of vegetables were most apparent in men who were overweight and those who smoked. In these groups, the risk of heart disease was reduced by 29% and 40% respectively.[31]

STROKE Many studies have also reported that a diet plentiful in fruit and vegetables guards against ischemic stroke. (An ischemic stroke occurs when a blood clot blocks an artery to the brain, most often because of prior narrowing and hardening of the arteries due to atherosclerosis.) In a combined analysis of eight studies enrolling 257,551 individuals who were followed for 13 years, researchers concluded that eating more than 5 servings of fruit and vegetables each day reduced the risk of suffering a stroke by 26%.[32]

HIGH BLOOD PRESSURE It's well established from randomized clinical trials that increasing your fruit and vegetable intake can lower blood pressure. In the Dietary Approaches to Stop Hypertension (DASH) study, people who were assigned a diet containing 9 daily servings of fruit and vegetables, in addition to 3 servings of low-fat dairy products, lowered their blood pressure significantly more than those who followed a typical American diet.[33]

WEIGHT GAIN A diet rich in fruit and vegetables can guard against heart disease by keeping your weight in check. In a report from the Nurses' Health Study, researchers learned that middle-aged women who increased their fruit and vegetable intake the most over a 12-year period were 24% less likely to be obese than their peers whose intake had decreased the most. What's more, women with the greatest increase in fruit and vegetable intake had a 28% lower risk of gaining a large amount of weight over the study period.[34]

WHAT MAKES FRUIT AND VEGETABLES HEART HEALTHY?

Because fruit and vegetables contain so many nutrients and phytochemicals, it's difficult to pinpoint any single component that contributes the most to reducing the risk of heart disease. Like so many other heart healthy foods, fruit and vegetables likely exert their protective effects though a number of beneficial nutrients. For starters, many fruit and vegetables are excellent sources of vitamin C, an antioxidant that aids in defending LDL cholesterol against oxidation. Fruit and vegetables also provide folate, a B vitamin that helps prevent an amino acid called homocysteine from accumulating in the bloodstream and damaging artery walls. Increasing your daily intake of fruit and vegetables is one of the best ways to boost your intake of potassium, a mineral that contributes to keeping your blood pressure at a healthy level. (For more information about potassium and its role, see Chapter 3, page 77.) And it goes without saying that an adequate intake of fruit and vegetables means an automatic increase in your daily fibre intake, including soluble fibre that can help lower LDL cholesterol.

But there's more to fruit and vegetables than their exceptional vitamin and mineral content. Many are also important sources of phytochemicals, believed to inhibit the formation of blood clots, lower LDL cholesterol, raise HDL cholesterol, and maintain proper blood vessel function. Phytochemicals studied for their potential to guard against heart attack and stroke include anthocyanins in berries, lycopene in tomatoes, and beta carotene in orange and dark green produce (think carrots and spinach!).

While most studies have looked at the effect of total fruit and vegetable intake and risk of heart disease, some have studied specific types of produce. A diet rich in berries has been shown to reduce blood clotting and boost HDL cholesterol in middle-aged adults with risk factors for heart disease. In this study, a daily intake of berries was also shown to significantly lower blood pressure, particularly in individuals with elevated blood pressure.[35]

Tomatoes also appear to protect the heart. In a study from Finland, researchers assigned 21 healthy adults with normal blood cholesterol levels to a low- or high-tomato diet for 3 weeks. The high-tomato diet included a daily serving of tomato juice (1²/₃ cup/400 ml) and ketchup (2 tablespoons/25 ml). After following the tomato diet, total blood cholesterol fell by 6% and LDL cholesterol dropped by 13%. Moreover, the high-tomato diet increased LDL cholesterol resistance to oxidation by free radicals.[36] (Oxidized LDL cholesterol poses a greater danger because it adheres more readily to artery walls.)

Eating more leafy greens might also ward off heart attack and stroke. A report in the *Journal of the National Cancer Institute* revealed that total fruit and vegetable intake was linked with a reduced risk of heart disease (as well as cancer), with green leafy vegetables offering the most protection. For every serving of leafy greens consumed per day, risk of heart disease decreased by 11%. Similarly, research from the Harvard School of Public Health revealed that leafy green vegetables are good for the heart. Scientists followed 84,251 women and 42,148 men for 14 and 8 years respectively and found that eating 1 daily serving of green leafy vegetables reduced the risk of heart disease by 23%.[37]

Top Fruit and Vegetables for Heart Health

Vitamin C	Folate	Potassium	Carotenoids	Polyphenols
Cantaloupe	Avocado	Apricots	Apricots	Blackberries
Grapefruit	Oranges	Banana	Cantaloupe	Blueberries
Kiwi	Orange juice	Cantaloupe	Mango	Boysenberries
Mango		Dates	Papaya	Cherries
Oranges	Artichoke	Honeydew	Peaches	Cranberries
Strawberries	Asparagus	Oranges	Pink grapefruit	Pomegranate
	Beets	Prunes	Nectarines	Purple grapes

Vitamin C	Folate	Potassium	Carotenoids	Polyphenols
Broccoli	Brussels sprouts		Watermelon	Strawberries
Brussels sprouts	Romaine lettuce	Spinach		Raspberries
Cauliflower	Spinach	Sweet potato	Carrots	
Red pepper		Swiss chard	Leafy greens	
Tomato juice		Tomato juice	Pumpkin	
			Red pepper	
			Sweet potato	
			Tomatoes	
			Tomato juice	
			Tomato sauce	
			Winter squash	

HOW MANY FRUIT AND VEGETABLE SERVINGS?

In terms of reducing your risk for heart disease, the evidence points to a daily intake of 7 servings of fruit and vegetables combined. That's certainly in line with the 2007 Canada's Food Guide recommendation of 7 to 10 servings per day. Most clients I see in my private practice don't come close to consuming 7 servings a day. The good news is that with a little planning, it's not difficult to boost your daily intake. When I advise clients on their diet, I encourage them to practise the following guidelines for fruit and vegetables:

- At breakfast, always include 1 or 2 fruit servings (e.g., 1/2 cup/125 ml of berries, 1 small banana, 1/4 cup/50 ml of dried cranberries or raisins, or 1/2 cup/125 ml of pure fruit juice).
- At lunch, be sure to add at least 1 vegetable serving (e.g., 1/2 cup/ 125 ml of baby carrots, 1 cup/250 ml of green salad, or 1/2 cup/125 ml of low-sodium vegetable juice).
- For between-meal snacks, eat at least 1 fruit serving (e.g., 4 dried apricots, 1 medium-sized orange or pear, or 1/2 cup/125 ml of unsweetened

applesauce) and 1 vegetable serving (e.g., $1/2$ cup/125 ml of raw veggie sticks).

- At dinner, include at least 3 vegetable servings (e.g., $1/2$ cup/125 ml cooked carrots, 5 asparagus spears, and 1 cup/250 ml of green salad).

What's a serving?

- 1 medium-sized fruit (apple, banana, nectarine, orange, peach, pear)
- $1/2$ grapefruit
- 1 cup (250 ml) cut-up fruit
- $1/2$ cup (125 ml) berries or grapes
- $1/4$ cup (50 ml) dried fruit
- $1/2$ cup (125 ml) unsweetened fruit juice
- $1/2$ cup (125 ml) cooked vegetables
- 1 cup (250 ml) salad greens
- $1/2$ cup (125 ml) vegetable juice

WHAT ABOUT JUICE?

To benefit your heart, you're much better off eating whole fruit and vegetables rather than drinking juice. Although studies suggest that pure, unsweetened fruit and vegetable juices can positively impact a number of risk factors for heart disease, the evidence for their cardio-protective effects is much weaker.

Fruit and vegetable juices lack the fibre found in their whole counterparts that can help lower cholesterol, control blood sugar, and promote a feeling of fullness. I am sure you'll agree that it's a lot less filling to drink a large glass of orange juice than it is to eat the two or three oranges you'd squeeze to make the juice.

Large portions of fruit juice also deliver extra calories in the form of natural sugar. Most fruit juices have anywhere from 120 to 140 calories per 1 cup (250 ml) serving—and some as many as 190. (One medium orange has only 62 calories!) In other words, drinking juice instead of eating the whole fruit could contribute to weight gain. My advice: If you drink juice, limit yourself to 1 food guide serving ($1/2$ cup/125 ml) per day. And be sure to buy 100% pure juices that do not have added sugar.

Commercial vegetable juice contains less sugar and fewer calories than fruit juice, but it's high in sodium. For instance, 1 cup (250 ml) of vegetable cocktail packs 690 milligrams of sodium—almost half of most people's daily requirement! If you have high blood pressure, look for low-sodium brands or invest in a juicer and make your own beverages from scratch.

QUICK TIPS TO INCREASE FRUIT AND VEGETABLE INTAKE

- Throw chopped banana, raisins, or dried cranberries into your bowl of whole-grain cereal.
- Purée frozen mixed berries with low-fat milk or soy beverage to make a breakfast shake.
- Add dried berries to muffin mixes and cookie batters. Try dried cherries, currants, cranberries, and blueberries for a change.
- At lunch, drink low-sodium vegetable juice instead of a diet soft drink or coffee.
- Pack leftover roasted vegetables in your lunch. Grilled red peppers, zucchini, onion, and portobello mushrooms make for a delicious sandwich.
- Use greens rich in beta carotene, such as Romaine lettuce, leaf lettuce, arugula, and spinach, for salads.
- Add spinach, kale, rapini, or Swiss chard to soups and pasta sauces.
- Bake, microwave, or boil sweet potatoes instead of white potatoes.
- Try strawberries marinated with balsamic vinegar and a sprinkle of sugar for dessert.
- Prepare individual snack-sized bags of dried apricots, raisins, and almonds for a mid-morning nibble.
- Serve carrot sticks, cherry tomatoes, bell pepper strips, and broccoli florets with hummus (chickpea dip) as an appetizer before dinner.
- Slice up bananas, apples, and pears and serve with a low-fat vanilla yogurt dip.
- Boost your energy with a glass of spicy tomato or vegetable juice.

Recipes

Cinnamon Pecan Baked Apples, page 368
Fig and Roasted Walnut Salad, page 259
Gazpacho, page 274
Mango Cashew Salad, page 260
Orange Ginger Smoothie, page 253
Spicy Sesame Swiss Chard, page 292
Squash and Apple Soup, page 280

Strawberry Rhubarb Muffins, page 360
Warm Spinach and Mushroom Salad with Goat Cheese, page 264

Tea: green and black

All teas are derived from the leaves of a plant called *Camellia sinensis*, and those leaves are rich in natural disease-fighting compounds called flavonoids. (Herbal tea, brewed from flowers, grasses, and herbs rather than *Camellia sinensis* leaves, lacks flavonoids.) This large family of compounds produced by plants can be further broken down into subclasses. The type of flavonoids found in fresh tea leaves are called catechins.

How tea leaves are processed determines the type of tea—green, black, or oolong—and the concentration of catechins. Fresh tea leaves have a very high concentration of catechins. Intentional breaking or rolling of the leaves during processing activates oxidation (fermentation), which destroys some of the catechins. If tea leaves are steamed or fired first, fermentation is halted and, as a result, catechins are retained. Teas are divided into three groups, based on the amount of fermentation the leaves undergo during processing:

- Tea leaves used to make white and green teas are steamed or fired to inactivate fermentation. Due to minimal oxidation, white and green teas have the highest concentration of catechins.
- Tea leaves used to make black teas are fully broken or rolled to maximize oxidation. The leaves are oxidized completely before drying, reducing their catechin content and giving black tea leaves their dark golden colour.
- Tea leaves destined to become oolong teas are broken to allow oxidation to an extent between white and green tea leaves and black tea leaves. Their catechin concentration is somewhere between those of green and black teas.

TEA AND HEART HEALTH

Many studies have examined the link between tea intake and risk of heart attack. Most studies show clear evidence that drinking at least 3 cups (750 ml) of tea per day reduces the risk of developing coronary heart disease. In a combined analysis of 17 studies, researchers found that a 3 cup

(750 ml) increase in daily tea consumption was associated with an 11% lower risk of heart attack. Since this review was published, several other studies have turned up positive findings for tea. A 7-year study of U.S. women found that the risk of heart attack, stroke, and death from heart disease was significantly lower in women who drank at least 4 cups (1 L) of black tea per day. In a study of 4807 Dutch men and women, aged 55 and older, those who drank more than 1½ cups (375 ml) of black tea per day were 43% less likely to suffer a heart attack than were non-tea drinkers.[38]

Drinking black tea on a regular basis might also safeguard people with existing heart disease. Researchers from Boston, Massachusetts found that among 1900 patients hospitalized for heart attack, those who reported being heavy tea drinkers—14 or more cups (3.5 L or more) per week—had a 44% lower death rate than non-tea drinkers. A moderate tea intake of less than 14 cups (3.5 L) per week was linked with a 28% lower risk of dying from heart disease.[39]

Green tea has also been shown to defend against heart disease. The Japanese dietary pattern is characterized by daily green tea, along with soy, fish, seaweeds, fruit, and vegetables. People who follow this dietary pattern to the greatest extent have a 23% lower risk of heart disease, despite the fact that it's also associated with a higher sodium intake and greater risk of hypertension. An 11-year study of 40,530 Japanese men and women without heart disease found that drinking 5 or more cups (1.25 L or more) of green tea per day, compared to less than 1 cup (250 ml), was linked with a 26% lower risk of dying from heart disease. In this study, regular green tea drinkers also had a significantly lower risk of stroke.[40]

Researchers have identified a few ways in which tea confers cardiovascular protection. Short-term studies have demonstrated the ability of catechins in tea to reduce blood clotting, shield LDL cholesterol from oxidation, reduce inflammation, and improve blood vessel function. Scientists assess the latter by measuring the function of the endothelium or inner lining of the blood vessels. Normally this lining releases nitric oxide, a substance that allows the blood vessels to dilate, or open. When the endothelium releases too little nitric oxide, blood vessels are more constricted and blood flow is reduced. Such dysfunction of the endothelium is considered a precursor to atherosclerosis. An easily done ultrasound measurement of the brachial artery, a major artery in the arm, gives a good indication of blood vessel function in the heart.

Catechins in tea exert their protective effect by enhancing the production of nitric oxide in the endothelium, thereby allowing blood vessels to dilate and relax. It's also thought that catechins block the synthesis of compounds that cause blood vessels to constrict. Two controlled studies showed that drinking 4 to 5 cups (1 to 1.25 L) of black tea daily for 4 weeks significantly improved endothelial function in people with existing heart disease and in people with elevated blood cholesterol.[41]

What about caffeine in tea?

The fact that caffeine temporarily increases blood pressure causes many people to worry that drinking tea and coffee can harm the heart. However, there is no evidence that drinking tea or coffee increases the risk of developing heart disease. You've just read how drinking tea can help fight heart disease, and the evidence suggests that coffee can do the same. Although drinking a caffeinated beverage acutely raises blood pressure (i.e., raises blood pressure very briefly after consumption), this elevation does not persist over time in healthy people. In fact, a recent report from the ongoing Nurses' Health Study found no evidence that daily coffee drinking increased a woman's risk of developing hypertension.[42]

Based on a review of the evidence, Health Canada contends that healthy adults are not at risk for adverse effects from caffeine, including cardiovascular effects, provided their daily intake is limited to 450 milligrams. (During pregnancy, women are advised to consume no more than 300 milligrams per day and some experts—including myself— suggest a stricter limit of 200 milligrams.)

That said, there are some people who should limit their daily caffeine intake. If you have hypertension or existing heart disease, I advise that you limit your daily caffeine intake to 200 milligrams (that's the amount in 4.4 cups/1.1 L of black tea). The fact that caffeine temporarily boosts blood pressure is a concern for people with hypertension, particularly folks who are under stress. That's because studies have demonstrated that the blood pressure–raising effects of caffeine and stress are additive. There's also evidence that regular tea and coffee drinking can increase homocysteine in the blood; at elevated levels, this amino acid can damage artery walls.

Use the chart below to help you manage your daily caffeine intake (as you'll see, tea contains significantly less caffeine than coffee).

Caffeine Content of Common Beverages and Foods (milligrams)

Coffee, brewed, 8 ounces (250 ml)	100
Coffee, instant, 8 ounces (250 ml)	66
Coffee, decaffeinated, 8 ounces (250 ml)	3
Espresso, 2 ounces (60 ml)	54
Starbucks coffee, venti, 20 ounces (591 ml)	415
Second Cup coffee, large, 20 ounces (591 ml)	391
Timothy's coffee, large, 18 ounces (532 ml)	245
Tim Hortons coffee, large, 20 ounces (591 ml)	270
Tea, black, 8 ounces (250 ml)	45
Tea, green, 8 ounces (250 ml)	30
Mountain Dew Energy, 20 ounces (591 ml)	91
Red Bull energy drink, 1 can, 250 ml	80
Diet cola, 1 can, 355 ml	50
Snapple Iced Tea, 16 ounces (473 ml)	42
Cola, 1 can, 355 ml	37
Dark chocolate, 1 ounce (30 g)	20

QUICK TIPS TO INCREASE TEA INTAKE

- Kick-start your day with a cup of freshly brewed white, green, or black tea.
- Serve freshly brewed iced tea (green or black) instead of water with lunch or dinner. Garnish with slices of lemon and sweeten to taste. (When making iced tea, double the strength of hot tea since it will be poured over ice.)
- Choose a cup of tea instead of a soft drink with your meal.
- Cook with tea. Add brewed tea to gravies, sauces, and marinades. Use tea as the liquid to braise meat.
- Use loose tea leaves as a flavourful rub for meat, fish, and poultry.

Dark chocolate

Earlier in this chapter, you read how including red wine, purple grapes, berries, and tea in your diet can help prevent heart disease. If you'll recall, these foods and beverages have a common ingredient: phytochemicals called flavonoids. Flavonoids have been shown to have antioxidant, anti-inflammatory, and anti-clotting properties, all of which are thought to protect the heart. These compounds also aid normal functioning of blood vessels by helping them dilate and relax.

Well, there's another flavonoid-rich food you can add to your heart healthy diet: dark chocolate!

The cocoa beans used to make dark chocolate are a rich source of catechins, the same type of flavonoids found in tea leaves. Dark chocolate's cardio-protective effects first made news in 2005, when Italian researchers demonstrated the chocolate's ability to lower blood pressure, reduce LDL cholesterol, and improve insulin sensitivity in 20 patients with never-treated hypertension. In the study, participants were given either a 3.3 ounce (100 g) bar of dark chocolate or a 3 ounce (90 g) bar of white chocolate each day for 15 days.[43] (White chocolate is not made from cocoa beans, so contains no flavonoids.)

Later in 2007, researchers from Germany published a study in the *Journal of the American Medical Association* suggesting you don't need to indulge in a large 100 gram portion (470 calories and 30 grams of fat!) of dark chocolate each day to notice a fall in blood pressure. In the current study, 1/5 ounce (6.3 g) of dark chocolate per day—only 30 calories' worth—was sufficient to lower blood pressure.

In the study, 44 adults, aged 56 to 73, were assigned to eat each day either 1/5 ounce (6.3 g) of dark chocolate or an equivalent 30-calorie portion of white chocolate for 18 weeks. Except for having prehypertension or hypertension, participants were otherwise healthy and were not taking blood pressure medications. Participants were instructed to maintain their usual diet and physical activity and abstain from all other cocoa products during the study. After 18 weeks, no one gained weight but only dark chocolate eaters experienced a decline in blood pressure. Everyone in the dark chocolate group had lower systolic or diastolic blood pressure and four people moved from hypertension to prehypertension.

Eating 30 calories of dark chocolate each day—the equivalent of about two Hershey's Kisses—lowered systolic pressure (the upper number) by 3 mmHg and diastolic pressure (the bottom number) by 2 mmHg. However, no one in the dark chocolate group achieved an optimal blood pressure reading. The researchers noted that while the magnitude of blood pressure lowering was small, it was noteworthy because, on a population level, such reductions would lower deaths from stroke and heart disease.[44]

Flavonoids in dark chocolate, like those in tea, are thought to reduce blood pressure by increasing the production of nitric oxide in the lining of blood vessels, which causes vessels to dilate. However, the findings from these two studies in no way imply that dark chocolate is a substitute for blood pressure–lowering medication. Do not substitute dark chocolate—or for that matter, any food or supplement—for medication prescribed by your doctor.

Another small study conducted among 32 post-menopausal women with high blood cholesterol showed that a high-flavonoid cocoa drink consumed daily for 6 weeks significantly improved vascular blood flow compared to a low-flavonoid drink.[45]

While the medical news for dark chocolate sounds positive, I certainly don't think it's a superstar food when it comes to fighting heart disease. Keep in mind these studies were short-term, lasting 15 days to 4 months. It's not known whether the blood pressure–lowering effect observed in the studies would persist over time. As well, study participants with elevated blood pressure were not yet taking medication. Once on medication, it's unknown whether dark chocolate would have an additional blood pressure–lowering effect. And not all findings have been positive: In a study of 40 patients with coronary heart disease, consuming a dark chocolate bar and cocoa drink daily for 6 weeks had no effect on blood vessel function.[46]

Even so, a small square of dark chocolate appears to be a heart healthy indulgence. It's certainly a healthier way to satisfy your sweet tooth than eating a box of Smarties or drinking a can of sugary pop. Just keep your portion size small to prevent weight gain!

QUICK TIPS TO INCREASE DARK CHOCOLATE INTAKE

- Read labels. Look for dark chocolate that contains at least 70% cocoa solids. The greater the percentage of cocoa solids, the more flavonoids are present.
- Enjoy a small square of dark chocolate after lunch to help curb sweet cravings later in the afternoon.
- Sip a mug of homemade hot dark chocolate by mixing cocoa powder with skim milk. Sweeten with a bit of sugar, if desired.

- Dip cut-up fruit in melted dark chocolate for a healthy dessert.
- Bake with unsweetened dark chocolate. Add chopped dark chocolate to muffins, loaves, and cookies.

Recipes

Chocolate Zucchini Muffins, page 346
Marbled Chocolate Banana Bread, page 356
Chocolate Fruit Fondue, page 367
Chocolate Cake with Crystallized Ginger, page 365
Chipotle Chili, page 312

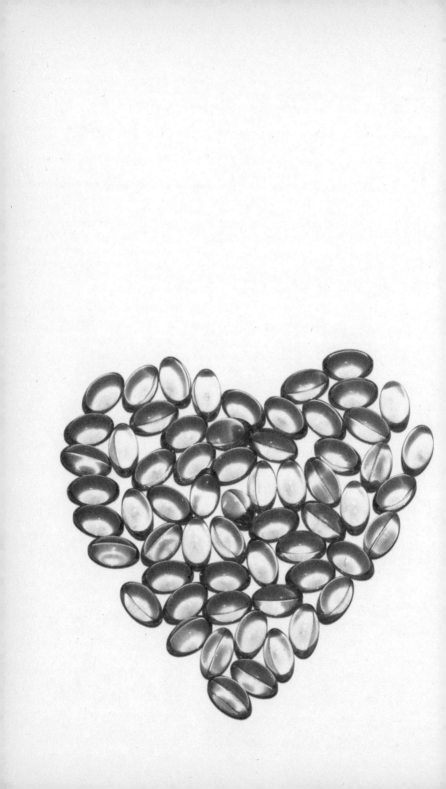

5

Heart healthy vitamins, minerals, and supplements

In the previous chapters, you've read about a number of foods and nutrients that scientists have consistently linked to a lower risk of developing coronary heart disease. Many of these foods owe their cardio-protective effects, in part, to certain vitamins or minerals they contain. For example, magnesium in whole grains is thought to guard against heart disease by regulating blood pressure and blood sugar. Vitamin C in fruit and vegetables might protect the heart by shielding LDL cholesterol from oxidation. And folate in legumes can contribute to a healthier heart by lowering elevated homocysteine levels in the blood.

Many people wonder if getting their nutrients in supplement form can reduce the risk of heart attack. In fact, many people pin their hopes on extra health insurance supplied by a vitamin supplement. After all, if a little of something is a good thing, then more must be better, right? Especially if your food intake isn't stellar? As it turns out, consuming a higher dose of certain nutrients does appear to offer protection from heart disease. But for other nutrients, supplements don't seem to do any good—and in some situations, certain vitamin supplements can be dangerous. In the following pages, you'll learn which supplements are worth considering and which ones you should stay clear of.

Antioxidant nutrients

An antioxidant is any substance that can prevent damage to cells and tissues in the body caused by harmful free radicals. Free radicals are unstable oxygen molecules that are formed naturally through the body's normal metabolic processes. Your body has a built-in system for scavenging and neutralizing free radicals before they do harm. However, if these systems become overwhelmed because your diet lacks antioxidant-rich foods and/or your body is producing too many free radicals, cellular damage can occur. One consequence of free radical damage is oxidized LDL cholesterol particles that contribute to the process of atherosclerosis.

Dietary antioxidants include vitamins C and E, beta carotene, and selenium. When it comes to preventing or treating heart disease, scientists have been most interested in vitamins C and E and beta carotene. Their interest was piqued when numerous observational studies showed that people with high intakes of fruit and vegetables and foods naturally rich in vitamin E had a lower risk of heart attack or death from heart disease. Since fruit and vegetables are excellent sources of antioxidants, researchers suspected they played a role in protecting the heart. Studies also revealed that people who chose to take antioxidant supplements had a lower risk of developing heart disease. However, people who take vitamin supplements may have many healthier lifestyle habits than people who don't use supplements. For example, supplement users may have a healthier diet, they may be non-smokers, and/or they may exercise more—all of which influence heart disease risk.

Nevertheless, such observations led researchers to test the theory that antioxidants taken as supplements would reduce the risk of developing heart disease. Several large, well-controlled studies have been conducted using vitamins C and E and beta carotene alone or in combination. Most clinical trials have had disappointing results: Antioxidant supplements appear to be no substitute for antioxidant-rich foods.

VITAMIN C AND BETA CAROTENE
Vitamin C

In contrast to the results of observational studies suggesting that diets plentiful in vitamin C–rich fruit and vegetables guard against heart disease, studies that assessed vitamin C supplements, mostly in combination with vitamin E, have found scant evidence of any cardiovascular benefit. My advice: Rely on 7 to 10 daily servings of fruit and vegetables to get your vitamin C.

Men and women need 90 and 75 milligrams respectively of vitamin C daily. If you're a smoker, you need to consume an additional 35 milligrams to help your body defend itself against free radicals formed from cigarette smoke. While these official recommended daily allowances (RDAs) meet your body's daily need for vitamin C, higher intakes may be required to guard against heart disease.

Vitamin C Content of Selected Foods (milligrams)

Papaya, 1	188
Red pepper, raw, 1	152
Orange juice, 1 cup (250 ml)	124
Broccoli, cooked, 1 cup (250 ml)	101
Strawberries, 1 cup (250 ml)	98
Brussels sprouts, cooked, 1 cup (250 ml)	97
Green pepper, raw, 1	96
Grapefruit juice, 1 cup (250 ml)	94
Pineapple, raw, 1 cup (250 ml)	74

Kiwi fruit, 1 medium	70
Orange, 1 medium	70
Vegetable juice cocktail, 1 cup (250 ml)	67

Source: U.S. Department of Agriculture, Agricultural Research Service. 2007. USDA Nutrient Database for Standard Reference, Release 20. Nutrient Data Laboratory Home Page, http://www.ars.usda.gov/nutrientdata

Beta carotene

If you're taking a beta-carotene supplement in the hopes of warding off a heart attack, you're wasting your time. Randomized controlled trials have found no evidence whatsoever that supplemental doses ranging from 20 to 50 milligrams per day are effective in preventing heart disease. In fact, taking high dose beta carotene supplements may be harmful if you're a smoker. Two large trials conducted in men at high risk for lung cancer (e.g., cigarette smokers, former smokers, or those with a history of occupational asbestos exposure) found that supplemental beta carotene increased lung cancer risk by 16% and 24% respectively.[1]

To date, an official recommended dietary intake for beta carotene has not been established. Experts contend that consuming 3 to 6 milligrams of beta carotene daily will maintain a blood level in the range associated with a lower risk of chronic diseases. A diet that provides 7 to 10 servings of fruit and vegetables per day and includes one bright orange vegetable daily should provide sufficient beta carotene as well as other disease-fighting carotenoids.

Beta Carotene Content of Selected Foods (milligrams)

Sweet potato, baked, 1 medium	16.8
Carrot juice, 1/2 cup (125 ml)	11.0
Pumpkin, canned, 1/2 cup (125 ml)	8.5
Pumpkin pie, 1 slice	7.4
Carrots, cooked, 1/2 cup (125 ml)	6.5
Spinach, cooked, 1/2 cup (125 ml)	6.3

Collard greens, cooked, 1/2 cup (125 ml)	5.8
Kale, cooked, 1/2 cup (125 ml)	5.7
Turnip greens, 1/2 cup (125 ml)	5.3
Carrots, raw, 1/2 cup (125 ml)	4.6
Cantaloupe, 1 cup (250 ml)	3.2
Winter squash, 1/2 cup (125 ml)	2.9

Source: U.S. Department of Agriculture, Agricultural Research Service. 2007. USDA Nutrient Database for Standard Reference, Release 20. Nutrient Data Laboratory Home Page, http://www.ars.usda.gov/nutrientdata

VITAMIN E

Evidence suggests that taking a vitamin E supplement can help lower the odds of developing heart disease. Two of the first studies to report that vitamin E supplements offered protection from heart disease appeared in the *New England Journal of Medicine* in 1993. These large studies found significant reduction in risk from heart disease among healthy men and women who took a daily 100 IU (international units) vitamin E supplement.[2] (These studies were not randomized controlled trials, the gold standard of scientific evidence. Rather, the researchers followed a large group of men and a large group of women for a period of years and gathered supplement and medical information at regular intervals. After a certain amount of time, the researchers determined who developed heart disease.)

More recently, the Women's Health Study, a long-term randomized trial, investigated the effect of a 600 IU vitamin E supplement taken every other day on the prevention of heart disease in almost 40,000 healthy American women aged 45 or older. Overall, vitamin E had no effect on dying from any cause. But when the researchers looked at different causes of death, they noted a significant 24% reduction in cardiovascular deaths among vitamin E users. What's more, women 65 and older taking vitamin E were 26% less likely to have a heart attack or die from heart disease than older women not taking the vitamin supplement.[3]

There's little evidence, however, that vitamin E is effective in preventing heart attacks in people with existing heart disease. Two large trials conducted in individuals with previous heart attack, stroke, or evidence of heart disease found that a daily vitamin E supplement did not change the risk of subsequent heart attack or stroke. The HOPE-TOO study, a Canadian-led randomized controlled trial published in March 2005, tested whether vitamin E could prevent heart attack, stroke, or cancer in 7000 older men and women with existing cardiovascular disease or diabetes. Participants were given 400 IU of vitamin E or a placebo for 7 years. At the end of the study, there were no differences in heart attacks, strokes, or cancer between the two groups.[4]

Vitamin E: more harm than good?

Some trials have found that high dose vitamin E supplements may actually cause health problems in people with existing heart disease. In 2005, researchers from The Johns Hopkins School of Medicine published a meta-analysis of 19 randomized controlled trials conducted on more than 135,000 men and women who took anywhere from 17 to 2000 IU of vitamin E each day. (A meta-analysis combines data from a number of smaller studies into one large study.) The investigators found that those individuals who took high dose vitamin E supplements (400 IU or more) for 1 year had roughly a 4% higher death rate than people who took a placebo. That amounted to an extra 39 deaths for every 10,000 people who were taking vitamin E.

The authors of this review concluded that high dose vitamin E supplements should be avoided. However, the nine trials in this meta-analysis were conducted in adults with chronic disease. In other words, the results may not apply to healthy people. As well, other scientists have criticized the statistical method used by the researchers to get their results. In fact, the Johns Hopkins researchers themselves noted that their results were probably due to chance and concluded that vitamin E offered no benefit for preventing deaths from any cause (e.g., heart disease, stroke, cancer).[5]

The HOPE-TOO study noted that vitamin E users (people with diabetes and/or existing heart disease) were 13% more likely to suffer heart failure, a condition in which the heart's ability to pump blood is weakened. How vitamin E might increase heart failure, or the risk of dying, is unclear. It is possible high doses of vitamin E might actually cause oxidative stress instead of reducing it. Excess vitamin E might also displace other fat-soluble nutrients, disrupting the body's natural balance of antioxidants. Some researchers believe that other forms of vitamin E, such as gamma-tocopherol found in walnuts, nuts, pecans, and sesame oil, may be more important for cancer prevention than alpha-tocopherol (the main type of vitamin E found in supplements).

Vitamin E: food or supplements?

My advice? Get the vitamin E you need by eating a variety of foods. Healthy men and women require 15 milligrams (22.0 IU) of vitamin E per day. If you have existing cardiovascular disease or diabetes, avoid high dose vitamin E supplements. If you do take a supplement, take no more than 100 IU per day (the meta-analysis that reported a higher risk of death at 400 IU found no harm at 100 IU).

And if you don't have heart disease or diabetes? If you're a post-menopausal woman, recent evidence suggests that taking 600 IU of vitamin E every other day may help prevent a heart attack and reduce the risk of dying from heart disease. But that's all we have to go on. If you're a male, there's no good evidence at this time to warrant popping a vitamin E pill to prevent heart disease. The ongoing Physicians' Health Study is expected to provide answers about the role of vitamin E and the prevention of heart disease in men in 2008 (at the time of writing, the study had yet to be published). As you'll see from the list below, many of the heart healthy foods discussed in Chapter 4 are naturally high in vitamin E.

Vitamin E Content of Selected Foods (milligrams)

Sunflower seeds, dry roasted, 1/4 cup (50 ml)	8.4
Almonds, 24 nuts (1 oz/30 g)	7.4
Sunflower oil, 1 tablespoon (15 ml)	5.6
Safflower oil, 1 tablespoon (15 ml)	4.6
Hazelnuts, 20 nuts (1 oz/30 g)	4.3
Carrot juice, 1 cup (250 ml)	2.7
Avocado, 1 fruit	2.7
Pine nuts, 1/4 cup (50 ml)	2.6
Peanut oil, 1 tablespoon (15 ml)	2.1

Spinach, cooked, 1/2 cup (125 ml)	1.9
Peanuts, 28 nuts (1 oz/30 g)	1.9
Olive oil, 1 tablespoon (15 ml)	1.9

Source: U.S. Department of Agriculture, Agricultural Research Service. 2007. USDA Nutrient Database for Standard Reference, Release 20. Nutrient Data Laboratory Home Page, www.ars.usda.gov/nutrientdata

THE BOTTOM LINE ON ANTIOXIDANT SUPPLEMENTS

The Heart and Stroke Foundation of Canada and the American Heart Association both agree that at this time the scientific evidence does not justify taking an antioxidant supplement, alone or in combination with other supplements, for the purpose of preventing heart disease. Relying on such supplements can give some people a false sense of security. An overwhelming amount of data points to the cardio-protective effects of antioxidant-rich foods, and no supplement can make up for a diet that lacks these heart healthy foods.

B vitamins: folate (folic acid), B6, and B12

You might have heard that taking a supplement of B vitamins, especially folate (folic acid), is good for your heart. The theory that these supplements help ward off heart attack stems from the fact that three B vitamins in particular—folic acid, B6, and B12—lower homocysteine levels in the blood. You'll often see the names folate and folic acid used interchangeably. Technically, folate refers to the vitamin when it's found naturally in foods and folic acid is the synthetic form of the nutrient that's added to supplements and fortified foods such as white flour, enriched pasta, and enriched corn meal.

Homocysteine is an amino acid made by the body during normal metabolism. If you recall from Chapter 1, many experts consider a high homocysteine level in the blood to be a risk factor for heart disease and stroke. The link between elevated homocysteine and heart disease was first proposed in 1969, when researchers noticed that children with inherited high homocysteine also had premature atherosclerosis. Since that time, many studies have suggested that excess homocysteine in your bloodstream increases the likelihood of developing heart disease. A combined analysis of 30 studies revealed that a 25% lower homocysteine level would translate into a 32% lower risk of heart disease in women and a 19% lower risk in men.[6]

Excess homocysteine is thought to do harm by damaging the lining of the arteries. Studies in the lab have demonstrated the ability of homocysteine to cause oxidative stress, inflammation, blood clotting, and blood vessel dysfunction.

The amount of homocysteine in your bloodstream is strongly influenced by your diet, as well as genetics. When it comes to diet, the strongest contributors to a normal homocysteine level are folate and vitamins B6 and B12. These three B vitamins help break down homocysteine in the body so it doesn't accumulate. Even marginal deficiencies of these nutrients—due to poor dietary intake or the inability of the body to absorb the vitamins—can lead to a high homocysteine level. Numerous studies have clearly shown that taking a supplement of folic acid, alone or in combination with vitamins B6 and B12, lowers homocysteine levels. And the higher a person's homocysteine level, the greater the reduction. Studies have used daily doses of folic acid ranging from 0.5 to 5 milligrams, although 0.8 to 1 milligram appears to provide maximal homocysteine lowering. (The recommended daily intake for folate for men and women is 0.4 milligram.)

The fact that folic acid is an effective, simple, and inexpensive way to lower blood homocysteine has raised the prospect that the supplement could actually prevent the development of heart disease. But so far, large randomized controlled trials have failed to find any beneficial effects of B vitamins in lowering the risk of coronary heart disease. (The exception: One study reported a 25% lower risk of stroke in people taking B vitamins.[7]) The most recent findings came from the Women's Antioxidant and Folic Acid Cardiovascular Study, a randomized controlled trial involving 5442 women at high risk for heart disease who were given a daily B vitamin supplement (2.5 milligrams of folic acid, 50 milligrams of B6, and 1 milligram of B12) or a placebo (dummy pill). After 7 years, the researchers found that taking B vitamins did not lower the risk of cardiovascular events (e.g., heart attack, stroke, coronary artery bypass surgery) even though the women's homocysteine levels dropped significantly.[8]

An earlier report combined the findings from 177 studies involving 16,958 participants that compared the effect of folic acid supplements on risk of heart disease events. The researchers concluded that folic acid supplements were no better than placebos in reducing the risk of cardio-vascular events or stroke in people with pre-existing heart disease or kidney disease.[9]

It's unclear why the B vitamin homocysteine-lowering trials conducted to date have not demonstrated any benefit. One possibility is that the introduction of mandatory folic acid food fortification in 1998 has meant that B vitamin supplements have a lesser effect on homocysteine levels than expected. It's also possible that B vitamins simply have no effect on your risk of heart disease. Keep in mind that all trials have been conducted in high-risk individuals—people with documented heart disease or kidney disease. The effect of long-term folic acid supplementation on the risk of heart disease in healthy people is unknown.

SHOULD YOU TAKE A B VITAMIN SUPPLEMENT?

The Heart and Stroke Foundation of Canada does not feel there is enough evidence to recommend an amount of folic acid, B6, or B12 for the prevention of heart disease. At this time, the association also does not recommend routine testing of homocysteine levels in healthy people because there is no evidence that lowering high homocysteine guards against heart disease. It is important, however, that you increase your intake of B vitamins from food sources to help meet your recommended daily intakes.

Recommended Daily Allowance (RDA) of Folate

	RDA milligrams (micrograms)
Men and women, all ages	0.4 (400)
During pregnancy	0.6 (600)
During breastfeeding	0.5 (500)
Daily upper limit*	1.0 (1000)

*The daily upper limit is the highest level of intake from a supplement that is considered safe for almost all individuals.

Best food sources: cooked lentils, kidney beans, black beans, Brussels sprouts, cooked spinach, asparagus, artichoke, avocado, orange juice, enriched pasta

Recommended Daily Allowance (RDA) of Vitamin B6

	RDA (milligrams)
Men and women, 19–50 years	1.3
Men, 50+	1.7
Women, 50+	1.5
During pregnancy	1.9
During breastfeeding	2.0
Upper daily limit	100

Best food sources: beef, chicken, salmon, tuna, bran cereal, whole-grain cereals, avocado, bananas, baked potato

Recommended Daily Allowance (RDA) of Vitamin B12

	RDA (micrograms)
Men and women, all ages	2.4
During pregnancy	2.6
During breastfeeding	2.8
Upper daily limit	None established

Best food sources: meat, poultry, fish, eggs, milk, yogurt, cheese, fortified soy products (e.g., soy beverages, veggie burgers, veggie dogs, soy ground round), fortified rice beverages

Even if taking a folic acid supplement doesn't prevent a future heart attack, I think it is a wise idea for people—and particularly women of childbearing age—to take a multivitamin that contains 0.4 milligram of folic acid along with the other B vitamins. The evidence is clear that women who are planning a pregnancy or who could become pregnant can reduce the risk of neural tube defects in their developing baby by taking 0.4 milligram of folic acid. (A neural tube defect occurs when the brain and spinal cord fail to close properly during the early weeks of pregnancy.) Even though there's plenty of folate in lentils and cooked spinach (hardly everyday foods for most people!), your body absorbs only about half of the B vitamin from foods. Synthetic folic acid, on the other hand, is nearly 100% absorbed.

Evidence also suggests that taking a multivitamin with folic acid may help reduce the risk of certain cancers. Folate is involved in the synthesis, repair, and normal functioning of DNA, the genetic material in all cells. There's some indication that a folate deficiency can cause damage to DNA that may lead to cancer. A handful of studies have linked diets low in folate with an increased risk of breast, colon, and pancreatic cancers. In a study of women aged 55 to 69 years, those who took a daily multivitamin containing folic acid for more than 15 years had a markedly lower risk of developing colon cancer. Another study that followed 14,000 people for 20 years found that men who did not drink alcohol and whose diets provided the recommended daily intake of folate were less likely to develop colon cancer.[10]

It's pretty easy to meet your daily vitamin B6 requirements from your diet since, as you'll notice from the list above, it's found in a wide variety of foods. When it comes to B12, however, some people find it a challenge to meet their daily needs from diet. With the exception of fortified soy products and rice beverages, B12 occurs naturally only in animal foods. So if you are a strict vegetarian, you need to supplement your diet with vitamin B12.

As we get older, our bodies become less efficient at absorbing B12 from foods. Stomach acid must cleave the vitamin from the food proteins it's attached to, but many older adults produce inadequate amounts of stomach acid. As a result, less B12 is absorbed. Adults aged 50 and older are advised to get their daily B12 from a supplement such as a multivitamin or from fortified foods. (B12 in these forms does not require stomach acid for absorption.)

If you have elevated homocysteine and you decide to take a folic acid supplement, do not take more than 1000 micrograms per day and be sure the supplement also contains vitamin B12. If you are B12 deficient, a folic acid supplement will mask that condition and your blood tests for B12 will appear normal. A hidden, untreated B12 deficiency can lead to irreversible nerve damage. Older adults and vegetarians are at greater risk for this deficiency. While many folic acid supplements contain vitamin B12, there are also B complex supplements that contain folic acid in addition to other B vitamins, including B12.

Controversy about folic acid supplementation

Recently, there's some concern that high doses of folic acid might do more harm than good. In a randomized controlled trial of 1021 men and women who previously had precancerous polyps removed from their colon, those who took a folic acid supplement (1 milligram) got just as many new polyps as those who took placebo pills. People in the folic acid group had higher rates of advanced tumours and multiple tumours, although this could have been a chance finding (i.e., the evidence wasn't what researchers call statistically significant). This finding raised the possibility that, if taken early, folic acid may prevent polyps from forming but, if taken once polyps form, folic acid in large amounts could accelerate tumour growth.[11]

If you have a history of colon cancer, or precancerous colon polyps, I advise you to avoid taking high dose folic acid supplements.

Vitamin D

Vitamin D's role in promoting calcium absorption for bone health and in helping to prevent osteoporosis is well recognized. Now, there's growing evidence that this vitamin might also guard against heart disease. In most observational studies, death rates from cardiovascular disease rise at higher latitudes (e.g., Canada and the northern United States), increase during the winter months, and are lower at high altitudes. This pattern fits with the observation that vitamin D deficiency is more common at higher latitudes, during long, dark winters, and at lower altitudes.

We rely on sunshine for our main source of vitamin D. When our skin is exposed to the sun's UVB rays for short periods of time, it synthesizes vitamin D. But during our long winter, there isn't enough UVB radiation to produce this vitamin in our skin. And in the summer, the sensible use of sunscreen blocks production by more than 90%. While vitamin D is found in foods such as fortified milk, oily fish, and egg yolks, the amount we consume from diet is considered insufficient to maintain good health.

Vitamin D is thought to protect the heart in a number of ways. It helps maintain normal immune function and normal blood pressure, assists in keeping heart cells healthy, and reduces inflammation in the body. Studies have linked low blood vitamin D levels to greater inflammation (i.e., higher C-reactive protein levels), impaired fasting glucose, metabolic syndrome, and hypertension—all risk factors for heart disease.

What's more, recent studies have revealed that people who are deficient in vitamin D do indeed have a higher risk of heart attack and coronary heart disease. In one study of 18,255 healthy men aged 40 to 75 years who were followed for 10 years, men who were vitamin D deficient were twice as likely to suffer a heart attack than those with sufficient vitamin D levels, even after controlling for other risk factors such as blood cholesterol, body weight, and family history of heart disease. Even men with intermediate blood vitamin D levels were at increased risk of a heart attack.[12]

Another study conducted in 3,248 men and women scheduled for a coronary angiography procedure noted that after almost 8 years of follow-up, patients in the lowest category of blood vitamin D level had a higher risk of dying from heart disease. (See Chapter 1, page 21, for information about the coronary angiography procedure.) Those with low vitamin D levels were also more likely to have elevated blood markers of inflammation, oxidative stress, and blood clotting.[13]

Studies certainly suggest that vitamin D deficiency may be an independent risk factor for heart disease. Perhaps you're wondering if you should take a vitamin D supplement to help prevent a future heart attack. At this time, there is no evidence that taking a daily vitamin D pill will lower the odds of developing heart disease. We'll have to wait for the results of randomized controlled trials to give us that answer.

TAKE A VITAMIN D SUPPLEMENT: 1000 IU PER DAY

Heart health benefits aside, there are other reasons why you should be taking a daily vitamin D supplement. First, foods don't supply sufficient vitamin D to maintain adequate blood levels of the nutrient. Second, Canadians don't produce enough vitamin D from sunlight between October and March. In fact, it's estimated that as many as 50% of North American adults, young and old, are deficient in vitamin D. Studies have also revealed that many children lack a sufficient level of the vitamin.

Third, and very important, there's now strong evidence that vitamin D helps reduce the risk of certain cancers, evidence that prompted the Canadian Cancer Society in 2007 to recommend that adults consider taking 1000 IU (international units) of vitamin D each day in the fall and winter. Older adults, people with dark skin, those who don't go outdoors often, and those who wear clothing that covers most of their skin should take the supplement year-round. The Canadian Cancer Society's vitamin D recommendation does not extend to children since, so far, research has focused only on adults.

Bottom line: It's prudent to supplement your diet with 1000 IU of vitamin D each day. Not only might it guard against heart disease, it might also cut your risk of developing osteoporosis and certain cancers. Choose a vitamin D supplement that contains vitamin D3, which is more potent than vitamin D2. To determine the dose you need to buy, add up how much you're already getting from your multivitamin and calcium supplements, and make up the difference. It can be difficult to hit 1000 IU on the nose since vitamin D is typically sold in 400 IU and 1000 IU doses. Not to worry, though, if your intake slightly exceeds 1000 IU. The current safe upper limit is set at 2000 IU per day—which vitamin D experts feel is far too low. In fact, many doctors advise a vitamin D intake of 2000 IU per day.

You can ask your doctor to test your blood for vitamin D; if you're deficient, you may be advised to supplement with 2000 IU of vitamin D each day. People at risk for vitamin D deficiency include older adults (as we age, the skin cannot synthesize vitamin D as efficiently), people with limited sun exposure, people with dark skin (the pigment melanin reduces the skin's ability to produce vitamin D), and people who are obese (fat deposits under the skin sequester vitamin D and alter its release into the bloodstream).

Magnesium

The mineral magnesium is needed for more than 300 biochemical reactions in the body. Among its many important roles, magnesium keeps your heart rhythm steady, maintains normal blood pressure, and helps regulate blood sugar—all of which influence your heart health.

A number of studies point to magnesium's ability to guard against type 2 diabetes, a major risk factor for heart disease. The ongoing Nurses' Health Study and the Health Professionals' Follow-up Study have been following 85,060 healthy women and 42,872 healthy men since the 1980s. One report from these studies revealed that, over time, the risk of developing type 2 diabetes was greater in men and women with a lower magnesium intake. The Iowa Women's Health Study followed a group of post-menopausal women since 1986. After 6 years of follow-up, the researchers found that the risk of diabetes was lower in women who consumed the most whole grains, fibre, and magnesium. The Women's Health Study examined almost 40,000 healthy women and reported that among women who were overweight, the risk of type 2 diabetes was significantly greater among those with a lower magnesium intake. A recent analysis of seven studies that investigated the link between magnesium from foods and magnesium from supplements concluded that increasing intake by 100 milligrams per day could lower the risk of type 2 diabetes by 15%.[14]

How does magnesium work to help prevent type 2 diabetes? It's thought that the mineral regulates blood sugar control by influencing the release and activity of insulin, the hormone that clears glucose from the bloodstream. Sufficient levels of magnesium may help keep insulin resistance in check (this condition often precedes type 2 diabetes). Studies have also examined the possible benefit of magnesium supplements on blood sugar control in people with diabetes. In a 16-week study of 63 people with below-normal blood magnesium levels, those who took a 300 milligram magnesium supplement each day had higher blood levels of magnesium and improved blood sugar control.[15]

Many studies have revealed that a higher intake of magnesium-rich foods such as whole grains, legumes, and vegetables is associated with a lower risk of developing high blood pressure.

Furthermore, there is evidence that magnesium may help reduce the risk of coronary heart disease and protect from consequences of heart disease. Researchers have observed lower death rates from heart disease in populations that routinely drink "hard" water, which is higher in magnesium than "soft" water. (Soft water is treated to remove minerals, with the exception of naturally occurring sodium.) As well, studies have associated higher blood levels of magnesium with a lower risk of coronary heart disease. There's also evidence that low body stores of magnesium increase the likelihood of abnormal heart rhythms (arrhythmia), a potentially fatal complication of heart attack.

If you have heart disease, consuming more magnesium may improve your prognosis. One study conducted in people with stable heart disease found that, compared to the placebo treatment, magnesium supplementation (365 milligrams taken twice daily) improved tolerance and duration during an exercise stress test. Those taking magnesium supplements were also less likely to experience chest pain.[16] It's thought that magnesium helps maintain the normal functioning of blood vessels during exercise by allowing vessels to dilate, or relax.

HOW MUCH MAGNESIUM?

Dietary surveys suggest that many North Americans don't consume the recommended amount of magnesium. While symptoms of magnesium deficiency are rarely seen in Canada, many experts have expressed concern about the prevalence of marginal, or suboptimal, magnesium stores in the body.

Recommended Daily Allowance (RDA) of Magnesium

	RDA (milligrams)
Children, 1–3 years	80
Children, 4–8 years	130
Boys and girls, 9–13 years	240
Boys, 14–18 years	410
Girls, 14–18 years	360
Men, 19–30 years	400
Women, 19–30 years	310
Men, 31+ years	420
Women, 31+ years	320
During pregnancy	350–360
During breastfeeding	310–320
Daily upper limits	(milligrams)
Children, 1–3 years	65
Children, 4–8 years	110
Children, 9–13 years	350
Teenagers, 14–18 years	350
Men and women, 19+ years	350

The best way to increase your intake and maintain normal body stores of magnesium is to boost your intake of many of the heart healthy foods discussed in Chapter 4. Whole grains, nuts, legumes, leafy green vegetables, and dried fruit are excellent sources of the nutrient. The chart below lists some of the top food sources of magnesium.

Magnesium Content of Selected Foods (milligrams)

Wheat bran, 2 tablespoons (25 ml)	46
Wheat germ, 1/4 cup (50 ml)	91
Almonds, 24 nuts (1 oz/30 g)	84
Brazil nuts, 8 nuts (1 oz/30 g)	64
Peanuts, 28 nuts (1 oz/30 g)	51
Sunflower seeds, 1 ounce (30 g)	100
Black beans, cooked, 1 cup (250 ml)	121
Chickpeas, cooked, 1 cup (250 ml)	78
Kidney beans, cooked, 1 cup (250 ml)	80
Lentils, cooked, 1 cup (250 ml)	71
Navy beans, cooked, 1 cup (250 ml)	107
Soybeans, cooked, 1/2 cup (125 ml)	131
Tofu, raw, firm, 1/2 cup (125 ml)	118
Dates, 10	29
Figs, dried, 10	111
Green peas, cooked, 1/2 cup (125 ml)	31
Spinach, cooked, 1/2 cup (125 ml)	81
Swiss chard, cooked, 1/2 cup (125 ml)	76

Source: Canadian Nutrient File, 2007b, Health Canada. Retrieved June 2008 from: http://205.193.93.51/cnfonline/newSearch.do?applanguage=en_CA. Adapted and Reproduced with the permission of the Minister of Public Works and Government Services Canada, 2008

DO YOU NEED A MAGNESIUM SUPPLEMENT?

If a blood test indicates you have very low magnesium stores, increasing your intake of heart healthy foods may not be enough to restore your magnesium levels to normal. A daily magnesium supplement will be necessary. As well, some people may benefit from extra magnesium because of particular conditions. For instance, certain diuretics used to treat high blood pressure (e.g., Lasix, hydrochlorothiazide) cause magnesium to be excreted in the urine; in poorly controlled diabetes, increased magnesium loss in the urine is associated with elevated blood sugar. Older adults are at risk for magnesium deficiency because they tend to consume less of the mineral in their diets than younger adults and because magnesium absorption decreases with age.

Even if you don't fall into one of the above categories, you may feel your magnesium intake is below par despite your best efforts to eat more heart healthy foods. In this case, you might consider taking a magnesium supplement. But keep in mind, when it comes to promoting healthy blood pressure, studies show that magnesium-rich foods do the trick, not supplements. And those foods also supply other nutrients and antioxidants linked to heart health. While magnesium supplements may be helpful in boosting your intake, be sure to include magnesium-rich foods in your daily diet. And if you're following my advice from the previous chapter, you're already doing so!

About magnesium supplements

Magnesium supplements combine magnesium with another substance, so you'll find magnesium oxide, magnesium citrate, magnesium carbonate, magnesium fumarate, and magnesium sulphate. It's the amount of elemental magnesium in a supplement (listed on the label) and its bioavailability that influence the mineral's effectiveness. Bioavailability refers to how much magnesium is absorbed in the intestines and is ultimately available to be used by your body's cells and tissues. Research suggests that magnesium oxide has a lower bioavailability than other forms of magnesium.

Magnesium supplements are typically sold in 200 or 250 milligram doses. Unless you have been diagnosed with a magnesium deficiency, you shouldn't need more than this amount if you're also including magnesium-rich foods in your diet. If you take calcium supplements, a simple way to boost your intake of magnesium is to buy calcium pills with magnesium added. Calcium/magnesium supplements are sold in a 2:1 or 1:1 ratio of calcium to magnesium. In other words, a 2:1 cal/mag supplement will usually supply 300 milligrams of calcium and 150 milligrams of magnesium. If you take such a calcium supplement twice daily to meet your needs, you'll be consuming 300 milligrams of magnesium, close to the recommended daily intake. Supplement manufacturers often promote a 2:1 ratio as being ideal for absorption despite the fact there is no credible research to support this.

High doses of magnesium supplements can cause diarrhea and abdominal cramping. Do not exceed the safe upper limit of 350 milligrams of supplemental magnesium per day.

Coenzyme Q10

Coenzyme Q10 is a fat-soluble vitamin-like substance made by every cell in the body. Because the body produces it, coenzyme Q10 is not considered an essential nutrient and there is no recommended daily intake for it. The highest concentrations occur in heart, liver, kidney, and pancreas cells, but it's also found in lipoproteins that transport cholesterol and fat in the bloodstream. Beyond what's synthesized in the body, we get some coenzyme Q10 from our diet. The richest food sources include meat, poultry, fish, soybean oil, canola oil, and nuts. We consume moderate amounts from fruits, vegetables, eggs, and dairy products. It's estimated we take in less than 10 milligrams of coenzyme Q10 each day from dietary sources.

Coenzyme Q10 supplements are available in drug stores and health food stores in doses ranging from 30 to 100 milligrams, far more than what we consume from diet. (Interestingly, coenzyme Q10 is widely used in Japan as part of the treatment for cardiovascular disease. In fact, most coenzyme Q10 supplements sold in North America are supplied by Japanese companies.)

Coenzyme Q10's role in producing energy in cells and its antioxidant powers have led researchers to study its effectiveness at preventing and treating heart disease. Test tube studies have demonstrated that coenzyme Q10 inhibits the oxidation of LDL cholesterol. (If you'll recall, the oxidation of LDL cholesterol by free radicals is considered an important step in the development of atherosclerosis.) It's also thought that coenzyme Q10 regenerates vitamin E in lipoproteins after the vitamin neutralizes harmful free radicals. (Vitamin E is another fat-soluble antioxidant that helps prevent the oxidation of lipoproteins such as LDLs.)

Research hints that coenzyme Q10 supplements may help improve heart health in people with heart disease. Studies examined the effect of coenzyme Q10 in addition to conventional medical therapy in patients with chronic stable angina (chest pain) and found that the supplement (60 to 600 milligrams per day) improved exercise tolerance during an exercise stress test and reduced or delayed electrocardiograph changes associated with angina.[17]

Several small studies suggest that taking a coenzyme Q10 supplement could be beneficial in treating hypertension. Two recent trials reported reduced blood pressure in patients taking 120 milligrams of coenzyme Q10 per day.[18] Some, but not all, research suggests that a daily 200 milligram coenzyme Q10 supplement can improve the functioning of the inner lining of blood vessels (the endothelium) in patients who have both diabetes and high blood cholesterol.[19]

HOW MUCH COENZYME Q10?

There is no consensus on how much coenzyme Q10 is beneficial for heart health. The evidence isn't strong enough to support making a general recommendation; however, what I can tell you are the amounts used in clinical studies that have reported beneficial effects.

- For angina, a dose of 50 milligrams of coenzyme Q10 taken three times per day has been used.
- For reducing the risk of future heart problems in patients who suffered a recent heart attack, a dose of 60 milligrams taken twice daily has been used.
- To prevent statin-induced muscle pain, studies have given patients 100 to 200 milligrams per day.
- For treating high blood pressure, researchers have given study participants 120 to 200 milligrams per day in divided doses (e.g., 60 milligrams twice per day).

There have been no reports of adverse effects from taking coenzyme Q10 supplements. Studies suggest that a very small number of people may experience upset stomach, nausea, diarrhea, or reduced appetite with daily doses greater than 100 milligrams. Some of these side effects can be minimized if high doses are divided and taken two or three times per day.

One word of caution if you take the prescription anticoagulant medication warfarin (Coumadin): There have been reports that concurrent use of the drug and coenzyme Q10 reduced the blood-thinning effect of warfarin. If you take warfarin, do not take coenzyme Q10 supplements without first consulting your doctor.

DO YOU NEED A COENZYME Q10 SUPPLEMENT?

While studies have not investigated the ability of coenzyme Q10 supplementation to prevent the development of heart disease, I often see clients in my private practice who take a daily supplement, particularly those who are prescribed statin drugs to lower cholesterol. A number of studies have shown that statins decrease blood levels of coenzyme Q10, which makes sense since coenzyme Q10 circulates in the blood on LDL cholesterol particles. However, it's unclear whether statins reduce the concentration of coenzyme Q10 found in body tissues. There's also preliminary research that supports a role for coenzyme Q10 in decreasing muscle pain caused by statins. Despite more research being needed to confirm if coenzyme Q10 supplements might benefit those taking cholesterol-lowering statins, many people take the supplement as a safeguard.

Supplementing might also offset the natural decline in coenzyme Q10 stores that occurs with aging and that is thought to contribute to reduced energy metabolism in many tissues, especially the heart and skeletal muscles.

Garlic

The heart disease–fighting properties of garlic are attributed to a variety of powerful sulphur-containing chemicals, in particular allicin and allyl sulphides. Many of these are also responsible for garlic's distinctive smell. In addition to sulphur compounds, fresh and cooked garlic also adds vitamin C, B6, manganese, and selenium to your diet.

Interest in garlic's potential to guard against heart disease began when researchers noticed that people living near the Mediterranean—where garlic is a common ingredient in meals—had lower rates of death from cardiovascular disease. Since then, many studies have investigated garlic's effect on such risk factors for heart disease as blood cholesterol, blood pressure, and blood clot formation.

In laboratory studies, garlic and its sulphur compounds have been shown to inhibit the action of HMG-CoA reductase in the liver, a critical enzyme involved in cholesterol synthesis.

As a result, more than 40 clinical trials have examined the effects of raw garlic and garlic supplements on blood cholesterol. The results of many trials suggest that garlic supplements modestly lower total cholesterol, LDL (bad) cholesterol, and blood triglycerides over the short term (1 to 3 months). However, similar cholesterol-lowering effects have not been found in studies lasting 6 months. A recent randomized clinical trial from Stanford University Medical School enrolled 192 adults with moderately high LDL cholesterol levels for 6 months and found that raw garlic and garlic supplements were no better at lowering cholesterol than placebo pills.[20]

Despite the conflicting findings around garlic's cholesterol-lowering properties, the herb might protect the heart in other ways. Most studies show garlic and garlic supplements can significantly impede the clumping together (aggregation) of platelets in the blood, one of the first steps in the formation of blood clots that can lead to a heart attack or stroke. Some, but not all, studies suggest that garlic might help lower blood pressure. In test tube studies, garlic's sulphur compounds have been shown to have antioxidant powers and to reduce the oxidation of LDL cholesterol. Garlic may also help reduce inflammation, a process thought to play an important role in the development of heart disease.

Studies that have attempted to assess the effect of garlic supplements on the progression of atherosclerosis in humans have turned up mixed results. One study from Germany investigated the effect of a 900 milligram garlic supplement and, after 4 years, found that, in women, the amount of plaque in the arteries was significantly greater in those taking the placebo pill than in those taking the garlic supplement; however, in men, there was no difference between those taking garlic and those taking the placebo.[21] (I should point out that this study was funded by a garlic supplement company.)

One small study from the University of California at Los Angeles Medical Center conducted in patients with heart disease found that taking 4 millilitres of aged garlic extract per day (Kyolic brand) slowed progression of calcified plaque in the arteries by more than 65% compared to the placebo-taking group.[22] (Fatty plaques are made of fat, cholesterol, and calcium. Computerized tomography (CT) heart scans can detect the amount of calcium in those plaques. Evidence indicates that the more calcification you have, the worse your heart disease. Even the presence of very small amounts of calcium might indicate that you could go on to develop heart disease.)

The bottom line: It's unclear whether garlic supplements can reduce atherosclerosis and it's not yet known whether supplementation can prevent heart attack or stroke.

SHOULD YOU TAKE A GARLIC SUPPLEMENT?

Based on the evidence to date, taking a garlic supplement might help you lower LDL cholesterol and triglyceride levels at least for the short term. Several types of garlic supplements are available, each providing differing amounts and types of sulphur compounds depending on how they are manufactured.

- *Supplements of powdered or dehydrated garlic* are made from garlic cloves that are sliced then dried at a low temperature to preserve an enzyme that triggers the production of allicin, which in turn stimulates the production of other active sulphur compounds. The most commonly used doses range from 600 to 900 milligrams per day.
- *Supplements of aged garlic extract* are made by aging garlic cloves for up to 20 months in a water and ethanol solution. This aging process reduces the content of allicin and sulphur compounds that cause garlic's strong odour. Aged garlic extract is usually standardized to contain a guaranteed amount of S-allyl-L-cysteine, a powerful sulphur compound believed to lower LDL cholesterol and inhibit blood clotting. Doses used in studies typically range from 2.4 to 7.2 grams per day.
- When it comes to *fresh garlic*, 4 grams (roughly one clove) per day have been used in cholesterol-lowering studies.

More garlic is not always better. Consuming large amounts—as supplements or raw—can have side effects, the most common being unpleasant breath and body odour. More uncomfortable and potentially serious adverse effects include irritation of the digestive tract, heartburn, flatulence, nausea, vomiting, and diarrhea. A hefty dose of garlic can also possibly increase the risk of bleeding; if you're having surgery, avoid using fresh garlic and garlic supplements for the 7 days prior to the procedure.

There's also potential for garlic to enhance the blood thinning effects of prescription drugs such as warfarin (Coumadin) or of other supplements such as fish oil, vitamin E, ginkgo biloba. Be sure to inform your health care provider if you are taking a garlic supplement, especially if you are on anticoagulant medication.

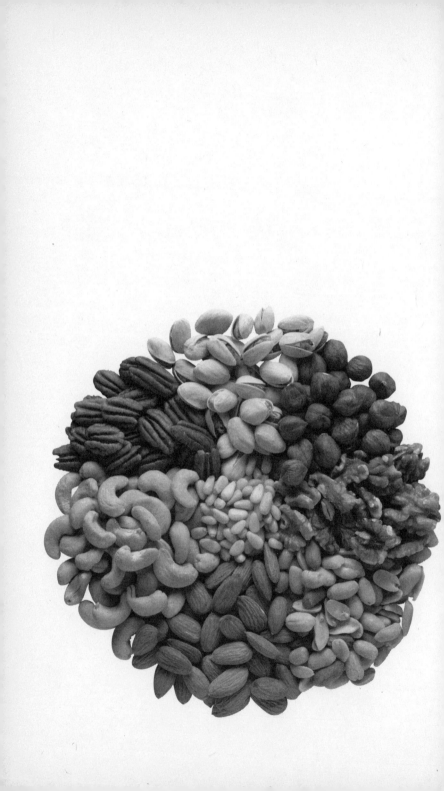

6

Diet plans to help prevent heart disease

In the previous chapters, you learned how individual foods and nutrients impact your risk for heart disease by influencing risk factors such as LDL cholesterol, blood triglycerides, blood pressure, blood sugar, and even inflammation in the body. You learned that excess saturated and trans fats and dietary cholesterol can boost LDL cholesterol, too much sugar can increase triglycerides, and high intakes of sodium and alcohol can raise blood pressure. I also explained how soluble fibre–rich foods and nuts help lower LDL cholesterol, and how fruit and vegetables and legumes help reduce elevated blood pressure.

Now it's time to combine all of those heart healthy foods and nutrients into a meal plan that can help you improve your cholesterol level, lower blood pressure, and ultimately, reduce your risk for heart disease. As I mentioned earlier, preventing heart disease is not just about eating fewer fatty animal foods or adding a handful of almonds to your afternoon snack. Scientific studies have demonstrated that protection comes from the additive effect of eating many heart healthy foods—while limiting those that increase heart disease risk. Adopting and consistently following a heart healthy dietary pattern is the best way to modify risk factors and guard against heart disease.

In this chapter, you'll learn about three diets—all scientifically proven to significantly and positively modify risk factors for heart disease. Two of these have even been shown to reduce your 10-year risk of developing heart disease. Each diet is slightly different, so you can choose the one best suited to your food preferences and lifestyle. Before you read about each heart healthy diet, it's important to review the main nutritional approaches that lower blood pressure, reduce blood cholesterol and triglycerides, raise HDL cholesterol, and improve blood glucose control.

Dietary and Lifestyle Factors that Improve Risk Factors for Heart Disease

Lower blood pressure	Lose weight
	Reduce sodium
	Increase potassium
	Reduce refined sugars and starches
	Reduce alcoholic beverages
Lower LDL cholesterol	Reduce saturated and trans fats
	Limit dietary cholesterol
	Increase soluble fibre
	Add nuts
	Add plant protein (e.g., soy)
	Add plant sterols
Lower triglycerides	Lose weight
	Reduce sugars
	Reduce alcoholic beverages
	Add fish and fish oil

Raise HDL cholesterol	Lose weight
	Regular aerobic exercise
	Moderate alcohol (1–2 drinks per day maximum)

Reduce fasting blood glucose	Lose weight
	Reduce refined starches
	Reduce sugars
	Emphasize low glycemic carbohydrates
	Moderate portion size of starchy foods
	Regular aerobic exercise

The DASH (Dietary Approaches to Stop Hypertension) diet

For years, researchers have studied the effects of single nutrients—such as calcium, magnesium, and potassium—on lowering of blood pressure. While these minerals are important for the regulation of blood pressure, studies using supplements have been inconclusive. The DASH randomized controlled trials have shown that if you get your nutrients from a combination of certain foods—a dietary pattern—the effects on blood pressure are dramatic.

The DASH trial hit the news in 1997 when the landmark study, published in the *New England Journal of Medicine*, demonstrated the potent blood pressure–lowering effect of a specific heart healthy eating plan, called the DASH diet. The diet is low in saturated fat, cholesterol, and total fat, and carbohydrate-rich in that it emphasizes fruit, vegetables, whole grains, and low-fat dairy products (e.g., it emphasizes unrefined carbohydrate–rich foods rather than refined starches and sugars).

In that first DASH trial, 459 adults with prehypertension or hypertension were randomized to follow one of three diets for 8 weeks: (1) a control diet (i.e., a typical North American diet), (2) a diet rich in fruit and vegetables, or (3) a "combination" diet rich in fruit, vegetables, and low-fat dairy products with reduced saturated fat and total fat (i.e., the DASH diet). Sodium intake and body weight were maintained at a constant level during the study.

As you might have already guessed, the DASH diet significantly lowered blood pressure compared to the control diet and reduced blood pressure to a greater extent than the fruit and vegetable diet. Blood pressure lowering was similar for men and women. Individuals on the DASH diet who had mild hypertension achieved a reduction in blood pressure similar to that obtained by drug treatment. What's more, blood pressure reductions occurred within 2 weeks of starting the plan and were maintained for the duration of the study. It's also important to note that the DASH diet resulted in substantial blood pressure lowering in the absence of weight loss. The 2100-calorie DASH diet was not designed to promote weight loss but, rather, to examine the impact of a dietary pattern on blood pressure.[1]

The researchers then decided to study the blood pressure–lowering effects of different levels of sodium while following the DASH diet. The DASH-Sodium trial, published in 2001, tested effects at three different sodium levels—3300, 2400, and 1500 milligrams per day. A total of 412 participants were assigned to either the control diet or the DASH diet, eating foods with high, intermediate, or low sodium levels for 30 days.

The DASH eating plan resulted in significantly lower systolic blood pressure readings at each sodium level. The low-sodium DASH diet produced greater reductions in blood pressure than either the DASH diet alone or the low-sodium control diet. Although people with hypertension lowered their blood pressure the most, those with normal blood pressure also had big reductions.[2]

The DASH diet can do more than lower your blood pressure: It's also effective in reducing blood cholesterol. Compared to the control diet, the DASH diet significantly decreased total and LDL cholesterol levels and did not increase blood triglycerides.[3] (A high-carbohydrate diet can raise blood triglycerides, particularly if it contains mostly refined carbohydrate foods. In the case of the DASH diet, carbohydrate was supplied mainly by whole grains, fruit, vegetables, and legumes.)

Another study tested the effectiveness of the DASH diet in improving risk factors in 116 men and women with metabolic syndrome (this condition involves a number of risk factors for heart disease and type 2 diabetes; for more information, see Chapter 2, page 50). Volunteers were prescribed one of three diets for 6 months: (1) a control diet, (2) a weight-reducing diet emphasizing healthy food choices, or (3) the DASH diet with reduced calories. Compared to people on the control diet, those following the lower-calorie DASH diet decreased their blood pressure, reduced triglycerides and fasting blood glucose, and raised their HDL (good) cholesterol level.[4]

The DASH diet has also been studied to determine its long-term impact on the risk of developing heart disease. Recently, researchers examined adherence to a DASH-style diet in 88,517 healthy women. After 24 years of follow-up, women whose diets most closely resembled the DASH diet were 24% less likely to develop heart disease compared to those who strayed the most from the eating plan. Adhering to a DASH-style diet was also associated with a lower risk of stroke.[5]

WHAT DOES THE DASH DIET LOOK LIKE?

The DASH diet provides food choices that are high in fibre, calcium, magnesium, and potassium, which have all been associated with lower blood pressure. It's also low in refined carbohydrates and saturated fats, which can cause salt retention and elevated blood pressure. The DASH diet is easy to follow: Just increase your fruit and veggies, use low-fat dairy, and cut your saturated fat and sodium intake.

Following the DASH Diet (2100 calories)

Food group	Daily servings	Serving size	What's in it?
Grain products	6–8	1 slice (30 g) bread 1/2 pita pocket 1 ounce (30 g) ready-to-eat breakfast cereal 1/2 cup (125 ml) cooked rice, pasta, hot cereal	Fibre, energy
Vegetables	4–5	1 cup (250 ml) raw leafy vegetables 1/2 cup (125 ml) cooked vegetable 1/2 cup (125 ml) vegetable juice	Potassium Magnesium Fibre
Fruit	4–5	1 medium-sized fruit 1/4 cup (50 ml) dried fruit 1/2 cup (125 ml) fresh/ frozen fruit 1/2 cup (125 ml) 100% fruit juice	Potassium Magnesium Fibre

Food group	Daily servings	Serving size	What's in it?
Non-fat or low-fat milk and milk products	2–3	1 cup (250 ml) skim or 1% milk 1 cup (250 ml) non-fat or 1% yogurt 1 1/2 ounces (45 g) 7% cheese	Calcium Protein
Meat, poultry, fish	6 or less	1 ounce (30 g) cooked meat, poultry, fish 1 whole egg (limit to 4 per week) 2 egg whites	Protein Magnesium
Nuts, seeds, legumes	4–5 per week	1/3 cup (75 ml) nuts 2 tablespoons (25 ml) nut butter 2 tablespoons (25 ml) seeds 1/2 cup (125 ml) cooked dry beans	Magnesium Potassium Protein, fibre
Fats and oils	2–3	1 teaspoon (5 ml) vegetable oil 1 teaspoon (5 ml) soft margarine 1 tablespoon (15 ml) salad dressing 2 tablespoons (25 ml) low-fat salad dressing 1 tablespoon (15 ml) mayonnaise	The DASH diet has less than 30% of calories from fat.
Sweets and added sugars	5 or less per week	1 tablespoon (15 ml) sugar 1 tablespoon (15 ml) jam or jelly 1/2 cup (125 ml) sorbet 1 cup (250 ml) lemonade	

Source: U.S. Department of Health and Human Services. National Institutes of Health. National Heart, Lung, and Blood Institute. Available at: www.nhlbi.nih.gov/health/public/heart/hbp/dash/new_dash.pdf

If you're a male or very active, you might need more than 2100 calories a day to sustain your energy level. On the flip side, if you're overweight, you might need to drop your calorie intake, especially if you're a female. Even a small weight loss—as little as 5% to 10% of your body weight—can lower your blood pressure. The following chart lists the number of daily servings for various calorie levels.

DASH Eating Plan: Number of Daily Servings for 1600, 2600, and 3100 calories (cal)

	Number of servings per day		
	1600 cal	2600 cal	3100 cal
Whole grains	6	10–11	12–13
Vegetables	3–4	5–6	6
Fruit	4	5–6	6
Non-fat or low-fat milk and milk products	2–3	3	3–4
Lean meat, poultry, fish	3–6	6	6–9
Nuts, seeds, legumes	3/week	1/day	1/day
Fats and oils	2	3	4
Sweets and sugars	0	≥2	≥2

Source: U.S. Department of Health and Human Services. National Institutes of Health. National Heart, Lung, and Blood Institute. Available at: www.nhlbi.nih.gov/health/public/heart/hbp/dash/new_dash.pdf

The OmniHeart diets

The OmniHeart study (Optimal Macronutrient Intake Trial for Heart Health) evaluated three diets that followed the same principles as the DASH diet—i.e., low in saturated fat and good sources of calcium, magnesium, and potassium—with some modifications. The researchers' aim was to improve on the DASH diet: They tweaked the amount of protein and unsaturated fat to see if doing so would yield greater heart benefits in 164 adults with prehypertension and hypertension.

The diets tested were as follows: (1) a carbohydrate-rich diet similar to the DASH diet, (2) a diet rich in protein (almost half from plant sources), and (3) a diet rich in unsaturated fat (mostly as monounsaturated fat). The researchers shifted calories from carbohydrates to increase the protein and unsaturated fat contents of the two modified DASH-style diets. The following chart shows where the calories came from.

OmniHeart Diets: Carbohydrate, Protein, and Fat (% calories)

	Carbohydrate diet	Protein diet	Unsaturated fat diet
Carbohydrate	58	48	48
Protein	15	25	15
Total fat	27	27	37
Monounsaturated fat	13	13	21
Polyunsaturated fat	8	8	10
Saturated fat	6	6	6

All diets provided 2100 calories per day and were low in saturated fat and cholesterol (140 milligrams per day). Each diet also provided a daily intake of 30 grams of fibre, 4700 milligrams of potassium, 500 milligrams of magnesium, 1200 milligrams of calcium, and no more than 2300 milligrams of sodium.

Study participants followed their respective diets for 6 weeks. The results of the study were impressive. All diets lowered blood pressure, improved LDL cholesterol, and reduced the risk of developing heart disease by as much as 16 to 21%. But the protein and unsaturated fat diets were even more effective than the carbohydrate-rich diet at reducing certain risk factors and the 10-year risk of heart disease. Compared with the carbohydrate diet, the protein diet went further in lowering blood pressure among those with hypertension and reducing LDL cholesterol and triglycerides. (The carbohydrate diet had no effect on blood triglycerides.) Compared with the carbohydrate diet, the unsaturated fat diet went further in lowering blood pressure, reducing triglycerides, and increasing HDL cholesterol.[6]

As you read earlier, the DASH study showed that a carbohydrate-rich diet that emphasizes fruit, vegetables, and low-fat dairy products and is low in saturated fat and cholesterol substantially lowers blood pressure and LDL cholesterol. Building on this finding, the OmniHeart study demonstrated that partial replacement of carbohydrate with protein (half from plant foods) or with unsaturated fat (mostly monounsaturated fat) can further reduce blood pressure, LDL cholesterol, and heart disease risk. The OmniHeart diets allow you to incorporate more flexibility into a DASH-style eating plan.

WHAT DO THE OMNIHEART DIETS LOOK LIKE?

As you'll see below, the protein diet emphasized more plant protein from legumes, nuts, seeds, and soy foods than the other two diets, and meat, poultry, and fish were increased slightly. The unsaturated fat diet incorporated the liberal use of olive oil, canola oil, and margarines made from olive oil. To reduce calories from carbohydrate, the protein and unsaturated fat diets replaced some fruit and vegetables with protein or unsaturated fat, contained fewer sweets, and provided smaller portions of grain foods.

Following the OmniHeart Diets (2100 calories)

Food group	Protein diet Daily servings	Unsaturated fat diet Daily servings	Serving size
Grain products (mostly whole grains)	5	4	1 slice (30 g) bread 1/2 pita pocket 30 g ready-to-eat breakfast cereal 1/2 cup (125 ml) cooked rice, pasta, hot cereal

Food group	Protein diet Daily servings	Unsaturated fat diet Daily servings	Serving size
Vegetables	5.5	5	1 cup (250 ml) raw leafy vegetables 1/2 cup (125 ml) cooked vegetable 1/2 cup (125 ml) vegetable juice
Fruit	4	5	1 medium-sized fruit 1/4 cup (50 ml) dried fruit 1/2 cup (125 ml) fresh/ frozen fruit 1/2 cup (125 ml) 100% fruit juice
Non-fat or low-fat milk and milk products	2.5	2	1 cup (250 ml) skim or 1% milk 1 cup (250 ml) non-fat or 1% yogurt 1 1/2 ounces (45 g) 7% cheese
Lean meat, poultry, fish	6	4	1 ounce (30 g) cooked meat, poultry, fish 2 egg whites
Nuts, seeds, legumes	3	1	1/4 cup (50 ml) nuts 2 tablespoons (25 ml) nut butter 2 tablespoons (25 ml) seeds 1/2 cup (125 ml) cooked dry beans
Fats and oils	3.5	12	1 teaspoon (5 ml) vegetable oil 1 teaspoon (5 ml) soft margarine 1 tablespoon (15 ml) salad dressing 2 tablespoons (25 ml) low-fat salad dressing 1 tablespoon (15 ml) mayonnaise

Food group	Protein diet Daily servings	Unsaturated fat diet Daily servings	Serving size
Sweets and added ugar	2.5	1.5	1 teaspoon (5 ml) sugar 1 teaspoon (5 ml) jam or jelly 1/2 cup (125 ml) sorbet

Source: www.omniheart.org. Available at: www.omniheart.org/OmniDiets.pdf

OMNIHEART DIET TIPS TO INCREASE PROTEIN

- Include a serving of legumes, nuts, or seeds or lean meat, skinless chicken, or fish in at least 2 meals.
- Have a serving of skim or 1% milk or yogurt at 3 meals, or 2 meals and 1 snack.
- Use egg whites or egg substitutes at breakfast and other meals.
- Top whole-grain cereal with 1/4 cup (50 ml) of nuts.
- Spread unsalted nut butter on whole-grain toast.
- Add different types of legumes to salads and main dishes.
- Try vegetarian soy-based meat substitutes in sandwiches, chili, pasta sauces, and other dishes.
- Control calories by limiting desserts to 3 small servings per week or less and limiting added fats and oils to 3 1/2 teaspoons (17 ml) per day.

OMNIHEART DIET TIPS TO INCREASE UNSATURATED FAT

- Have 1 teaspoon (5 ml) per day of olive oil– or canola oil–based margarine on whole-grain bread.
- Have 1 to 2 tablespoons (15 to 25 ml) of salad dressing made with olive or canola oil and vinegar in a daily salad.
- Add 1 teaspoon (5 ml) of olive or canola oil or a margarine made with these oils to vegetables at dinner.
- Use olive oil or canola oil to sauté vegetables.
- Eat 1/4 cup (50 ml) of unsalted nuts rich in monounsaturated fats each day (e.g., almonds, peanuts, pecans).

- Regulate calories by limiting desserts to 2 small servings per week or less and limiting grains to 4 servings per day.

The portfolio diet

The portfolio diet studies have successfully demonstrated that eating a combination of certain foods can have a dramatic cholesterol-lowering impact that's as effective as certain medications. Dr. David Jenkins, Canadian Research Chair in Metabolism and Nutrition at the University of Toronto and St. Michael's Hospital, has been studying such a combination of cholesterol-lowering foods for the past 8 years. His portfolio diet is low in saturated fat and cholesterol and includes foods you've learned about in Chapter 4—namely, soy protein, almonds, soluble fibre, and plant sterols.

Each individual component of Dr. Jenkins' dietary portfolio has a proven track record in reducing blood cholesterol. By adding only one of these foods to a low-fat diet, you can expect to lower your LDL cholesterol by about 5%. But Dr. Jenkins' research has shown that combining all four of these foods in the diet has a much more powerful effect on lowering cholesterol.

In a study published in 2005, the Toronto researchers evaluated the cholesterol-lowering abilities of three diets: (1) low–saturated fat diet, (2) a low–saturated fat diet combined with a statin drug, 20 milligrams per day of lovastatin (Mevacor), and (3) the portfolio diet. After 4 weeks, the low–saturated fat, low–saturated fat plus statin, and portfolio diet groups achieved reductions in LDL cholesterol of 8%, 30.9%, and 28.6% respectively.[7]

While these results are impressive, this study was tightly controlled. The portfolio diet foods were given to study participants at weekly clinic visits so adherence to the diet was extremely high. But most people don't have researchers shopping for, preparing, and measuring their food portions. Is it feasible for normal, busy folks to follow the portfolio diet in the real world, and get similar results? According to a 2006 study, the answer is yes.

In that study, 66 men and women with elevated LDL cholesterol (greater than 4.1 mmol/L) were instructed to follow the portfolio diet for 12 months. For 2 months prior to starting, participants followed a low–saturated fat and low-cholesterol diet. At the outset, they were instructed to consume a certain amount of almonds, soy protein, viscous fibre, and plant sterol–enriched margarine each day. Participants shopped for and prepared their own foods, with the exception of the special margarine that was supplied to them (I mentioned earlier that plant sterol–enriched foods are not available in Canada at this time.)

Significant reductions in blood cholesterol were seen after 3 months on the diet and were sustained for 1 year. LDL cholesterol dropped by 13% on average, a reduction that translates into a 26% lower risk of heart disease. The more closely participants followed the diet, the better their results. Those who were the most compliant, roughly one-third of participants, lowered their LDL-cholesterol by 29%.[8]

The portfolio diet does more than lower LDL cholesterol. A recent 1-year study found that following the diet significantly lowered blood pressure, starting within the first 2 weeks. The researchers attribute this result to the diet's daily inclusion of almonds, soy protein, and soluble fibre. The portfolio diet was also found to lower levels of C-reactive protein in the blood (a marker of inflammation) as effectively as the statin drug lovastatin (Mevacor).[9]

WHAT DOES THE PORTFOLIO DIET LOOK LIKE?

Like the other heart healthy diets described in this chapter, the portfolio diet is low in saturated fat, trans fat, and dietary cholesterol. But unlike the other diet plans, the portfolio diet is pretty much a vegetarian diet. The plan limits the use of low-fat dairy products, egg whites, poultry, and fish and does not allow red meat. Wherever possible, soy foods and legumes are substituted for animal foods.

The diet also adds a portfolio of four cholesterol-lowering foods to your daily menu: soluble fibre, nuts, soy protein, and plant sterols. (See Chapter 4 for tips on how to add these foods to your daily diet.) Margarine enriched with plant sterols is an important component of the Jenkins' portfolio diet. At this time, Health Canada has not approved the sale of plant sterol–enriched margarines. (In the U.S., you'll find it sold as Take Control margarine from Unilever.) Plant sterols can also be obtained in supplement form (e.g., Swiss Vegapure).

The Portfolio Diet Daily Food Checklist (2000 calories per day)

The most important food groups in this diet are in bold.

Food group	Daily servings	What's a serving?
Soluble fibre (20 g/day)	7 (3 g/serving)	1/2 cup (125 ml) oat bran, dry 2/3 cup (150 ml) oats, dry 1 slice (30 g) oat bran bread 1/4 cup (50 ml) barley, dry 2 teaspoons (10 ml) psyllium husk (Metamucil) 2 cups (500 ml) eggplant
	(1 g/serving)	1/2 cup (125 ml) okra
Soy protein (45 g/day)	7 (6.25 g/serving)	1 cup (250 ml) soy beverage 1/4 cup (50 ml) firm tofu 4 soy deli slices 1 soy burger 1 soy hot dog
Other vegetable proteins (12–16 g/day)	1	1/2 cup (125 ml) cooked beans, lentils, or chickpeas 1 cup (250 ml) instant lentil soup or vegetarian chili
Almonds (42 g/day)	1.5 (28 g/serving)	24 nuts (1 oz/30 g)
Plant sterols (2 g/day)	5 (0.4 g/serving)	1 teaspoon (5 ml) fortified margarine (Flora Pro-activ, Take Control)
Fruit and vegetables	10	1 cup (250 ml) raw leafy vegetables 1/2 cup (125 ml) cooked vegetables 3/4 cup (175 ml) vegetable or fruit juice 1 medium-sized fruit 1/4 cup (50 ml) dried fruit 1/2 cup (125 ml) fresh or frozen fruit
Monounsaturated oils and margarines	4	1 teaspoon (5 ml) olive or canola oil margarine
	(5 g/serving)	1 teaspoon (5 ml) olive or canola oil
Sweets	2	1.5 teaspoons (7 ml) jam or jelly

Food group	Daily servings	What's a serving?
Foods not encouraged		
Fat-free or low-fat dairy	0 to 2 servings/ week	1 cup (250 ml) milk 1 cup (250 ml) yogurt
Egg whites and egg substitutes	0 to 3 servings/ week	1/4 cup (50 ml) of egg whites or egg substitutes
Poultry and fish	0 to 3 servings/ week	3 ounces (85 g) cooked poultry or fish
Red meat	None allowed	

Source: Dr. David Jenkins, University of Toronto

A TYPICAL DAILY MENU ON THE PORTFOLIO DIET

- Breakfast: include soy milk, oatmeal cereal with chopped fruit and almonds, oatbran bread, plant sterol–enriched margarine, and jam
- Lunch: include soy cold cuts, oat bran bread, lentil soup or vegetarian chili, and fruit
- Dinner: include stir-fry with vegetables, tofu, fruit, and almonds
- Snacks: include nuts, raw vegetables, low-fat yogurt (no more than 2 times per week), and soy milk thickened with Metamucil

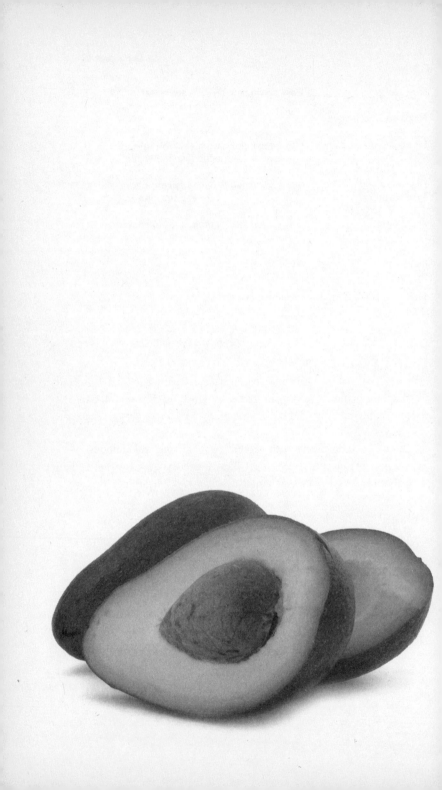

7
Shopping for heart healthy foods

Many of the heart healthy foods described in this book are relatively straightforward to shop for. It's easy to spot fresh fruit and vegetables in the produce section, omega-3 rich seafood at the fish counter, unsalted nuts in the bulk food bins, and vegetable oils packed with monounsaturated fats in the salad dressing aisle. But some foods require careful label reading to ensure you're making choices low in saturated and trans fats, sodium, and added sugars. You'll need to read ingredient lists on breads and cereals to choose products made from a whole grain and offering a good source of fibre. And you need to be careful not to opt for foods just because they're stamped with a healthy logo. This chapter will arm you with plenty of information and tips to help you select heart healthy foods—both fresh and prepackaged—at the grocery store.

Before you grocery shop

Before you head to the supermarket, you need to have a plan. It will save you time while shopping as well as return trips for a forgotten item. Knowing what you need to buy, where to find it, and what to look for will reduce the temptation to add less healthful foods to your grocery cart. Sticking to a plan can also save you money by helping you buy only the things on your list, and reminding you what items you have grocery coupons for.

MAKE A GROCERY LIST

There are a few different ways to organize your shopping list. Some people group similar items together. Others arrange the categories of their grocery list according to the order in which foods are found in the store; your master list might have headings such as *canned goods, dairy case, frozen foods,* and so on. Another strategy is to organize your list by food groups. Here's an example of what a heart healthy grocery list might look like:

- *Vegetables & fruit:* avocado, apples, oranges, frozen blueberries, dried cranberries, asparagus, spinach, carrots
- *Grain products:* whole-wheat bread, large flake oatmeal, Kellogg's All Bran Buds with Psyllium, brown rice, whole-wheat penne noodles, quinoa
- *Milk & milk alternatives:* skim milk, plain 1% yogurt, unflavoured soy milk, light sour cream, part-skim cheddar cheese
- *Meat & alternatives:* ground turkey, canned salmon, firm tofu, canned black beans, plain unsalted almonds, peanut butter
- *Fats & oils:* extra-virgin olive oil, canola oil margarine
- *Other:* dark chocolate, green tea

You might want to add a few other categories for foods that don't fit anywhere, such as *condiments, non-food items,* and *health and beauty products.* Do whatever keeps you organized the best. Once you've found a winning template, consider creating a master form on the computer that you can print and post on the fridge, adding to it during the week as needed.

DON'T SHOP WHILE HUNGRY

Make sure you have a meal or snack before heading off to the store. We all know what happens when we rush to the store on an empty stomach—we come home with more food items than planned, some of them not so healthy. Eating before you shop will limit impulse purchases.

GET FAMILIAR WITH YOUR STORE'S LAYOUT

Knowing how the grocery store is laid out can you save time—and prevent unnecessary trips down the junk food aisle. Healthy, fresh foods such as fruit and vegetables, dairy products, and fresh meats, poultry, and fish are usually placed around the perimeter of the store. Just stick to the outer aisles and you'll find plenty of nutritious foods. The unhealthy, processed foods—cookies, potato chips, soft drinks, fruit drinks, boxed pasta mixes, and such—are usually in the middle aisles. And beware of feature items at the end of shopping aisles. Often these foods are full of extra calories from fat or sugar.

Not all foods on your shopping list will be found round the perimeter of the grocery store. A heart healthy diet can absolutely include packaged foods, provided you choose carefully. That means reading nutrition labels and ingredient lists.

What healthy food symbols do and don't tell you

The majority of Canadians say they want food labels to clearly identify healthy products. Food companies have listened. During the past 4 years, companies such as Sobeys, General Mills, Kraft Canada, PepsiCo, and President's Choice (Loblaw) have initiated on-package food symbols that highlight healthier choices. While a colourful logo can help you quickly spot a food product that's better for you, it doesn't always mean a food is nutritious. Packages of Kraft Dinner and President's Choice Rice Chips and bottles of Gatorade and Diet Pepsi are stamped with "good for you" decals, but health foods they're not.

On-package labelling programs certainly have benefits. They promote awareness of health and nutrition within the grocery store and encourage the food industry to develop healthier products. But the increase in industry-driven labelling programs with logos of assorted sizes, shapes, and colours can be a source of confusion to shoppers. Labelling programs are intended to help you choose products that meet designated criteria, thereby earning the right to bear the company's "healthy choice" icon. Confusion arises because companies don't use the same nutrient criteria when evaluating their products. Some focus on the presence of a vitamin, mineral, or dietary fibre. Others focus on the absence of nutrients such as calories, fat, cholesterol, or added sugars. A few products earn their stripes because they deliver a functional benefit, such as hydration, from ingredients proven to be effective (e.g., Gatorade).

Not all food companies have designed their own logo program based on internally developed criteria. Sobeys developed a line of products called Compliments Balance-équilibre, which fit the Heart and Stroke Foundation of Canada's nutrient criteria and display the foundation's Health Check symbol. The not-for-profit Health Check program is the only third-party labelling program in grocery stores in Canada. Participating food companies submit their products for review in relation to criteria that are based on Canada's Food Guide and that include reduced fat, saturated fat, cholesterol, and sodium levels. If a product passes the test, the company pays the foundation a licensing fee in order for eligible products to carry the red and white Health Check symbol.

Because there are no universal criteria, a "healthy choice" logo on one company's product might not meet another company's guidelines. And many products would not meet the Heart and Stroke Foundation's nutrient criteria. For example, roughly 50% of PepsiCo's Smart Spot products would not earn a Health Check mark.

Here's a look at the various labelling programs and what they mean to your diet:

- *Heart and Stroke Foundation of Canada's Health Check*. Different food categories must meet different criteria based upon Canada's Food Guide to Healthy Eating. For instance, dairy products must be lower in fat and a good source of calcium; fresh meat and poultry must be lean (10% or less fat); breads must be low in fat and a source of fibre; soups must be low in fat and reduced sodium, and a source of vitamins A and C or iron or calcium or fibre. Sodium levels are evaluated for all food categories.

Check *for* **Health Check**™

In early 2008, the Heart and Stroke Foundation tightened its nutrient criteria to reflect changes made to the revised Canada's Food Guide (2007). Stricter criteria are now in place for fat, trans fat, sugar, sodium, and fibre. For example, in addition to meeting other nutrient guidelines, the trans fat content of packaged foods must now be no more than 5% of the total fat content, cold breakfast cereals must contain no more than 6 grams of sugar (excluding sugars from pieces of fruit), and frozen dinners must supply no more than 720 milligrams of sodium.

- *Sobeys Compliments Balance-équilibre.* All products use criteria from the Heart and Stroke Foundation's Health Check program.

- *President's Choice Blue Menu.* Products must contain no hydrogenated oils, no artificial colour or flavours, no added MSG (monosodium glutamate) or flavour enhancers, and limited preservatives. In addition, products must meet one of the following criteria: lower in fat, lower in calories, high in fibre, lower in sodium, a source of omega-3 fats, or a source of soy protein.

- *General Mills Goodness Corner.* This icon-based information system identifies products that have one or more nutritional qualities, including whole grain, 1 gram of sugar, low fat, source of fibre, high fibre, and excellent source of iron.

- *Kraft's Sensible Solution.* A product qualifies for a green Sensible Solution flag if (1) it contains a meaningful amount of nutrients such as calcium, fibre, or whole grain or delivers a benefit such as heart health or hydration while staying within specific limits on calories, fat, sodium, and sugar (e.g., Post Shreddies, Minute Rice) or (2) it meets criteria for "reduced," "low," or "free" in calories, fat, saturated fat, sugar, or sodium (e.g., Jello Light, Kraft Miracle Whip Light Dressing).

- *PepsiCo's Smart Spot.* To display the green Smart Selections Made Easy symbol, products must meet one of three criteria: (1) the product is low in fat, saturated fat, and cholesterol, contains no trans fat, and has no more than 480 milligrams of sodium and 25% calories from added sugar per serving (e.g., Quaker Corn Bran Squares, Quaker Chewy

Granola Bars), or (2) the product delivers a benefit from natural or fortified ingredients and is proven to be effective (e.g., Gatorade, Aquafina Water), or (3) the product contains at least 25% fewer calories, fat, sugar, or sodium than the original version (e.g., Diet 7UP, Baked! Cheetos).

As "healthy choice" symbols continue to spring up on food packages, read the company's explanation to learn what the logo means. Most programs state on the package why a product has earned its symbol. If you can't find an explanation, visit the company's website. The bottom line: Just because a product is part of a company-driven logo program, it still might not be the healthiest choice. You need to read the Nutrition Facts box to determine if a product is suitable for your diet.

Deciphering the Nutrition Facts box

Mandatory nutrition labelling is relatively new in Canada. As of December 12, 2005, most prepackaged foods were required by law to carry a Nutrition Facts box listing the calories and the amounts of total fat, saturated and trans fats, cholesterol, sodium, carbohydrate, fibre, sugars, protein, calcium, iron, and vitamins A and C for a specified serving. Small food companies were given until the end of 2007 to add nutrition information to their packages.

Nutrition Facts Per 1 cup (264g)	
Amount	**% Daily Value**
Calories 260	
Fat 13g	**20%**
Saturated Fat 3g + Trans Fat 2g	**25%**
Cholesterol 30mg	
Sodium 660mg	**28%**
Carbohydrate 31g	**10%**
Fibre 0g	**0%**
Sugars 5g	
Protein 5g	
Vitamin A 4% • Vitamin C 2%	
Calcium 15% • Iron 4%	

Nutrition labels make it easier for you to compare brands of similar products and assess the nutritional value of foods—and that can help you follow a heart healthy diet. But you need to know what the numbers mean, what to watch out for, and how to put the facts and figures into practice. The following tips will to help you sort through—and decipher—label information that's relevant to your diet.

SERVING SIZE INFORMATION This is the place to start and that's why it's listed first. The nutrient amounts that follow are based on 1 serving of the food. The serving size is given in familiar household units—cups, tablespoons, or a portion of the food (e.g., $1/4$ pizza, 1 slice of bread)—and is followed by the metric equivalent.

For something that seems so simple, serving size information can sometimes be tricky. What you consider to be 1 serving can actually be 2 or more. Products to watch out for include fruit juice, snack personal-size pizzas, pita bread, flatbreads, and bagels. The nutrition information for many whole-grain bagels is given for half a bagel; if you eat the whole bagel, you'll need to double the numbers. The bottom line: A serving size is not necessarily the whole package. Read the serving size and know how much you typically consume.

When comparing two brands of a similar food, make sure you're comparing nutrient numbers for identical serving sizes. For instance, most brands of salad dressing list numbers for 1 tablespoon (15 ml), but some specify 2 tablespoons (25 ml) as a serving.

CALORIES This number tells you how much energy you get from 1 serving of the food. The number of servings you consume determines how many calories you actually take in. How you prepare a food will also influence the calories you consume. Packaged rice and pasta dishes (most brands are too high in sodium to be heart healthy!) and muffin and cake mixes require that you add ingredients such as margarine, oil, milk, or eggs. To know how much you are consuming, always check calories and nutrient amounts under the "as prepared" heading.

By itself, the calorie count means little. Calorie requirements are different for everyone, depending on age, body size, gender, activity level, and whether you're pregnant or breastfeeding.

TOTAL FAT; SATURATED AND TRANS FAT The combined amount of saturated, polyunsaturated, monounsaturated, and trans fats is listed next as total fat. If you're looking for a lower fat product, compare brands on grams of total fat per serving. But, as you've learned, a food product with a lot of fat grams isn't necessarily unhealthy. For instance, vinaigrette salad dressings, packages of nuts, and nut butters contain heart healthy monounsaturated fats. What's most important is to look at the next lines of information, which give the grams of saturated and trans fats—the two fats linked to a higher risk of heart disease because they raise LDL cholesterol.

The upper daily limit of saturated plus trans fat you should consume depends on your calorie intake. Current guidelines recommend consuming no more than 10% of daily calories from these so-called bad fats. For a 2000-calorie diet, that means no more than 22 grams of saturated plus trans fat per day. (The math: 2000 calories × 10% = 200 calories; since 1 gram of fat = 9 calories, then 200 ÷ 9 = 22 grams.)

CHOLESTEROL I told you earlier that, since your liver manufactures most of the cholesterol in your bloodstream, dietary cholesterol has little or no effect on most people's blood cholesterol. Even so, current guidelines recommend limiting your daily intake to 300 milligrams per day.

SODIUM Your upper daily sodium limit should be 2300 milligrams. If all of your meals aren't based on packaged foods (which they shouldn't be if you're eating a heart healthy diet), don't panic over a big sodium number for one food. A serving of tomato juice with 700 milligrams of sodium is okay as long as you eat lower sodium foods for the rest of the day. On the other hand, you might want to pass on a frozen dinner that delivers a whopping 1500 milligrams of sodium. (I advise choosing low-fat frozen dinners that contain no more than 200 milligrams of sodium per 100 calories.)

CARBOHYDRATE, FIBRE, AND SUGARS Next on the label comes grams of total carbohydrate: all of the starch, fibre, and sugar that's in 1 serving of the food. If you have diabetes and your diet requires you to count carbohydrates, this is useful information. Otherwise, the numbers that follow—fibre and sugars—are more important.

Women should strive for 25 grams of fibre per day; men, 38 grams. Women and men over 50 should consume 21 and 30 grams, respectively, of fibre daily. Look for foods with at least 2 grams of fibre per serving; breakfast cereals should deliver at least 5 grams per serving. Just because a package claims "made with whole grains" doesn't mean it has much fibre. General Mills Whole Grain Chocolate Lucky Charms has a measly 1 gram of fibre per serving. One serving (13 crackers) of Christie Vegetable Thins Multigrain has no fibre at all.

The sugar numbers include both naturally occurring sugars (e.g., fruit or milk sugars) and refined sugars added during food processing (e.g., sucrose, glucose-fructose, honey, corn syrup). If you're limiting added sugars, you need to read the ingredient list. Look for names such as sucrose, dextrose, glucose, fructose, honey, molasses, malt, corn syrup, rice syrup, cane juice, invert sugar, and fruit juice concentrate. You might be surprised to see how many types of sugar appear on the ingredient list of just one product!

PROTEIN If you eat a mixed diet that contains meat, poultry, fish, eggs, legumes, soy, and dairy you're more than likely meeting your daily protein requirements. Since protein helps keep you feeling full longer after eating, choose snack foods that provide a little protein, such as granola bars and trail mix.

% DAILY VALUE Fat, saturated plus trans fat, carbohydrate, fibre, sodium, vitamins A and C, calcium, and iron are also expressed as percentage of Daily Value. Daily Value is based on a recommendation for a healthy diet and represents the contribution (from 0 to 100%) 1 serving of a food makes towards the particular nutrient's recommended intake.

Use the % Daily Value to see whether nutrients you are trying to consume more of (fibre, vitamins A and C, calcium, and iron) have high percentages in a food product. If you want to boost your fibre intake and are comparing two brands of a breakfast cereal, choose the one with the highest % Daily Value for fibre per similar serving size. If you want to buy a yogurt that provides the most calcium, choose the brand with the highest % Daily Value for calcium. If one serving of food has a 15% Daily Value or more for fibre, vitamins A and C, calcium, or iron, it's considered a high source of these nutrients; a % Daily Value of 25% or more means it's an excellent source.

It's not always wise to strive for a higher % Daily Value. In the case of saturated plus trans fat and sodium, choose food products with a lower percentage. Foods with a 5% Daily Value or less for fat, cholesterol, and sodium are considered low in these nutrients. Foods with a 10% Daily Value or less for saturated plus trans fat are also low in these bad fats.

READ INGREDIENTS LISTS

All packaged foods must list ingredients in order, from greatest to least amount used. The first few ingredients usually make up the bulk of the food. Often, the fewer the ingredients the better, especially if there are a lot of unhealthy extras. If you're limiting added sugars, look for sucrose, dextrose, glucose, fructose, honey, molasses, malt, corn syrup, cane juice, and fruit juice concentrate. Ingredient lists are useful for people with food allergies or intolerances who must avoid certain ingredients. And scanning the ingredient list is often the only way you can tell if products are made from whole grains.

Understanding nutrition and health claims

Manufacturers can make a nutrition claim on labels to help sell products. Claims like "low in fat," "light," "sodium free," or "zero trans fat" refer to 1 serving of the food. If you devour a box of low-fat cookies, your snack might not be low in fat after all. To make a claim, products must meet nutrient criteria set out by Health Canada. Here are a few common claims and what they mean (per serving):

- "Sodium Free"—less than 5 milligrams of sodium
- "Cholesterol Free"—less than 2 milligrams of cholesterol and low in saturated fat; cholesterol-free products are not necessarily low in total fat
- "Low Fat"—3 grams or less of fat
- "Low in Saturated Fat"—2 grams or less of saturated and trans fat combined
- "Trans fat free"—less than 0.2 grams of trans fat and low in saturated fat
- "Reduced"—at least 25% less of a nutrient than in the original product (e.g., reduced fat, reduced sodium)
- "Calorie-reduced"—at least 25% fewer calories than the original food (the food to which the product is compared)
- "Source of Fibre"—at least 2 grams of fibre
- "High in Fibre"—at least 4 grams of fibre
- "Very High in Fibre"—at least 6 grams of fibre
- "Good Source of Calcium"—165 milligrams or more of calcium
- "Light"—as a nutritional characteristic, allowed only on foods that are either "reduced in fat" or "reduced in calories"; as a sensory characteristic, such as taste or texture, must be explained on the label (e.g., "light in colour")

Just as you shouldn't choose a food solely on the basis of a healthy logo or checkmark, you shouldn't choose one based only on a nutrition claim. Read the Nutrition Facts box and ingredient list to get the whole picture. Because a food is stamped "zero trans fat" doesn't mean it's low in sodium or refined sugars. Potato chips deep-fried in non-hydrogenated corn oil may be better for your arteries, but they won't do your waistline any favours.

DIET AND HEALTH CLAIMS

Food companies are also allowed to highlight a relationship between diet and disease on packages, providing they meet regulations about nutrient content. The following five claims have been permitted since 2003:

- A healthy diet low in sodium and high in potassium and reduced risk of high blood pressure.
- A healthy diet with adequate calcium and vitamin D and reduced risk of osteoporosis.
- A healthy diet low in saturated and trans fat and reduced risk of heart disease.
- A healthy diet rich in vegetables and fruit and reduced risk of some types of cancers.
- The non-carcinogenic benefits of non-fermentable carbohydrates in gums and hard candies.

Making healthy choices in the grocery store

Now it's time to walk down the aisles of the grocery store and fill your cart with heart healthy foods. Applying your nutrition knowledge of fats, sugars, whole grains, and sodium along with your label-reading skills should make it easier to identify these foods. Your first stop in the supermarket should be the produce section. These foods don't have nutrition labels, but they're rich in cardio-protective nutrients such as beta carotene, vitamin C, folate, magnesium, potassium, and phytochemicals.

THE PRODUCE SECTION
- Fill your cart with a variety of colourful fruit and vegetables. Choose orange and dark green produce for folate and beta carotene. When in season, buy polyphenol-rich berries.

- Pass up wilted vegetables and overripe fruit, even if they cost less. One exception: Overripe bananas can be used in whole-grain muffin and pancake batters and smoothies.
- Choose grapefruit and oranges that are heavy for their size as they'll have more juice. (If you take heart medication, check with your pharmacist to be sure it doesn't interact with grapefruit or grapefruit juice.)
- Check prepackaged produce carefully for quality.
- Pre-washed, pre-cut fresh veggies such as baby carrots, broccoli florets, cauliflower, shredded cabbage, grated carrot and cubed butternut squash, and packaged salad greens may cost more, but they can save you time in the kitchen.
- Choose brands of frozen vegetables without added salt; avoid those that are frozen in sauce.
- If possible, choose canned vegetables that are low in sodium or contain no added sodium.
- When buying canned fruit, choose brands that are packed in water or their own juice. Avoid canned fruit packed in syrup because it has added sugar.
- Choose 100% unsweetened fruit juices; avoid fruit drinks and punches, which have plenty of added sugar. Try antioxidant-packed juices such as cranberry, pomegranate, and blueberry. Remember, 1 fruit serving is equivalent to 1/2 cup (125 ml) of juice!
- Wash and cut some fresh fruit and veggies as soon as you get home. Store them in small containers or bags in the front of the fridge for easy-to-grab snacks.
- You'll also find excellent sources of vegetarian protein, such as tofu, veggie burgers, and soy deli slices, in the produce section.

THE DAIRY CASE

- Buy skim or 1% milk rather than 2%, whole milk (3.3% MF), and cream. This decreases the saturated fat and calories but keeps all other nutrients the same. Look for the grams of total fat and saturated fat per serving as you compare similar products.
- When buying soy beverages, choose a brand that is unflavoured (less added sugar) or unsweetened (no added sugar) and calcium-enriched. Check the Nutrition Facts box for the % DV for calcium—it should say

25% to 30%. Most brands are enriched with calcium along with vitamin D, B12, and other nutrients.

- Buy evaporated skim milk instead of cream or light cream for coffee.
- Buy yogurt with a milk fat content of 1% or less. Choose low-fat (7% MF) or fat-free sour cream over full-fat sour cream (14% MF).
- More often, choose cheese made from skim or part-skim milk. The label will state a milk fat content of less than 20%. Choose 1% or fat-free cottage cheese.
- If you use butter, do so sparingly and buy small quantities. Butter is made from milk fat. It's high in saturated fat and contains dietary cholesterol, which can contribute to atherosclerosis.
- Choose margarine over butter. Margarine is made from vegetable oil. It is much lower in saturated fat than butter and contains no cholesterol. Buy a soft tub brand that is trans fat–free (non-hydrogenated). To increase your intake of monounsaturated fat, choose one that's made from olive oil or canola oil.
- Buy whole eggs that are enriched with omega-3 fats (from flaxseed or fish oil). Buy pure egg whites (sold in cartons next to the fresh eggs) to dilute the cholesterol content of whole-egg dishes such as omelets and scrambled eggs.
- Don't buy food past its expiration date. The "sell-by" date refers to how long the grocery store can keep the product for sale on the shelf. However, the product is still safe and wholesome past this date. Milk cartons carry "sell-by" dates. If milk has been properly refrigerated at 40 degrees Fahrenheit (4.5 degrees Celsius) or below, it generally stays fresh for up to 3 days after this date. The "use-by" date is intended to tell you how long you can keep the product at top eating quality in your home.

THE MEAT AND FISH COUNTER

- Buy lean cuts of meat and pork. Look for the words *round* or *loin* in the name for beef and *loin* or *leg* when buying pork. In Canada, all cuts of beef are lean (except for short ribs) when trimmed of visible fat. Choose lean or extra lean ground meat.
- Choose chicken and turkey breast because they often have less fat and fewer calories than other meats. Remove the skin before eating. Buy extra lean ground turkey and extra lean ground chicken.

- Read meat packages to determine how many servings you get. For instance, since 1 serving of meat is 3 ounces (90 g), then a package that contains 1 pound (454 g) of steak should serve five people!
- Take advantage of sales on bulk family packs, then divide and freeze portions for later use.
- Buy enough fresh or frozen fish to serve as meals twice per week (canned fish counts too). Salmon, trout, Arctic char, herring, and sardines are excellent sources of omega-3 fatty acids.
- If you want the convenience of frozen fish sticks, look for products that are free of trans fat and have no more than 500 milligrams of sodium per 3 to 4 ounce (85 to 113 g) serving. If the serving size is larger, sodium numbers can be slightly higher.
- If you eat canned tuna regularly, choose "light" or "flaked" tuna rather than "white" or "albacore." Light tuna has less mercury than albacore tuna.
- Leaner deli meats include turkey, chicken breast, roast beef, and lean ham. Avoid fatty sausage, salami, and bologna.

THE BREAD AND CRACKER SECTION

- Read the ingredient list. Look for whole-wheat flour, whole-rye flour, rye meal, or another whole grain—such as whole spelt flour, flaxseed, oats, kamut, quinoa, barley, or brown rice—to be listed as the first ingredient.
- Choose whole-grain bread that has at least 4 grams of fibre and no more than 400 milligrams of sodium per 2 slices (1 slice is 30 to 35 grams). Check serving sizes. For most people, a serving size of bread is 2 slices. Yet some nutrition labels give you the calories, fibre, and sodium for 1 slice.
- Choose crackers made from a whole grain (i.e., the first ingredient listed). Read the Nutrition Facts table on boxes of crackers and choose a brand that is low in saturated plus trans fat. Compare brands on sodium.

THE CEREAL AISLE

- Choose a cereal that is made from a whole grain (i.e., the first ingredient listed) and is low in sugar and high in fibre.
- Look for ready-to-eat breakfast cereals that have at least 5 grams of fibre and no more than 6 to 8 grams of sugar per 1 serving. (Cereals with

dried fruit can be higher in sugar due to their natural sugar content.)

- Ready-to-eat cereals high in cholesterol-lowering soluble fibre include Kellogg's All Bran Buds with Psyllium, Kellogg's Guardian, and Nature's Path Smart Bran.
- Hot cereals high in soluble fibre include oatmeal and oat bran. Keep in mind that steel-cut and large flake oats are low glycemic foods. (Instant oatmeal has a high-glycemic index.)
- If you do buy instant oatmeal—it's still a good source of soluble fibre— choose the regular, unflavoured version to cut added sugar (however, it will have added sodium). Add your own fruit for sweetness.

HEALTHY CHOICES IN OTHER AISLES

- Buy whole-wheat, whole-spelt, or kamut pasta and brown rice to boost the whole-grain content of your meal plan.
- Stay clear of pasta and rice mixes that come in a package. These side dishes add a hefty dose of sodium, and sometimes fat, to your meal. What's more, very few brands are 100% whole grain.
- Stock up on canned beans for quick vegetarian meals. Buy lentils, black beans, soy beans, chick peas, kidney beans, etc.
- Oils can go rancid quickly, so avoid the urge to buy an economy-sized bottle of vegetable oil. Buy small bottles and store them in a cool, dark cupboard (walnut, sesame, and flax oils should be kept in the fridge).
- Buy bottled salad dressings made with olive or canola oil. Read labels to compare amounts of sodium and sugar.
- Stop by the bulk food section to pick up dried fruit and unsalted nuts for snacks.
- Buy unsalted nut butters to add monounsaturated fat to your diet.

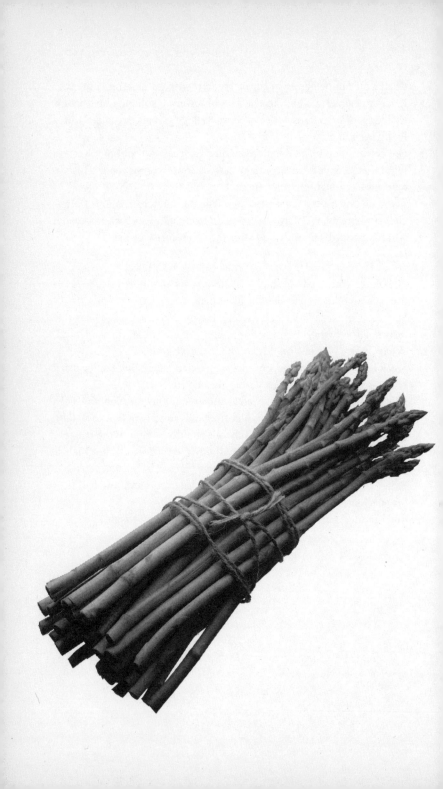

8

Heart healthy dining out

Most of us know a Big Mac has roughly 500 calories and a medium order of french fries delivers close to 400. Fast food restaurants do a pretty good job of making nutrition information accessible through in-store brochures and company websites. But if asked to cite how many calories come with a plate of nachos, a steak dinner, or a bowl of pasta, you might be hard pressed to answer. Most full-service restaurant chains don't display calorie information on menus or have nutrition brochures available upon request. Only a few chains are able to direct consumers to an online nutrition guide.

While Health Canada has created strict labelling guidelines for packaged foods, critics disapprove of the lack of nutrition information in restaurants. In 2006, Member of Parliament Tom Wappell introduced Bill C-283, which called for improvements to nutrition labelling, but it was defeated. The bill would have required restaurant menus to disclose calories and amounts of saturated plus trans fat and sodium. On a positive note, in 2008, the Canadian government called on the foodservice industry to voluntarily reduce trans fat in cooking oils and spreads to at most 2% of total fat content and in other foods to no more than 5% of total fat content by June 2009.

The implication of all this for us, and the restaurants, hits home with an example: If you knew that a chicken fajita dinner serves up 1429 calories, 38 grams of fat, and a whopping 4550 milligrams of sodium, you might reconsider your order—especially if you're watching your waistline or managing your blood pressure. Given that the typical Canadian eats out an average of 11 times every 2 weeks, this information could make a significant difference to your health.

In 2005, The Canadian Restaurant and Foodservices Association established a voluntary nutrition information program for its members. The program required that, by the end of that year, participating chains provide nutrient values for self-selected menu items through on-site pamphlets—their availability prominently displayed on menus—and company websites. Most participating fast food chains have lived up to their promise, but the majority of full-service restaurants have not.

Calories, fat, and sodium in restaurant meals

In the fall of 2007, I teamed up with *The Globe and Mail* and CTV's *Canada AM* to commission an independent lab analysis of popular restaurant meals at four national chains: Milestones, Kelsey's, The Keg, and Jack Astor's. Our findings: Just about every menu entree came in over 1000 calories. Sodium ranged from a low of 245 milligrams (for a lightly dressed salad) to a high of 4550 (chicken fajitas). Add in an appetizer, a beverage, and a dessert, and calorie counts climbed to over 2000. On top of being piled high with calories, the meals we analyzed also provided in excess of the Recommended Daily Allowance of fat, saturated fat, and sodium.

To put the following numbers in perspective, consider that the average adult needs about 2000 calories, no more than 65 grams of fat and 20 grams of saturated fat, and, at most, 2300 milligrams of sodium per day.

Milestones

	Calories	Fat (g)	Saturated fat (g)	Sodium (mg)
Appetizer: Milestones Hot Spinach/Artichoke Dip (1/2 portion)	389	21.7	8.2	608.5
Roasted Chicken Penne Asiago	1205	59.5	17.7	1869
Iced tea, 10 ounces (300 ml)	107	0	0	64
Mexican Chocolate Cake with ice cream (1/2 portion)	355	20.5	9	31.6
Total for meal	**2056**	**101.7**	**34.9**	**2573.1**

Dips are supposed to be fattening, so no surprise here. But who'd have thought that a pasta entree—with chicken breast, roasted tomatoes, and spinach—could deliver as many calories and as much fat as two Big Macs? And thanks to the Asiago cheese and cream, you're getting almost a full-day's portion of artery-clogging saturated fat. This meal clocks in at 2056 calories and provides more than a day's worth of sodium and almost 2 days' worth of saturated fat.

Kelsey's

	Calories	Fat (g)	Saturated fat (g)	Sodium (mg)
Appetizer: Kelsey's Loaded Nachos (1/2 portion)	1008.5	55	19	1992
Chicken Fajitas	1429	38.5	17.4	4450
Regular Beer, 1 pint (473 ml)	204	0	0	19
Total for meal	**2641.5**	**93.5**	**36.4**	**6461**

Eat this meal and be prepared to power walk for at least 6 hours on the treadmill to burn off the calories. And no, the sodium numbers are not a typo. Salty chips and fajita seasoning make this meal a health hazard for anyone with high blood pressure. In just one meal, you're getting a day's worth of fat, two days' worth of saturated fat, and nearly three days' worth of sodium.

The Keg

	Calories	Fat (g)	Saturated fat (g)	Sodium (mg)
Appetizer: Scallops & Bacon (1/2 portion)	103	3.8	1.2	446
Sourdough bread w/ butter (1/4 portion)	178	3.2	1.8	419
Keg Classic Dinner	1161	55	22.7	1664
Red wine, 9 ounces (270 ml)	217	0	0	0
Chocolate Mousse Pyramid	261	16.3	11.3	31.4
Total for meal	**1920**	**78.3**	**37**	**2560.4**

On this hypothetical date, you share an appetizer, have two pieces of bread, sip on a glass of wine, order the New York Keg Classic Dinner—a 10-ounce steak served with Caesar salad, vegetables, and a Keg-Size baked potato—and then follow with dessert. The damage? Far more calories, fat, and sodium than anyone needs in one meal. Eat out like this once a week and you'll gain 20 pounds (9 kg) per year.

Jack Astor's

	Calories	Fat (g)	Saturated fat (g)	Sodium (mg)
Appetizer: Roasted Garlic Bruschetta (2 pieces)	325	15.5	2.8	884
Key West Salad w/ Chicken, dressing on the side	273	11.1	1.8	245

White wine, 6 ounces (180 ml)	146	0	0	0
Total for meal	**744**	**26.6**	**4.6**	**1129**

If you're careful, you can order a meal that doesn't send your diet in a tailspin. This entree salad with grilled chicken, avocado, and roasted nuts—drizzled with only 1 tablespoon (15 ml) of dressing—comes in at a respectable 273 calories. Even with 2 pieces of bruschetta, this meal is pretty decent on calories and fat. The only downside: half a day's worth of sodium in one meal.

We also sent three different so-called "kid-friendly" meals to the lab for a nutrient breakdown. It turns out kids' meals didn't fare much better than adult meals, which is surprising, given that 26% of Canadian children aged 2 to 17 are considered overweight or obese and that type 2 diabetes among youth is on the rise. To help you put the following numbers in perspective, Health Canada recommends:

- Low active boys aged 4 to 9 should consume about 1600 calories per day. Low active girls aged 4 to 9 should consume roughly 1480 calories daily. (Kids are considered "low active" if they participate in 30 to 60 minutes of moderate activity, like walking, per day.)
- Kids should consume no more than 17 grams of bad fats (saturated plus trans fat) each day.
- Children aged 1 to 3 should need only 1000 milligrams of sodium per day; kids aged 4 to 8 require 1200 milligrams.

Kelsey's Kid's Meal

	Calories	Fat (g)	Saturated fat (g)	Sodium (mg)
Chicken Tenders (comes w/ fries, apple juice, ice cream)	1369	51.6	8.5	2767.5

Hard to believe that one "pint-sized" meal delivers enough calories to fuel a child's day, not to mention one-and-a-half day's worth of sodium. Your child would have to eat 6 Wendy's Kids' Meal Hamburgers to consume that many calories and fat grams.

The Keg Kid's Meal

	Calories	Fat (g)	Saturated fat (g)	Sodium (mg)
Half-rack Ribs (comes w/ fries, Caesar salad, veggies & dip, milk, ice cream)	921	45.7	14.8	1243

The Keg deserves a pat on the back for serving salad and raw veggies with every kid's meal. But thanks to the fatty ribs, this meal serves up almost a full day's worth of saturated fat. The grilled chicken or sirloin steak meals are sure to have less calories, fat, and sodium.

Jack Astor's Kid's Meal

	Calories	Fat (g)	Saturated fat (g)	Sodium (mg)
Pasta w/ Cheese Sauce (comes w/ soft drink and a cookie)	822	28	12	1049.4

At least this kid's meal doesn't come with fries. But 822 calories' worth of white flour, margarine, cheese, and sugar does not make for a healthy meal. With half a day's worth of calories and three-quarters of a day's supply of saturated fat, this meal is a splurge.

To be fair, some restaurants do provide healthy alternatives for kids. The Keg and Jack Astor's offer grilled chicken and lean sirloin steak served with salad and vegetables. Red Lobster offers broiled fish and crab legs with veggies. And some menus offer rice, baked potatoes, and corn instead of greasy fries.

Tips for ordering in restaurants

To order heart healthy meals requires learning the language of restaurant menus. Menu items that are fried, basted, braised, au gratin, crispy, scalloped, pan-fried, pan-seared, sautéed, stewed, stuffed, and butter-brushed are usually high in fat, saturated fat, and calories. Instead, look for words that indicate low-fat cooking techniques such as baked, broiled, grilled, steamed, poached, roasted, and lightly sautéed or stir-fried. If you're uncertain about a dish, ask your waiter how it's prepared.

Sometimes healthier items are marked *light* or *heart healthy* on menus, and the server should be able to provide nutritional information to back up the claims. Even if there isn't a lower fat item on a menu, you might be able to order a healthy meal if you, so to speak, read between the menu lines. For example, if a menu features a creamy broccoli soup, there's a good chance it's possible to order a side of steamed broccoli even though it's not officially offered. In general, the higher the quality of the restaurant, the more likely the chef will cater to special requests. The following strategies will help you eat well in any restaurant.

TIPS TO CUT FAT, ESPECIALLY SATURATED AND TRANS FATS

- When ordering grilled meat, fish, or chicken, ask that the food be grilled either without butter or prepared lightly with only a little olive oil.
- Choose tomato-based pasta dishes rather than creamy ones. Tomato sauces are much lower in calories than cream-based alfredo sauces and contain virtually no saturated fat. (Alfredo and rose sauces are made with whipping cream, which delivers a hefty amount of saturated fat.) A serving of tomato sauce counts as a vegetable serving too.
- When ordering soup, stick with broth-based soups instead of cream-based soups and chowders. To increase your intake of magnesium- and fibre-rich legumes, choose minestrone, lentil, and bean soups most often.
- Order sandwiches made with whole-grain breads instead of high-fat croissants or white breads.
- If you have a choice of sides, order steamed veggies, salad, baked potato, or steamed brown rice instead of french fries.
- Ask for salsa with a baked potato instead of butter, sour cream, cheese, or bacon. Salsa is fat-free and very low in calories.
- If you do want french fries on occasion, ask what kind of cooking oil is used. Make sure it is trans fat–free.
- Order sandwiches without butter or "special sauce." Ask for mustard, which adds flavour but virtually no calories.

- Watch out for healthy-sounding salads. Salad entrees that come laden with cheese, bacon, and plenty of dressing can have more fat and calories than an all-dressed burger.
- Order salad dressings, sauces, and sour cream on the side. That way you can control how much you use.
- Request low-fat items even if they are not on the menu—fat-reduced salad dressings, salsa for a baked potato, or fresh fruit for dessert.

TIPS TO CUT EXCESS SUGARS

- Wash your meal down with water, unsweetened iced tea, or milk. Avoid unnecessary sugar calories in pop, fruit drinks, and fruit juices.
- If you're craving dessert, opt for something healthy like fresh berries or fruit.
- If you really want the rich dessert, share it with a friend. Remember, half the dessert means half the sugar and half the calories (and half the saturated fat too!).

TIPS TO REDUCE SODIUM

- Stay clear of menu items described as pickled, marinated, smoked, barbecued, smothered (in sauce), teriyaki, and, of course, salted or salty, or that include soy sauce, broth, miso, gravy, or bacon as an ingredient. These are indicators of higher sodium meals.
- Avoid using the salt shaker. Taste a few bites before you automatically salt your meal. Chances are your meal doesn't need an extra dash of sodium.
- Order dressings, gravies, and condiments on the side. Salad dressings, barbecue sauce, ketchup, mustard, and pickles can add considerably to the sodium content of a meal. Request them to be separate from your meal and use them sparingly.
- When ordering pizza or a burger, skip the cheese or bacon, which not only adds saturated fat, but piles on the sodium too. If you can't fathom pizza without mozzarella, ask for half the amount of cheese that's typically used.
- Request that your meal be prepared without added salt, MSG (monosodium glutamate), or sodium-containing ingredients such as soy sauce and broths.

TIPS TO SLIM DOWN PORTION SIZE

- Don't eat it all—take half of your meal home. Ask the server to bring a doggie bag with your meal. When the meal is served, portion off the extra and put it away. If it's sitting on your plate you're more likely to eat it!
- Instead of a large entree, order two appetizers or an appetizer and a salad as your meal. Consider sharing an entree with a friend. Many steak dinners weigh in at 8 to 10 ounces—a perfect share size.
- Cut down on starchy side dishes. Skip the bread basket if the meal comes with rice, potatoes, or pasta. Or ask for extra vegetables instead of the potatoes or rice. Don't want a huge bowl of pasta? Ask for a half-portion.
- Slow your pace. After every bite, put down your knife and fork and chew your food thoroughly. Stop eating when you feel full, not stuffed. Remember it takes 20 minutes for your brain to get the signal that your stomach has had enough food.

You need to be assertive when dining out. Remember you're paying for your meal. If you don't know what's in a dish or don't know the serving size, ask. If you're eating at a family-style restaurant or fast food outlet, you can also check the restaurant's website in advance to determine healthier choices.

Choosing healthy ethnic cuisine

Enjoying ethnic cuisine is a great way to add interesting flavours and variety to your diet. And many ethnic dishes contain heart healthy foods such as beans, nuts, whole grains, fresh vegetables, and fish. The trick is to know which menu items are the healthier choices. Here are a few strategies to help you dine healthfully on foods from around the world.

CHINESE CUISINE

- Stay clear of high-fat items such as General Tsao's Chicken. Beware of lemon and orange chicken and beef dishes that are often breaded and fried, and therefore higher in fat.

- Look for the words *steamed, boiled, Jum* (poached), *Kow* (roasted), and *Shu* (barbecued).
- Limit items that are deep-fried, crispy, batter-dipped, breaded, and fried.
- Choose dishes made with small portions of beef, chicken, or pork. Ask for dishes to be prepared with extra veggies. Chicken wings, duck, and spare ribs are high in saturated fat.
- Opt for seafood, fish, and tofu dishes to reduce your intake of saturated fat and increase your intake of soy and omega-3 fatty acids.
- Ask for brown rice instead of white.
- Order clear soups instead of egg drop soup.
- Use chopsticks to slow down your eating. Chopsticks also help you eat less of the sauce than you might otherwise eat when using a fork.
- Keep in mind that most Chinese dishes are made with high-sodium soy sauce, so avoid using soy sauce at the table.
- If you're sensitive to MSG (monosodium glutamate), ask that your meal be prepared without it.

FRENCH CUISINE
- Beware of appetizers with salty ingredients such as olives, capers, and anchovies. Choose lower sodium starters such as steamed mussels or a green salad.
- Pass on the French onion soup, which is high in sodium and saturated fat. Order a lentil or bean soup, if available.
- Instead of hollandaise, mornay, béchamel, or Béarnaise sauce (all high in saturated fat), look for menu items made with bordelaise or other wine-based sauces.
- Substitute creamy *au gratin* potato side dishes with lightly sautéed vegetables.
- If you don't want to splurge on calories for dessert, order fresh berries instead of crème caramel or chocolate mousse.

ITALIAN CUISINE
- Beware of larger-than-life pasta portions. At some family-style restaurants, a serving of pasta can easily yield 4 cups (1 L), which is the equivalent of 8 slices of bread! If you're trying to control your weight, order a half-portion of pasta.

- Choose plain bread or bruschetta instead of garlic-buttered or cheese-topped breads.
- When ordering soup, choose fibre-rich lentil, bean, vegetable, or minestrone.
- Best bets for salads include mista, arugula, and spinach. Caprese and Caesar salads are higher in saturated fat (thanks to the cheese) and calories. Order salad dressing on the side to reduce your calorie and sodium intake.
- Dip your bread in heart healthy extra-virgin olive oil instead of butter, which is full of saturated fat.
- Choose lower fat tomato-based sauces such as marinara, primavera, arrabbiata, and puttanesca.
- Limit your intake of high-fat dishes made with rich cream sauces such as alfredo, carbonara, rosé, and vodka. Save these dishes, high in saturated fat, for a special occasion.
- Choose dishes with grilled chicken, seafood, and fish. Mussels or clams in a tomato-based broth are excellent choices. Veal is also lean, especially if you choose a dish that is baked, not fried.
- Avoid dishes with sausage, excessive amounts of cheese, and breaded meats.
- Order thin-crust pizza with veggies and chicken. Ask for part-skim mozzarella—some restaurants may have it. Or order a cheese-less pizza.

MEXICAN CUISINE

- Since many menu items contain generous portions of cheese and sour cream, it can be challenging to eat heart healthfully at a Mexican restaurant … but not impossible!
- Detour around the basket of deep-fried tortilla chips. Instead request plain, fresh tortillas for dipping in salsa.
- If available, order corn tortillas instead of the usual refined (white) wheat flour version. Corn tortillas are lower in fat and calories, and they are often made from whole-grain corn.
- Best bets for starters include ceviche (raw fish marinated in lemon juice) and soups, including gazpacho, black bean, and vegetable.
- Best bets for entrees include chicken or black bean burritos, soft chicken tacos, fajitas, and stuffed and baked tamales (corn tortillas).
- Load your tacos, burritos, or fajitas with salsa instead of sour cream.

- Ask for black beans instead of refried beans, which are often fried in lard or some other type of fat.
- Limit higher fat items such as nachos and cheese, taco salad, and deep-fried tortilla dishes such as chimichangas and taquitos.
- Go heavy on the black beans and veggies, which add fibre to your meal.

THAI CUISINE

- Choose the lighter, stir-fried dishes over dishes made with coconut milk (a rich source of saturated fat).
- Ask that cooking be done with vegetable oil rather than coconut or palm kernel oil.
- Instead of fried spring rolls, order cold fresh spring rolls.
- Best bets for starters include clear soups such as tom yam goong (hot and sour shrimp soup). Tom ka gai and tom yam hed soups are higher in fat because they're made with coconut milk. Green mango salad and seafood salad are also good choices.
- Avoid dishes with fried noodles (mee krob, radnar talay) and fried rice. Order steamed rice to accompany your meal.
- Healthier dishes include satay, grilled or sautéed chicken, fish, or meat (but keep portions small) and sautéed tofu.
- To limit your saturated fat and boost your intake of omega-3 fats, look for seafood as your main protein source.
- Use chopsticks to slow your eating pace.
- For dessert, order lychees (a small round fruit) instead of deep-fried ice cream or banana fritters.

JAPANESE CUISINE

- Best bets for starters include seaweed salad, edamame (boiled or steamed soybeans), clear soups (miso and suimono), and tofu in broth. Sashimi (raw fish), sushi (raw fish and rice), udon and soba (buckwheat) noodles in broth are low-fat choices.
- Best bets for entrees include grilled (yakimono) dishes such as yakitori, teriyaki chicken, and salmon.
- Higher fat menu items include tempura (shrimps and vegetables deep-fried in a light batter), shabu-shabu (thinly sliced prime rib cooked in broth and served with dipping sauce), and tonkatsu (deep-fried breaded pork cutlet).

- If you're trying to lower your sodium intake, ask for your food to be prepared without high-sodium marinades, sauces, and salt. Miso soup is also high in sodium.

INDIAN CUISINE

- Best bets for starters include lentil soup, mulligatawny soup, and raita (sliced cucumber in yogurt).
- Avoid deep-fried appetizers such as samosas and pakoras.
- Opt for roti, chapati (thin, dry whole-wheat bread), or naan (leavened, baked bread) instead of fried and stuffed breads. Roasted papads (thin crispy lentil wafers) are also good choices.
- Lower fat dishes include dhal (lentils), chicken or fish tandoori (marinated in spices and cooked in a clay oven), chicken or beef tikka (roasted with mild spices), kebabs, and chicken or vegetable biryani (rice dishes with spices).
- Ask for curry dishes that are made with a yogurt base. To reduce saturated fat, limit curries made with coconut milk or cream.

GREEK CUISINE

- If you're counting calories and sodium, ask for salad dressing, olives, and feta cheese to be served on the side. That way you'll control how much fat and sodium you add to your Greek salad.
- Best bets for starters include dolmades (grape leaves stuffed with rice and served cold), octopus (grilled or marinated and served cold), steamed mussels, and pita with hummus (chickpea dip) and tzatziki (yogurt dip).
- Appetizers to avoid include spanakopita or spinach pie (layers of phyllo dough brushed with butter and filled with cheese, oil, and egg) and crispy calamari that's been breaded and fried.
- Best bets for entrees include chicken or pork souvlaki. With the exception of extra salt from the marinade, shish kebabs are the healthiest items on a Greek menu. Other good choices include grilled chicken, lamb, and fish.
- Stay clear of moussaka (casserole with layers of ground meat and fried eggplant covered with a buttery sauce). If you really must order this high-fat meal, consider sharing it with a friend and ordering extra vegetables and steamed rice.

- Instead of a higher fat gyro sandwich, order a souvlaki-stuffed pita. To make a gyro, restaurants put a moulded mixture of compressed meat, breadcrumbs, and onions on a vertical spit and roast it.
- As for dessert, you're better off ordering fruit. Pastries like baklava are made with buttery phyllo dough and plenty of sugar. A good-sized portion can set you back 550 calories, 21 grams of fat, and 8 teaspoons (40 ml) of sugar. If you want to splurge, split this treat with a friend.

Tips for ordering a heart healthy breakfast

The tips I've given you so far have focused on ordering healthier lunch and dinner items on restaurant menus. But what about breakfast? I routinely see clients in my private practice who travel for business and pleasure and have to order breakfast in a hotel or a diner. Breakfast menus can be loaded with calories, saturated fat and, most definitely, sodium. I'll bet you didn't realize that Denny's French Toast Slam serves up 1180 calories, 27 grams of saturated fat, and 2520 milligrams of sodium! And many baked goods such as muffins and pastries harbour cholesterol-raising trans fat.

The following strategies will help you navigate fat and sodium traps when ordering breakfast away from home.

- Start your meal with a bowl of fresh fruit or berries. If fresh fruit is not available, order a small-sized 100% fruit juice. (Remember orange juice is a good source of the B vitamin folate.)
- Order whole-grain toast instead of white and ask for it unbuttered, then spread on peanut butter (monounsaturated fat) or jam instead. Resist the temptation to have high-fat pastries such as croissants, muffins, or Danishes.
- Ask for a whole-grain cereal like Bran Flakes, Shreddies, or low-fat granola. Order skim or 1% milk. Some restaurants might even offer soy beverage for cereal.
- To start your day with a good source of soluble fibre, order a bowl of hot oatmeal. Top it with fresh berries or raisins instead of brown sugar.
- If you feel like eggs, request an egg white omelet with vegetables—fried in vegetable oil instead of butter.
- When given a choice between side (strip) bacon and Canadian (back or peameal) bacon, choose the latter since it's lower in saturated fat.

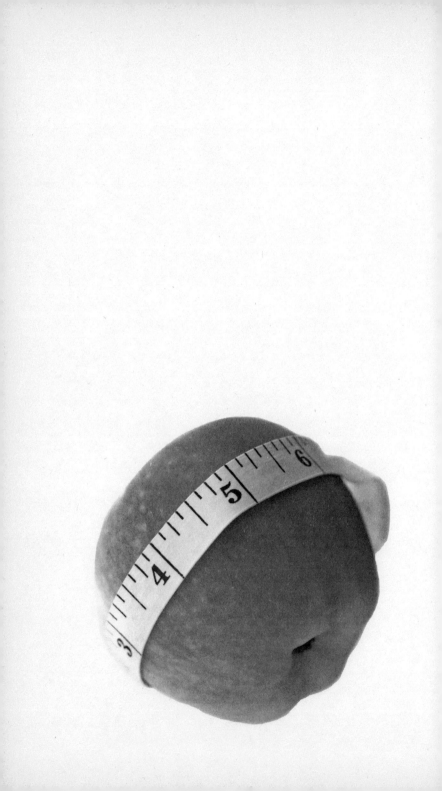

9

Maintaining a healthy weight

Over the last 30 years, a growing number of Canadians have become overweight or obese. Today it's estimated that 60% of adults and 26% of children fall into one of these categories. What's shocking is the dramatic rise in obesity we've witnessed since 1978. The biggest increase has occurred among kids aged 12 to 17, where the rate tripled from 3% to 9%. For adults, the most striking upsurge occurred among those aged 25 to 34 and those who were 75 or older.[1]

Being overweight is not just a matter of appearance. There is compelling evidence that carrying excess weight puts you at risk for a number of health problems, including type 2 diabetes, high LDL cholesterol and triglycerides, elevated blood pressure, inflammation, and metabolic syndrome. Clearly, overweight and obesity increases the likelihood of developing coronary heart disease.

How healthy is your weight?

Most people rely on the bathroom scale to decide on whether they're happy with their body weight. But to get a more accurate picture of your health, there are other numbers you need to consider—though I certainly don't advocate throwing out your scale. Weighing-in helps motivate people to stick to a weight-loss plan. And as you'll learn later in this chapter, it's also a very important way to stay on top of small weight gains before they accumulate. Think about it: It's much easier to lose an extra 3 pounds than 10 or more.

But as useful as the scale may be, it doesn't tell you everything you need to know about your weight as it relates to health risk. Determining how much body fat you have—and where you carry it—is important not only for weight control, but also for identifying your risk for heart disease.

BODY MASS INDEX (BMI)

If you're between the ages of 18 and 65, BMI is a height and weight formula that gives a pretty reliable snapshot of your body fat. The easiest and quickest way to determine your BMI is to use an online calculator; you'll find one on my website (www.lesliebeck.com). Your body mass index is calculated by dividing your weight (in kilograms) by your height (in metres squared).

Doctors and dietitians use the BMI to classify your body weight and assess your risk for disease as follows:

- BMI values less than 18.5 are considered underweight and increase a person's risk for conditions such as osteoporosis, nutrient deficiencies, and eating disorders.
- BMI values from 18.5 to 24.9 are defined as healthy or normal weight and linked with a lower risk of health problems.
- If your BMI falls between 25 and 29.9, you're classified as overweight.

What's Your Body Mass Index (BMI)?

1.	Determine your weight in kilograms (kg) (Divide your weight in pounds by 2.2)	Weight (kg)
2.	Determine your height in centimetres (cm) (Multiply your height in inches by 2.54)	Height (cm)
3.	Determine your height in metres (m) (Divide your height in centimetres by 100)	Height (m)
4.	Square your height in metres (m^2) (Multiply your height in metres by height in metres)	Height (m^2)
5.	Now, calculate your BMI (Divide #1, your weight (in kg), by #4, your height in m^2)	BMI

- A BMI of 30 or greater is considered obese. As your BMI goes up, so does your risk for type 2 diabetes, heart disease, high blood pressure, gallbladder disease, sleep apnea, and some forms of cancer.

Keep in mind, though, that sudden or considerable weight gains or weight losses may also indicate health risk, even if this occurs within the "normal" BMI category.

The body mass index can also be calculated for children and teenagers, but its interpretation depends on age and gender. At each checkup, the doctor should calculate your child's BMI-for-age percentile, which indicates how his or her measurements compare to other children's in the same age group. Regular measuring of BMI allows you to monitor your child's weight over time, and also gives the doctor an opportunity to discuss healthy eating and exercise habits with your son or daughter.

An increasing BMI over time is definitely linked with a greater risk of developing heart disease. Researchers followed 13,230 healthy men, average age of 51, for 8 years to see who developed coronary heart disease, heart attack, or stroke. At the end of the study period, a higher BMI was associated with an increased risk of heart disease. Compared to men whose BMI remained stable for the 8 years, those whose BMI increased by 0.5 to 2.0 points were 40% more likely to have heart disease.[2]

Another study, which followed 29,122 healthy men aged 40 to 75 for 3 years, revealed that in middle-aged men, BMI predicted the risk of being diagnosed with coronary heart disease; for older men, the association between BMI and risk of heart disease was much weaker. Among men younger than 65, those with a BMI between 25 and 29 were 72% more likely to develop heart disease than men with a BMI of less than 23. Men whose BMI was over 33 had more than a 3-fold higher risk of heart disease than lean men. In men older than 65, the waist-to-hip ratio was a much better predictor of heart attack.[3] (Keep reading to learn how to calculate your waist-to-hip ratio.)

BMI, Weight Classification, and Risk of Heart Disease

BMI = Weight (kg) ÷ Height (m^2)

	Weight classification	Risk of heart disease
<18.5	Underweight	
18.5–24.9	Healthy weight	Least
25.0–29.9	Overweight	Increased
≥30.0	Obese	High

The BMI is not without drawbacks. For starters, it doesn't tell you where you're carrying your body fat, which is important in determining the risk of coronary heart disease. It also doesn't distinguish between body fat weight and muscle weight. Athletes and heavily muscled people may have a high body mass index but very little fat (muscle weighs more than fat on the scale).

WAIST CIRCUMFERENCE

If you want to know where your body fat is located, and how that fat is affecting your heart health, you need to measure your waist. Simply take a measuring tape and measure your waist at the narrowest part of your trunk, about 1 inch (2.5 cm) above your belly button, without holding the tape too tightly or too loosely. (Resist the urge to suck in your stomach!)

Excess fat around the abdomen (apple shape) is associated with greater health risk than fat located on the hips and thighs (pear shape). When it comes to health, not all fat cells are alike. Whereas body mass index measures overall fat, your waist circumference is a good measure of abdominal fat. The fat round your middle consists of *subcutaneous fat*, the fat just beneath the skin that you can pinch, and *visceral fat*, a type of deep fat that packs itself around your organs. It's visceral fat that's considered dangerous to your health because it secretes chemicals that increase the body's resistance to insulin and cause inflammation throughout the body.

A waist circumference of 37 inches (94 cm) or greater for men and 31.5 inches (80 cm) or greater for women increases the likelihood of type 2 diabetes, high blood pressure, elevated cholesterol, heart attack, stroke, metabolic syndrome, and some cancers. Lower thresholds for waist circumference are recommended for Asian populations because studies suggest health risk increases for them at lower levels of body weight than in Caucasian populations.

Increased girth predicts a person's risk of disease and death better than BMI alone. For instance, the combination of a normal BMI and an increased waist circumference is thought to double the risk of certain diseases. A number of studies have determined that your waist measurement or waist-to-hip ratio is a much better predictor of heart attack risk than BMI.[4] That's why the Canadian guidelines to assess body weight now use both BMI and waist circumference.

Your Waist Circumference and the Risk of Heart Disease

		Risk of heart disease
Men	<37 inches (<94 cm)	Lower
	≥37 inches (≥94 cm)	Increased
Women	<31.5 inches (<80 cm)	Lower
	≥31.5 inches (≥80 cm)	Increased

WAIST-TO-HIP RATIO (WHR)

The waist-to-hip ratio is simply your waist measurement divided by your hip measurement. It's another index of body fat distribution used by doctors and researchers. However, some studies suggest it's less accurate than waist circumference at predicting health risk. Even so, it does a much better job of predicting the risk of heart disease in men and women. Canadian researchers studied 27,000 men and women from 52 countries and found that those who had suffered a heart attack had a significantly higher waist-to-hip ratio than people in the non–heart attack group. In fact, the waist-to-hip ratio was 3 times stronger than BMI in forecasting the risk of heart attack.[5]

Your Waist-to-Hip Ratio (WHR) and the Risk of Heart Disease

WHR = Waist circumference ÷ hip circumference

		Risk of heart disease
Men	≤0.9	Lower
	>0.9	Increased
Women	≤0.8	Lower
	>0.8	Increased

10 strategies for losing weight

If you've determined you need to lose excess weight, especially around your belly, there's no time like the present to get started. Numerous studies have documented the effect of weight loss on risk factors for heart disease: You'll reduce your blood pressure, lower cholesterol and triglycerides, raise HDL (good) cholesterol, reduce C-reactive protein (a marker of inflammation in the body), and help control your blood sugar. And you don't have to lose a lot of weight to reap health benefits. Researchers have demonstrated that losing a moderate amount of weight—as little as 5% to 10% of body weight—is enough to lower blood pressure and prevent impaired fasting glucose from progressing to type 2 diabetes.

It's beyond the scope of this book to outline a weight-loss plan (you'll find four meal plans for weight loss in my book *The No-Fail Diet*). But in Chapter 6, page 163, you'll find a 1600-calorie version of the DASH diet that can help you lose weight while lowering blood pressure and cholesterol. The strategies below will help you shed excess weight permanently, regardless of which heart healthy diet you choose to follow. (A heart healthy weight-loss plan is not a low carbohydrate diet that shuns whole grains and fruit!)

1. *Set a realistic, measurable goal.* If your body mass index is over 25, determine what your weight needs to be in order for your BMI to fall in the healthy zone. Make your weight goal a 3 to 5 pound (1.5 to 2 kg) weight range, rather than one single number. It's not realistic to always hit the exact same weight on the scale. After all, you need a little wiggle room for holidays and entertaining.

   Consider setting mini goals. Rather than keeping your eye on a long-term goal such as losing 25 pounds (11.3 kg), set your sights on smaller goals to help you stay motivated and maintain momentum. Breaking your weight-loss goal into 5 to 10 pound (2 to 4.5 kg) blocks allows you to experience success along the way. And mini goals don't have to be centred on weight loss. They can be daily, weekly, or monthly goals that challenge you to exercise more, eat more leafy green vegetables, eat more fish rich in omega-3 fatty acids, or drink more water.

   Aim to lose weight at a safe rate of 1 to 2 pounds (0.5 to 1 kg) each week. Rapid weight loss from a very low-calorie diet actually makes it harder to maintain your weight loss. When you put your body through a period of starvation by drastically cutting calories, you burn muscle and trigger hormonal changes in your body that cause it to be more efficient at storing fat. When you inevitably abandon the diet, your metabolism is slower, making it easier to gain your weight back.

2. *Reduce calories to 1200 to 1900 calories per day.* A good general target is 1400 to 1600 calories per day for women and 1600 to 1900 calories for men. Women are genetically programmed to store more body fat because of high levels of estrogen—the hormone that keeps fat on a woman's body, making it easier to get pregnant. Research shows that a woman burns 5% to 10% fewer calories for the body's metabolic needs than a man of the same height and weight. Men can consume more calories and lose weight because they burn more calories at rest due to their larger muscle mass. The more muscle you have on your body in relation to fat, the higher your resting metabolism. Your resting metabolism is the amount of energy required to keep your heart beating, your lungs breathing, your brain and liver functioning, and your cells alive at complete rest.

   Cut calories by eliminating sugary drinks and sweets as well as fatty, salty foods such as fast food meals, french fries, and potato chips.

Reduce portion sizes of meat and starchy foods such as rice, pasta, and potatoes. Instead, fill your plate with heart healthy vegetables that fill you up with fewer calories. Replace snacks of pretzels, crackers, and muffins, which supply lots of calories in even a small portion, with less energy-dense foods such as fruit and raw vegetables. If you're in the habit of snacking after dinner, replace those calories with a cup of tea, herbal tea, or calorie-reduced hot chocolate. Keep a food diary for 7 days before you embark on losing weight to see where your extra calories are sneaking in.

3. *Plan your meals and snacks in advance.* If you come home from work tired and hungry without a plan for dinner, chances are you'll order in. Or graze your way through the evening. On the weekend, plan a weekly menu of healthy meals and snacks. If planning a week's worth of meals seems too daunting, only look ahead to the next day. I have many clients who keep their food journal one day in advance—they find it serves as a plan they're more likely to stick with. To ensure you keep to your plan, make time for grocery shopping (make a list in advance!) and batch cook on the weekend.

4. *Assess your portion size.* I recommend that you measure your food portions during the first 2 weeks of following a weight-loss plan. Get to know what 1/2 cup (125 ml) or 1 cup (250 ml) of cooked brown rice or 3 ounces (90 g) of salmon looks like on your plate. In Chapter 6, pages 162 and 166, I've outlined serving sizes for the various food groups on the DASH and OmniHeart diets. Refer to these lists to learn the serving size equivalencies of different foods.

Tips to reduce portion size:

- Buy small packages of food at the grocery store. Economy-sized boxes of cookies, crackers, pretzels, and potato chips encourage overeating. If you resist the "more for less" thinking, you'll end up eating less. If you're serving dessert for guests, buy (or make) only what you plan to serve. Lingering leftovers can tempt even the most dedicated dieter into overeating.
- Serve smaller portions at mealtime. If you sit down to a plate overflowing with food, the chances are high that you'll finish it.

Most of us have a tendency to clear our plates, a habit that's rooted in childhood. If you don't serve yourself at dinner, ask whoever does to put less food on your plate.

- Use smaller plates. This trick really works. Instead of using a dinner plate, serve yourself on a luncheon-sized plate (7 to 9 in/18 to 23 cm in diameter). The plate looks full and you'll end up eating less food. I vividly remember one client telling me the only thing she did differently to shed 10 pounds was to serve her dinner on a luncheon-sized plate. Ditto for glasses. Reserve large glasses for water and use smaller ones for low-fat milk (1 cup/250 ml) and 100% fruit juice (1/2 cup/125 ml).

- Plate your snacks. Never, ever snack out of the bag or box. When you continually reach into that bag of mini rice cakes or pretzels, you never really get a sense of how much you're eating. It just doesn't register. You end up eating far more than you should. Whether your snack is crackers and low-fat cheese, popcorn, or apple slices, measure out your portion and put it on a plate. And then pay attention to the fact that you're eating! In other words, don't snack while doing something else, like watching TV or checking emails.

5. *Eat breakfast, even if you're not hungry.* Studies show that people who eat the morning meal do a better job of keeping their weight in check than those who go without. Eating breakfast kick-starts your metabolism and helps you consume fewer calories over the course of the day. People who eat breakfast are less likely to mindlessly snack in the morning and overeat at lunch and dinner. If you don't feel hungry in the morning, eat something small—a low-fat yogurt, a soy milk smoothie, or even an apple. In short order, you'll wake up with an appetite for breakfast.

6. *Stop eating when you feel satisfied, not full.* Think about your hunger level prior to eating and how full you felt after eating. Listening to your body can help prevent you from eating too many calories. Use the following scale to assess how you feel before you eat, halfway through a meal, and after you finish eating. Your goal is to stop eating when you reach level 5 on the hunger scale.

Hunger Scale

1	You feel starving. You can't concentrate because you feel so empty. You need food now!
2	You feel hungry and know that your stomach needs food, but you could wait a few minutes before eating.
3	You feel slightly hungry. You could eat something, but you couldn't eat a large meal.
4	Your hunger has almost disappeared. You could eat another bite.
5	You are no longer hungry. You feel satisfied, not full.
6	You feel slightly full.
7	You feel overly full and uncomfortable. Your waistband is noticeably tighter.
8	You feel stuffed, bloated, even nauseous. Some people call this the "Thanksgiving Day" full.

If you eat too quickly, you're more likely to overeat and feel stuffed. To slow your pace—and eat less—put down your knife and fork after every bite and chew your food thoroughly. You'll also be less likely to overeat if you avoid distractions, such as watching television, checking email, or reading while eating. Reserve the kitchen or dining room table for meals to help you pay attention to what—and how much—you're eating.

7. *Keep a food journal.* I recommend this strategy to all of my clients because, quite simply, it works. Many studies have shown that people who keep food diaries lose more weight and keep more pounds off in the long run. A recently published study of 1500 overweight and obese adults—one of the largest weight loss studies ever—found that people who wrote down what they ate at least 5 days each week lost twice as much weight as those who didn't.[6]

During the first 4 weeks of following your meal plan, write down what you eat and how much you eat. Tracking every bite—for better or worse—that passes your lips forces you to see what you're really eating. It will highlight what needs tweaking in your diet and help keep you focused on your goals. You can also use your food diary to track your intake of heart healthy foods such as fish, nuts (keep portion size small!), legumes, whole grains, soluble fibre-rich cereals, fruit, and vegetables. Are you eating fish twice per week?

8. *Weigh in weekly, or daily.* According to the National Weight Control Registry, a U.S. database of over 5000 people who have lost a significant amount of weight and kept it off, 75% of participants say their success comes from weighing themselves at least once per week.[7] Weighing-in helps you measure your progress. Seeing your efforts reflected on the bathroom scale motivates you to stick to your plan. On the flip side, if the scale doesn't budge, or if the needle creeps up after the weekend, you'll more likely pay extra attention to following your plan. Avoiding the scale because you're afraid of what it might tell you is a sure-fire way to let small weight gains accumulate into big ones.

9. *Indulge once per week.* Putting a food on a forbidden list makes it more desirable and can make you feel deprived. When you're stressed, angry, or bored, you're more likely to crave what you can't have, a feeling that can lead to bingeing. Rather than eliminating the foods you love, plan a weekly splurge so you won't feel deprived. (I mean a single treat—a dessert, a chocolate bar, an order of french fries—not one day's worth of indulgences.)

   While a weekly treat will help you stick to your weight-loss resolution, I don't advise that you keep treats in the house. Successful dieters in the National Weight Control Registry say they stay on track by keeping high-fat foods out of the house and stocking their kitchen with healthy foods.[8]

10. *Don't be discouraged by weight-loss plateaus.* When your weight loss comes to a halt, without any change in diet, exercise, or other lifestyle factors, this is called a weight-loss plateau. It can be frustrating, but trust me when I tell you that plateaus are a natural part of the weight-loss process. They often occur when you reach a weight that you have not been below for quite some time. As you lose weight, your body requires fewer calories and your rate of weight loss may temporarily slow down.

It takes persistence and consistency to break through a plateau. The key is not giving up. If you say to yourself it doesn't matter what you eat because your weight isn't budging, you'll never break through that number on the scale. Do not eat less food in order to speed up your weight loss! The best way to work through a plateau is to notch up your exercise to burn more calories. If you've been doing the same workout for months, it's time to challenge your body. Consider cross training by adding different types of cardiovascular exercises to your weekly routine.

And if hitting a plateau or some other circumstance causes a momentary lapse, don't let it throw you off course. It's only natural to stray from your plan once in a while. Doing so doesn't mean you've ruined all your hard work. If you backslide, get on track again at the next meal. You'll be pleasantly surprised to learn that an occasional slip won't prevent you from achieving your goal.

Tips for maintaining your weight over the years

As I tell all of my weight-loss clients, the strategies that helped them lose excess weight are the same ones that will help them keep it off long-term. Obviously you can't go back to eating as much as you did when you were 20 pounds (9 kg) heavier; now that your body is smaller, it requires fewer calories to function each day. But if you've ever lost weight and gained it back, you probably know old habits can creep back in if you're not paying attention. That said, once you've achieved your weight goal, you might need to adjust your calorie intake slightly to prevent further weight loss. I advise my clients to experiment by adding food in 100-calorie increments: Each week, add 100 calories to your daily diet while monitoring your weight. If you find your weight increases, you need to reduce your calorie intake—or add more exercise. When adding 100 calories' worth of food to your diet, make sure to choose heart healthy foods.

What Do 100 Calories Look Like?

	Amount
Protein foods	
Cheese, cottage, 1%	1/2 cup (125 ml)
Chickpeas, cooked	1/3 cup (75 ml)
Fish, light tuna	3 ounces (90 g)
Fish, halibut, sole	2 1/2 ounces (75 g)
Fish, salmon	2 ounces (60 g)
Lentils, cooked	1/2 cup (125 ml)
Milk and milk alternatives	
Milk, skim or 1%	1 cup (250 ml)
Soy milk, plain, enriched	1 cup (250 ml)
Yogurt, 1% MF	1 cup (250 ml)
Starchy foods	
Bread, whole-grain	1 slice (30 g)
Cereal, 100% bran	1/2 cup (125 ml)
Oatmeal, cooked	3/4 cup (175 ml)
Pasta, whole-wheat, cooked	1/2 cup (125 ml)
Popcorn, air-popped	3 cups (750 ml)
Rice, brown, cooked	1/2 cup (125 ml)
Fruit	
Apple	1 medium
Apricots	3 whole
Blueberries	1 cup (250 ml)
Dates	5
Orange	1 large
Pear	1 medium
Raisins	1/4 cup (50 ml)
Strawberries	1 cup (250 ml)
Fats and oils	
Almonds, unsalted	14 whole
Avocado	1/2 medium
Peanuts, unsalted	17 whole (2 tbsp/25 ml)
Peanut butter	1 tablespoon (15 ml)
Sunflower seeds	2 tablespoons (25 ml)
Vegetable oil, olive or canola oil	2 teaspoons (10 ml)

It takes work to keep your weight stable. Even if you don't need to lose weight, metabolism slows with age, making it harder to maintain a healthy weight. For each year after the age of 30, women require 7 fewer calories per day and men need to drop their daily intake by 10. That might not sound like much, but it can make a difference to your weight if you're still eating the way you did in your 20s. For example, a 65-year-old man needs to consume 350 fewer calories each day than he did at age 30—that's roughly the number of calories most folks eat at breakfast.

Maintaining a healthy weight over the years requires commitment. You need to stay on top of your food intake, your activity level, and all of the behaviours that helped you achieve your goal. Here are the top strategies that will help prevent incremental weight gain.

- *Reassess portion sizes.* Pull out the measuring cups and spoons and gauge how much food you are eating. Make sure you're not eating more food than you think you are. It's easy for portion sizes to creep up over time.
- *Be aware of extra nibbles.* It is easy to turn a blind eye to that piece of cheese you popped in your mouth when making the kids' lunches, or the repeated tastings when cooking dinner. But the scale keeps track of every calorie. Those mindless bites and sips can add up significantly— to an entire meal's worth if you're not careful. To resist sampling while you cook, chew sugarless gum or sip on a glass of vegetable juice. If leftovers tempt you, cook only the amount you plan to serve.
- *Don't treat the weekend as a holiday.* A key to successful weight maintenance is consistency. Among my clients, the most successful are those who stick to their meal plans during the week and on the weekend. Research shows that people who don't give themselves a day or two off to cheat are 1.5 times more likely to avoid unwanted pounds.
- *Step on the scale regularly.* Weighing-in gives you feedback about how well you are maintaining your weight. Many studies have indicated that frequent monitoring is a critical factor in keeping weight stable. Frequent weighing provides an early warning system: By catching small increases quickly, you can take corrective action to prevent further gain. If you do weigh yourself daily, don't be discouraged by normal daily fluctuations; it's mostly due to water weight.
- *Exercise regularly.* Just as exercise helps you lose unwanted pounds, it is essential if you want to prevent gaining pounds. The majority of

participants in the National Weight Control Registry say they exercise regularly to maintain their weight loss. Most combine walking with another type of planned exercise such as aerobics classes, biking, or swimming. Regular exercise helps you stay trim by burning calories and increasing your metabolism. It also increases your motivation to eat a more healthful diet. If you've successfully lost weight, research suggests it takes close to 1 hour of moderate aerobic exercise 5 days per week to keep the pounds off.

You'll learn more about the type and amount of exercise you need to help reduce the risk of heart disease in Chapter 10.

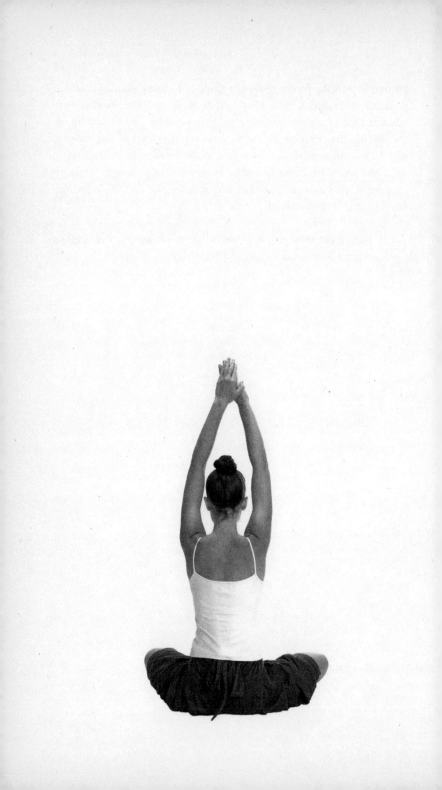

10

Exercise for preventing heart disease

If you recall, I told you earlier in this book that leading a sedentary lifestyle doubles the likelihood of suffering a heart attack. Indeed, physical inactivity is considered a major, independent risk factor for developing heart disease. Many studies have determined that people who are regularly active are less likely to succumb to heart disease and are 20% to 30% less likely than their sedentary peers to die from the disease. If you're inactive now, it's never too late to become physically active. Studies show that men and women who maintain exercise, or improve their fitness, have a lower risk of heart attack than individuals who remain unfit. What's more, there's mounting evidence that if you already have heart disease, routine exercise can improve your health. Research suggests that people with heart disease who exercise regularly are 25% to 30% less likely to die from any cause.

Physical activity helps bring down the odds of heart disease in plenty of ways: by lowering blood triglycerides, increasing HDL cholesterol, reducing blood pressure, and maintaining a normal blood glucose level. Regular exercise also helps prevent weight gain and promotes weight loss if you're overweight. In addition, working out—whether it's brisk walking or weight training—aids in dealing with stress and anxiety, which if left unmanaged can trigger hormones in your body linked to heart disease.

Canadian physical activity guidelines advocate moderate intensity exercise on most days of the week. Data suggest that if the entire population followed this advice, roughly one-third of deaths related to coronary heart disease could be prevented. That's pretty powerful. By now you might be wondering: How much exercise do I need to guard against heart disease and how hard do I have to work out? Current evidence indicates that 30 minutes of moderate intensity exercise is required on most days of the week to help reduce the risk of developing heart disease. That means you need to burn at least 1000 calories each week from exercise to reap its cardio-protective effects.

More vigorous intensity activities, which raise your heart rate to 50% to 85% of its maximum, may be especially beneficial to heart health. In a study of 12,516 middle-aged men, those who expended more than 1000 calories per week from vigorous forms of exercise had a 20% lower risk of developing heart disease than those who burned less than 500 calories per week. Another study found that, compared to men who did not run, those who ran for an hour or more each week were 42% less likely to be diagnosed with heart disease. In this study, walking also offered protection—a daily 30-minute brisk walk reduced the risk of heart disease by 18%.[1]

Activities that require moderate and vigorous effort are considered *cardio* or *aerobic* workouts (see below).

Moderate intensity activities	Vigorous intensity activities
Biking	Aerobics classes
Brisk walking	Basketball
Dancing	Fast swimming
Golf, if you don't use a cart	Hockey
Raking leaves	Jogging or running

Moderate intensity activities	Vigorous intensity activities
Swimming	Spinning classes
Tennis	Squash and racquetball
Water aerobics	

A balanced exercise program that keeps you healthy as you age should include three types of activities: cardiovascular, strength, and flexibility.

Cardiovascular exercises, 4 to 7 days per week

Group 1 activities	Group 2 activities	Group 3 activities
Cycling (indoor)	Aerobic dancing	Basketball
Jogging	Step aerobics	Handball
Walking	Hiking	Hockey
Rowing	In-line skating	Racquet sports
Stair-climbing	Skipping rope	Soccer
Cross-country skiing	Swimming	Volleyball
Distance cycling	Water aerobics	Circuit training

Group 1 activities provide constant intensity and are not dependent on skill; group 2 activities may provide constant or variable intensity, depending on your skill; group 3 activities provide variable intensity and are highly dependent on skill.

These aerobic or cardio activities help keep you slim and improve the fitness of your heart, lungs, and circulatory system. To improve your health and level of fitness, cardio workouts should involve continuously exercising large muscle groups (e.g., your legs), which then require more oxygen than usual. This challenges your cardiovascular system to deliver more oxygen to your working muscles. Not only do your legs get a workout, your heart and lungs get fit too!

If you're new to cardiovascular exercise, begin with activities that can be maintained continuously and don't require special skill (e.g., group 1 activities). The time you need to spend exercising depends on your effort. Moderate intensity exercises should be performed for at least 30 minutes and vigorous exercises for at least 20 minutes.

You don't have to get your 30 minutes all in one go. Research has demonstrated that as long as your total energy expenditure is the same, you can accumulate your 30 minutes (or more!) in shorter sessions and still reap the same cardiovascular benefits. A randomized controlled trial conducted in overweight women found that accumulating 20 to 40 minutes of exercise per day in 10-minute bouts—versus 20 to 40 minutes in one session—enhanced exercise adherence and promoted weight loss.[2]

CALCULATE YOUR TARGET HEART RATE ZONE

You're exercising hard enough if you're working out at 50% to 85% of your maximum heart rate (the maximum number of times your heart can beat in 1 minute). This is called your target heart rate zone. Beginners and older adults should aim to workout at 50% of their maximum heart rate. The most common way to estimate your maximum heart rate is to subtract your age from 220. However, this number can overestimate your maximum heart rate if you're under 40 and underestimate it if you're older. Researchers from the University of Colorado at Boulder recommend using the following formula:

$$\text{Maximum Heart Rate} = 208 - (0.7 \times \text{your age})$$

So if you're 40 years old, your maximum heart rate would be $208 - (0.7 \times 40) = 180$ beats per minute.

If you're new to exercise, you should work out at 50% to 70% of your maximum heart rate, which is calculated by multiplying your maximum heart rate by 0.5 and 0.7. Assuming you are 40 years old and have a maximum heart rate of 180, your target heart rate zone would be 90 to 126 beats per minute ($180 \times 0.5 = 90$ and $180 \times 0.7 = 126$).

If you already exercise regularly, you need to aim for 70% to 85% of your maximum heart rate. If your maximum heart rate is 180, you need to be working out in a target heart rate zone of 126 to 162 beats per minute.

There are a few ways to figure out your heart rate during exercise. You can spend around $200 and buy a heart rate monitor, which consists of a band you wear around your chest that transmits your heart rate to a wrist-watch. If you work out in a gym, you can use the heart rate grips on cardio machines; they work best if your hands are slightly damp with sweat and your grip is light.

Or you can do it the old-fashioned way. Using two fingers (your pointer and middle finger), find your pulse either on the inside of your wrist or on your neck. Look at the second hand of your watch and count the number of beats in 10 seconds (count from zero to 10), then multiply by 6 to get beats per minute. So, for example, during your exercise video, if your heart beats 24 times in 10 seconds, that means it's beating 144 times per minute.

Use the talk test

There's a much easier way to tell if you're slacking off or working too hard. If you can comfortably carry on a conversation while you exercise, you're not overdoing it. But if you don't become winded at all while talking, you need to increase the intensity.

Strength exercises, 2 to 4 days per week

Heavy yard work	Push-ups	Free weights (dumbbells, barbells)
Raking and carrying leaves	Chin-ups	Nautilus machines
Climbing stairs	Abdominal crunches	Cybex machines

Muscular strength, tone, and endurance are important to your overall health and physical fitness. Strength training (also called resistance training) improves your posture, prevents injuries, gives you definition, reshapes problem areas, increases your metabolism, and helps prevent osteoporosis. Research suggests that weight training can also ward off heart disease. A study from Harvard School of Public Health followed 44,452 healthy men for 12 years and revealed that men who worked out with weights for 30 minutes or more per week were 23% less likely to develop heart disease than men who did not weight train.[3] Training with weights increases muscle mass and can possibly increase resting metabolic rate, improve blood sugar control, and help lower blood pressure.

People with lower initial strength who work with weights will show greater improvement and at a faster rate than people who start out with higher strength levels. As you get stronger, it will become easier to lift the same amount of weight, or perform the same number of push-ups. Throughout your program, you must periodically (and gradually) increase the amount of work your muscles perform so that further improvements can be made. That means you need to increase the amount of weight you lift, or the number of push-ups and sit-ups you do.

Use the following guidelines for safe strength training:

- Warm up with 5 minutes of light aerobic activity and stretching to get your circulation going and your joints moving.
- Ask a personal trainer to show you the proper technique to protect your back and joints.
- Breathe regularly when doing an exercise.
- Rest for at least 1 day between strength training sessions.

REPS AND SETS

Repetitions (reps) refers to the number of times you do an exercise, such as a leg lunge. A set is a group of repetitions. Depending on your fitness goals, 1 to 3 sets per exercise is the norm.

Exercise Reps and Sets

Your goal	Reps	Sets	Frequency
Toning	12–15	3	3 times per week
Endurance	15–20	3	3 times per week
Strength (beginner)	6–8	3	3 times per week
Strength (novice)	4–8	5–6	5 times per week

You'll improve your muscular fitness by performing only 1 set of a given exercise, but research suggests that multiple sets are more beneficial for optimal gains in muscle strength and endurance. The amount of weight you lift will depend on your muscle strength and the number of reps you need to perform to achieve your goals. For example, if you want to tone your muscles, pick a weight that becomes difficult after 10 to 12 reps. The last 3 to 5 repetitions of the set should definitely challenge you. Your muscles should feel fatigued, but not painful.

If you are new to the world of strength training, I strongly recommend that you consult a certified personal trainer for your first few sessions. A personal trainer will instruct you on proper technique, specific exercises, and the appropriate amount of weight to use.

Flexibility exercises, 4 to 7 days per week

Gardening	Stretching exercise	Golf
Sweeping	Tai Chi	Bowling
Mopping	Yoga	Curling
Yardwork	Pilates	Dance
Vacuuming		

Being flexible means that your joints can move fluidly through a full range of motion. Gentle reaching, bending, and stretching keep your joints flexible and your muscles relaxed. The more flexible you are, the less likely you'll injure yourself while exercising. If you get into the habit of doing these exercises now, you'll be glad later on: Flexibility definitely enhances quality of life and independence for older adults.

Use the following guidelines for safe stretching:

- Warm up with light activity for 5 minutes before you stretch. This increases your body temperature and your range of motion. Or do your stretching after a cardio or weight workout.
- Stretch all your major muscle groups (back, chest, shoulders, arms, legs).
- Stretch slowly and smoothly without bouncing or jerking. Use gentle, continuous movement or stretch-and-hold (for 10 to 30 seconds), whichever is right for the exercise.
- Focus on the target muscle that you're stretching. Relax the muscle and minimize the movement of other body parts.
- Stretch to the limit of the movement, but not to the point of pain. Aim for a stretched, relaxed feeling.

- Don't hold your breath. Keep breathing slowly and rhythmically while holding the stretch.
- If you're not sure what to do, get help from a fitness expert at your health club. Or pick up a book on stretching at your local bookstore.

Tips to build in lifestyle activity

You can also get exercise in small ways during the day that won't increase your heart rate, but will burn calories. I call it the *lifestyle approach* to exercise. Short bouts of this type of exercise accumulate and can make a difference to your heart health and your waistline. Remember, your goal is to accumulate at least 30 minutes of moderate physical activity during the course of the day. Here are a few simple ways to build activity into your lifestyle:

- Walk whenever you can—get off the bus early, park at the back of the lot, walk part of the way to work, or take the dog for an extra-long walk.
- Get a pedometer and use it. This device clips on to your belt or waistband and counts the number of steps you take each day. To be healthy, you need to aim for 10,000 steps per day; for weight loss, you need to accumulate at least 12,000 to 15,000 steps.
- Use the stairs instead of the elevator, even if it's only partway.
- Take the stairs instead of the escalator at the shopping mall.
- Avoid using walking sidewalks at airports.
- Ride your bike, instead of driving, to visit a neighbourhood friend.
- Walk at lunch hour with co-workers or friends.
- Walk to deliver a message to a co-worker instead of sending an email.
- Play actively with your kids.
- Get up off the couch and stretch for a few minutes each hour.
- Ride a stationary bicycle while watching TV.
- On the golf course, carry or wheel your golf bag as you walk instead of riding in a cart.

Tips for sticking with exercise

The decision to get and stay physically fit requires a lifelong commitment of both time and effort. Exercising and eating healthfully must become things you do naturally every day, like brushing your teeth. And you need to be patient. Don't try to do too much too soon, or you'll give up before you get a chance to reap the rewards. Remember that some days will be harder than others. It's on those days that you need to focus on your goals and remind yourself why you're doing this.

- *Add variety.* If you perceive your workout as a chore, you more than likely won't stick with it. Keep it interesting by planning different types of cardio workouts each week: a power walk with a friend, a fitness class at the gym, a hike on the weekend. There is no rule that says you have to get on that treadmill 4 days a week to stay fit. If you find your weight training program is getting boring, change things up. Vary how often you do an exercise and the number of sets and reps you do. Find an alternate exercise that works the same muscles. Instead of doing your bicep curls with free weights, try doing them on a weight machine in the gym. Instead of doing 2 sets of bicep curls back to back, do only 1 set and then immediately do 1 set of triceps, followed by 1 set of shoulders. When you're done, repeat the circuit to complete your second set of each exercise.
- *Schedule your workouts.* Record your workout schedule in your BlackBerry, iPhone, day planner, or kitchen calendar. Book your exercise times just like you would any other appointment—and stick to those times. Remember that you are just as important as any other person that you schedule in during your day. If you can, arrange to exercise on the same days at the same time so that workouts become a natural part of your life, not something that happens only if you get around to it.
- *Find a workout partner.* You'll be more likely to exercise if you do it with a friend. If you're having trouble getting yourself out the door, ask a friend or family member to join you. Even if you don't feel like exercising, having someone to walk, jog, or bike with will increase your motivation and make the time fly by. Or try a group exercise class. Working out with people who share a common goal can be a big motivator.
- *Keep a fitness journal.* Recording your daily workouts and physical activity helps motivate you as you watch your fitness improve over time. Use your journal to reflect on what activities you've done for the past few weeks. Doing so provides a sense of accomplishment and encourages you to keep going.
- *Hire a certified personal trainer.* Working with a personal trainer motivates me to go to my weight workouts. I have someone waiting for

me, so I have to show up even if I don't feel like it. A trainer also makes me work harder than I would on my own, and seeing my progress inspires me to keep on exercising. I also enjoy the company as I work out.

You might want to hire a personal trainer only once or twice to show you the ropes and get you started. Or you might prefer weekly sessions to keep you focused. If you belong to a health club, there are bound to be a few personal trainers on staff. If you work out at home and would like the help of a personal trainer, the Certified Personal Trainers Network (www.cptn.com) can help you find a professional in your community.

When to check with your doctor first

Most healthy people can safely start an exercise program. However, if you're a male over 45 or a female over 55 and have not been regularly active, or have any health concerns, consult your doctor first. Regardless of your age, consult with your doctor if you have two or more of the following risk factors:

- high blood pressure
- high blood cholesterol
- diabetes
- you're a smoker
- family history of early onset heart disease (father before the age of 55 or mother before the age of 65)

Other reasons to visit your doctor before starting an exercise program include:
- You feel pain in your chest during physical activity.
- In the past, you have felt pain in your chest when you're not active.
- You sometimes lose your balance or become dizzy.
- You have a bone or joint condition that could be made worse by exercise.

PART 3

RECIPES THAT PREVENT HEART DISEASE

In this section of *Heart Healthy Foods for Life*, you'll learn how to transform disease-fighting foods into delicious, nutrient-packed meals that your whole family will enjoy. The recipes that follow will help you prepare meals that are low in saturated fat and sodium, high in fibre, and loaded with vitamins and minerals that guard against heart disease. Once you tackle a recipe or two, I think you'll find that preparing heart healthy dishes is easy and, even better, doesn't take a lot of time.

I've listed the 100-plus recipes by their heart healthy food ingredients, such as fish, whole grains, nuts, and monounsaturated fats, as well as by the recipe categories you're accustomed to seeing in most cookbooks. Each recipe is accompanied by a nutrient breakdown that includes calories, protein, total fat, saturated fat, carbohydrates, fibre, cholesterol, and sodium per serving. I've also highlighted recipes that are particularly good sources of heart healthy nutrients such as fibre, folate, magnesium, and potassium. The following definitions will help you interpret my recipe nutrient claims.

EXCELLENT SOURCE OF means ≥ 25% of the recommended daily intake

GOOD SOURCE OF means ≥ 15% of the recommended daily intake

LOW IN SODIUM means 140 milligrams or less of sodium per serving

LOW IN FAT means 3 grams or less of fat per serving

LOW IN SATURATED FAT means 2 grams or less of saturated fat per serving

LOW IN CHOLESTEROL means 20 milligrams or less of cholesterol per serving

HIGH SOURCE OF FIBRE means 4 grams or more of fibre per serving

VERY HIGH SOURCE OF FIBRE means 6 grams or more of fibre per serving

One of the best strategies to keep your heart healthy and manage your weight is to cook for yourself, rather than relying on restaurant meals, take-out food, and processed ready-to-eat meals. After tasting a few of these recipes, I think you'll agree—and get hooked on home-prepared meals. Enjoy!

Heart healthy recipes

Breakfasts 245

Salads and dressings 256

Soups 269

Side dishes (vegetables and grains) 283

Pasta and stir-fries 293

Meatless main dishes 307

Fish and seafood 320

Poultry and meat 330

Quick breads and muffins 342

Desserts 362

BREAKFASTS

Almond and Berry Yogurt Breakfast Parfait	245
Apple Cinnamon Hot Oats	246
Blueberry Almond Smoothie	247
Blueberry Maple Pancakes	248
Breakfast Banana Split	250
Cinnamon Flax French Toast	251
Cottage Cheese with Fresh Fruit	252
Orange Ginger Smoothie	253
Rainbow Egg White Omelet	254
Strawberry Almond Oat Bran Cereal	255

SALADS AND DRESSINGS

Chickpea and Black Bean Salad with Flaxseed Dressing	256
Crunchy Spinach and Sprouts Salad	257
Fig and Roasted Walnut Salad	259
Mango Cashew Salad	260
Mixed Berry Salad	261
Quinoa Tabbouleh	262
Roasted Beet Salad	263
Warm Spinach and Mushroom Salad with Goat Cheese	264
Wild Rice and Black Bean Salad with Cilantro Lime Dressing	265
Avocado Lime Dressing	266
Ginger Poppy Dressing	267
Honey Balsamic Dressing	268

SOUPS

Carrot Ginger Soup	269
Chicken Barley Soup	271
Curried Lentil Soup	273
Gazpacho	274
Hot and Sour Soup	275
Miso Soup	276

Roasted Parsnip and Pear Soup   277
Spicy Black Bean Soup   278
Squash and Apple Soup   280
White Bean and Vegetable Soup   281

SIDE DISHES (VEGETABLES AND GRAINS)
Caramelized Onions   283
Green Beans with Toasted Almonds   284
Grilled Balsamic Portobello Mushrooms   285
Grilled Corn on the Cob with Cajun and Lime Rub   286
Grilled Eggplant with Ginger Dressing   287
Orange Baked Squash   288
Roasted Squash with Ginger Orange Glaze   289
Roasted Vegetables   290
Sautéed Cherry Tomatoes with Garlic and Fresh Basil   291
Spicy Sesame Swiss Chard   292

PASTA AND STIR-FRIES
Beef Stroganoff   293
Chicken Mango Stir-Fry   295
Grilled Chicken and Mixed Vegetable Pasta   296
Honey Garlic Shrimp Stir-Fry   297
Lemon Sesame Chicken Stir-Fry   299
Pasta Salad with Tuna, Capers, and Lemon   300
Pasta with Salmon and Snap Peas   301
Roasted Vegetable Pasta   302
Sweet and Sour Tofu Stir-Fry   303
Tempeh Stir-Fry with Orange Garlic Sauce   305

MEATLESS MAIN DISHES
Almond-Crusted Tofu   307
Asparagus and Red Pepper Frittata with Goat Cheese   309
Chickpea Goulash   310
Chipotle Chili   312

Honey Garlic Soy Meatballs 313
Refried Bean Baked Tortilla 315
Roasted Vegetable Sandwich 316
Slow Cooker Stewed Lentils 317
Spicy Baked Tofu Bites 318
Thai Tofu Cutlets 319

FISH AND SEAFOOD

Grilled Salmon with Sesame Cilantro Pesto 320
Lemon Pepper Salmon Dip 321
Lemon Thyme Grilled Trout 322
Mussels Steamed in a White Wine Sauce 323
Pepper-Crusted Salmon 324
Seared Tuna Sandwich with Caramelized Onions 325
Smoked Salmon Sandwich with Capers and Red Onions 326
Sole with Tomatoes and Olives 327
Tilapia in a Tomato Fennel Sauce 328
Tuna Bruschetta 329

POULTRY AND MEAT

Grilled Honey Tarragon Turkey Breasts 330
Honey Garlic Pork Chops 331
Lemon Chicken 332
Moroccan Turkey Meat Loaf 333
Mustard-Glazed Chicken 334
Pork Loin Chops with Apple Chutney 335
Roasted Chicken Breasts with Curry Sauce 336
Slow Cooker Beef and Vegetable Stew 337
Slow Cooker Citrus Chicken with Potatoes 339
Turkey Burgers 340

QUICK BREADS AND MUFFINS

Apple Blueberry Bran Muffins 342
Carrot Walnut Bread 344

Chocolate Zucchini Muffins   346

Cinnamon Orange Loaf   348

Easy Beer Bread   350

Jalapeno Cornmeal Muffins   352

Lemon Poppy Seed Loaf   354

Marbled Chocolate Banana Bread   356

Pumpkin Quinoa Muffins   358

Strawberry Rhubarb Muffins   360

DESSERTS

Apple Raspberry Crisp with Maple Oat Topping   362

Broiled Grapefruit with Ginger Glaze   364

Chocolate Cake with Crystallized Ginger   365

Chocolate Fruit Fondue   367

Cinnamon Pecan Baked Apples   368

Dessert Crepes   369

Ginger Flax Cookies   371

Orange Fig Granola Bars   373

Pomegranate Poached Pears with Fresh Raspberries   375

Pumpkin Ginger Pie   376

Recipes Using Heart Healthy Foods

FISH (OMEGA-3 FATTY ACIDS: DHA AND EPA)

Grilled Salmon with Sesame Cilantro Pesto   320

Honey Garlic Shrimp Stir Fry   297

Lemon Pepper Salmon Dip   321

Lemon Thyme Grilled Trout   322

Mussels Steamed in a White Wine Sauce   323

Pasta Salad with Tuna, Capers, and Lemon   300

Pasta with Salmon and Snap Peas   301

Pepper-Crusted Salmon   324

Seared Tuna Sandwich with Caramelized Onions   325

Smoked Salmon Sandwich with Capers and Red Onions   326
Sole with Tomatoes and Olives   327
Tilapia in a Tomato Fennel Sauce   328
Tuna Bruschetta   329

FLAXSEED OIL (OMEGA-3 FATTY ACIDS: ALA)

Avocado Lime Dressing   266
Chickpea and Black Bean Salad with Flaxseed Dressing   256
Honey Balsamic Dressing   268

WHOLE GRAINS

Beef Stroganoff   293
Chicken Barley Soup   271
Chicken Mango Stir-Fry   295
Cinnamon Orange Loaf   348
Easy Beer Bread   350
Grilled Chicken and Mixed Vegetable Pasta   296
Honey Garlic Shrimp Stir-Fry   297
Jalapeno Cornmeal Muffins   352
Lemon Poppy Seed Loaf   354
Lemon Sesame Chicken Stir-Fry   299
Pasta Salad with Tuna, Capers, and Lemon   300
Pasta with Salmon and Snap Peas   301
Pumpkin Quinoa Muffins   358
Quinoa Tabbouleh   262
Roasted Vegetable Pasta   302
Strawberry Rhubarb Muffins   360
Sweet and Sour Tofu Stir-Fry   303
Tempeh Stir-Fry with Orange Garlic Sauce   305
Wild Rice and Black Bean Salad with Cilantro Lime Dressing   265

FLAXSEED (SOLUBLE FIBRE)

Apple Blueberry Bran Muffins   342
Apple Cinnamon Hot Oats   246

Chocolate Zucchini Muffins   346
Cinnamon Flax French Toast   251
Ginger Flax Cookies   371
Honey Garlic Soy Meatballs   313
Pumpkin Ginger Pie   376
Strawberry Rhubarb Muffins   360
Turkey Burgers   340

OATS AND OAT BRAN (SOLUBLE FIBRE)

Apple Blueberry Bran Muffins   342
Apple Cinnamon Hot Oats   246
Apple Raspberry Crisp with Maple Oat Topping   362
Blueberry Maple Pancakes   248
Breakfast Banana Split   250
Carrot Walnut Bread   344
Chocolate Zucchini Muffins   346
Moroccan Turkey Meat Loaf   333
Orange Fig Granola Bars   373
Strawberry Almond Oat Bran Cereal   255
Turkey Burgers   340

VEGETABLES

Asparagus and Red Pepper Frittata with Goat Cheese   309
Caramelized Onions   283
Carrot Ginger Soup   269
Crunchy Spinach and Sprouts Salad   257
Fig and Roasted Walnut Salad   259
Gazpacho   274
Green Beans with Toasted Almonds   284
Grilled Balsamic Portobello Mushrooms   285
Grilled Chicken and Mixed Vegetable Pasta   296
Grilled Corn on the Cob with Cajun and Lime Rub   286
Grilled Eggplant with Ginger Dressing   287
Lemon Sesame Chicken Stir-Fry   299

Orange Baked Squash   288

Rainbow Egg White Omelet   254

Roasted Beet Salad   263

Roasted Parsnip and Pear Soup   277

Roasted Squash with Ginger Orange Glaze   289

Roasted Vegetable Pasta   302

Roasted Vegetable Sandwich   316

Roasted Vegetables   290

Sautéed Cherry Tomatoes with Garlic and Fresh Basil   291

Slow Cooker Beef and Vegetable Stew   377

Slow Cooker Citrus Chicken with Potatoes   339

Spicy Sesame Swiss Chard   292

Squash and Apple Soup   280

Tuna Bruschetta   329

Warm Spinach and Mushroom Salad with Goat Cheese   264

White Bean and Vegetable Soup   281

FRUIT

Almond and Berry Yogurt Breakfast Parfait   245

Apple Raspberry Crisp with Maple Oat Topping   362

Blueberry Almond Smoothie   247

Breakfast Banana Split   250

Broiled Grapefruit with Ginger Glaze   364

Chocolate Fruit Fondue   367

Cinnamon Pecan Baked Apples   368

Cottage Cheese with Fresh Fruit   252

Mango Cashew Salad   260

Mixed Berry Salad   261

Orange Ginger Smoothie   253

Pomegranate Poached Pears with Fresh Raspberries   375

NUTS

Almond and Berry Yogurt Breakfast Parfait   245

Almond-Crusted Tofu   307

Blueberry Almond Smoothie   247
Breakfast Banana Split   250
Cinnamon Pecan Baked Apples   368
Green Beans with Toasted Almonds   284
Mango Cashew Salad   260
Strawberry Almond Oat Bran Cereal   255

LEGUMES

Chickpea and Black Bean Salad with Flaxseed Dressing   256
Chickpea Goulash   310
Chipotle Chili   312
Cinnamon Orange Loaf   348
Curried Lentil Soup   273
Refried Bean Baked Tortilla   315
Slow Cooker Stewed Lentils   317
Spicy Black Bean Soup   278
White Bean and Vegetable Soup   281
Wild Rice and Black Bean Salad with Cilantro Lime Dressing   265

SOY

Almond-Crusted Tofu   307
Honey Garlic Soy Meatballs   313
Hot and Sour Soup   275
Miso Soup   276
Spicy Baked Tofu Bites   318
Sweet and Sour Tofu Stir-Fry   303
Tempeh Stir-Fry with Orange Garlic Sauce   305
Thai Tofu Cutlets   319

DARK CHOCOLATE AND COCOA

Chocolate Cake with Crystallized Ginger   365
Chocolate Fruit Fondue   367
Chocolate Zucchini Muffins   346
Marbled Chocolate Banana Bread   356

OLIVES AND OLIVE OIL (MONOUNSATURATED FAT)

Grilled Chicken and Mixed Vegetable Pasta   296

Honey Balsamic Dressing   268

Roasted Vegetable Pasta   302

Roasted Vegetables   290

Sautéed Cherry Tomatoes with Garlic and Fresh Basil   291

Sole with Tomatoes and Olives   327

Heart Healthy Breakfasts

Almond and Berry Yogurt Breakfast Parfait

This parfait is an easy-to-prepare and tasty breakfast. Consider making it the night before and chilling it in the fridge overnight for a quick, healthy start to your day. This recipe can also double as a light dessert.

2 cups	low-fat (1% MF or less) plain or vanilla yogurt	500 ml
1 tbsp	honey	15 ml
1 tbsp	lemon zest	15 ml
2 cups	mixed berries, fresh or thawed from frozen	500 ml
1/2 cup	slivered almonds	125 ml

In a small bowl, combine yogurt, honey, and zest.

In 4 parfait glasses, layer berries, almonds, and yogurt mixture.

Refrigerate until ready to serve.

Serves 4.

Per parfait: 222 cal, 11 g pro, 9 g total fat (1 g saturated fat), 27 g carb, 4 g fibre, 2 mg chol, 93 mg sodium

Excellent source of: vitamin C, magnesium
Good source of: calcium, potassium
Low in sodium
Low in saturated fat
Low in cholesterol
High source of fibre

Apple Cinnamon Hot Oats

This high-fibre and high-protein breakfast will keep you feeling satisfied for hours, especially after a morning workout. It doesn't require much cooking time and it's an excellent source of cholesterol-lowering soluble fibre.

1 1/2 cups	rolled oats	375 ml
1	apple, peeled and finely diced	1
1 1/2 cups	low-fat (1% MF or less) milk or soymilk	375 ml
2 tbsp	dried cranberries	25 ml
1 tbsp	honey	15 ml
1 tsp	cinnamon	5 ml
1 tbsp	whole flaxseed	15 ml

In a small saucepan, combine oats, apple, milk, cranberries, honey, cinnamon, and flaxseed. Cover and simmer for 2 to 5 minutes, stirring constantly, until heated through and oats begin to soften.

Serve warm.

Serves 2.

Per 1 1/2 cup (375 ml) serving: 424 cal, 17 g pro, 7 g total fat (2 g saturated fat), 76 g carb, 9 g fibre, 9 mg chol, 86 mg sodium

Excellent source of: vitamin D, calcium, magnesium, iron, potassium
Low in sodium
Low in saturated fat
Low in cholesterol
Very high source of fibre

Blueberry Almond Smoothie

Almonds are an excellent source of monounsaturated fat, vitamin E, and magnesium—all of which promote heart health. That's why I've added them to this smoothie. While the recipe calls for blueberries, you can substitute any type of berry, such as raspberries or strawberries.

1 cup	low-fat (1% MF or less) milk or soymilk	250 ml
1/2 cup	orange juice	125 ml
1/4 cup	blueberries, fresh or frozen	50 ml
2 tbsp	sliced almonds	25 ml
2 tsp	maple syrup	10 ml
1	banana, peeled and chopped	1
1/2 tsp	vanilla extract	2 ml

In a blender, combine milk, orange juice, blueberries, almonds, maple syrup, banana, and vanilla. Purée until smooth.

Serve cold.

Serves 2.

Per 1 cup (250 ml) serving: 242 cal, 9 g pro, 9 g total fat (1 g saturated fat), 35 g carb, 3 g fibre, 6 mg chol, 62 mg sodium

Excellent source of: vitamin D, vitamin C, magnesium, potassium
Good source of: calcium
Low in sodium
Low in saturated fat
Low in cholesterol

Blueberry Maple Pancakes

These heart healthy pancakes use egg whites, whole-wheat flour, rolled oats, and oat bran, making them low in saturated fat and cholesterol and very high in fibre. If you're making these on the weekend, freeze any leftovers for reheating in the toaster when you need a quick breakfast mid-week.

Tip: If you've ever tried to fish out a piece of eggshell from a bowl of broken eggs, you know how tricky it can be. Since pieces of eggshell attract each other, simply use a larger piece to scoop out any bits in the bottom of the bowl.

4	egg whites	4
1 1/2 cups	whole-wheat flour	375 ml
1/2 cup	rolled oats	125 ml
2 tbsp	oat bran	25 ml
2 tsp	baking powder	10 ml
1/4 tsp	salt	1 ml
1/2 cup	blueberries, fresh or frozen	125 ml
1 cup	low-fat (1% MF or less) milk or soymilk	250 ml
2 tsp	maple syrup	10 ml
2 tsp	vanilla extract	10 ml
1 tsp	canola oil	5 ml

In a mixing bowl, whisk egg whites until they are white, fluffy, and hold their shape. Set aside.

In a separate large mixing bowl, combine flour, oats, oat bran, baking powder, salt, and blueberries.

Add milk, maple syrup, and vanilla to the flour and blueberry mixture. Mix until just combined. Be careful not to over mix.

Gently fold egg whites into batter; mix until just combined.

Meanwhile, heat oil in a skillet over medium heat. For each pancake, add approximately 1/2 cup (125 ml) of batter to the preheated skillet. When bubbles appear on the surface of the pancake, flip and continue to cook until lightly brown.

Makes 8 pancakes.

Serves 4.

Per 2 pancakes: 272 cal, 14 g pro, 4 g total fat (1 g saturated fat), 49 g carb, 7 g fibre, 3 mg chol, 398 mg sodium

Excellent source of: magnesium
Good source of: iron, potassium
Low in saturated fat
Low in cholesterol
Very high source of fibre

Breakfast Banana Split

This isn't the ice-cream-with-a-cherry-on-top kind of banana split, but it certainly is the heart healthy kind—made with toasted nuts, oats, low-fat yogurt, and a little bit of maple syrup. If you don't have time to toast the nuts and oats, not to worry. This "dessert for breakfast" will still taste great!

1 tbsp	walnuts pieces	15 ml
1/4 cup	rolled oats	50 ml
1	banana, sliced	1
1/2 cup	low-fat (1% MF or less) yogurt	125 ml
1 tbsp	maple syrup	15 ml
1/2 tsp	lemon zest	2 ml

Preheat oven to 375°F (190°C).

Combine walnuts and oats on a baking sheet. Bake for 5 to 7 minutes until lightly toasted and fragrant. Remove from oven; set aside to cool.

Meanwhile, in a small bowl, toss banana slices, yogurt, maple syrup, and lemon zest. Top with toasted walnuts and oats.

Serves 1.

Per serving: 367 cal, 14 g pro, 11 g total fat (1 g saturated fat), 59 g carb, 5 g fibre, 2 mg chol, 91 mg sodium

Excellent source of: magnesium, potassium
Good source of: calcium
Low in sodium
Low in saturated fat
Low in cholesterol
High source of fibre

Cinnamon Flax French Toast

This easy French toast recipe uses egg whites instead of a whole egg, making it virtually cholesterol free! Choose 100% whole-grain bread for an added boost of fibre.

Tip: A drizzle of maple syrup and fresh blueberries, or no added sugar jam, tastes great on this French toast.

4	egg whites, whisked	4
2 tbsp	low-fat (1% MF or less) milk or soymilk	25 ml
2 tbsp	ground flaxseed	25 ml
2 tsp	cinnamon	10 ml
1 tsp	orange zest	5 ml
2 tsp	canola oil	10 ml
4	slices whole-grain bread	4

In a shallow dish, whisk together egg whites, milk, flaxseed, cinnamon, and orange zest until frothy.

Meanwhile, heat oil in a skillet over medium heat.

Dip slices of bread into egg mixture and place in hot skillet. Cook over medium heat until lightly brown, turning once.

Serves 2.

Per 2 slices: 281 cal, 15 g pro, 10 g total fat (1 g saturated fat), 35 g carb, 7 g fibre, 1 mg chol, 425 mg sodium

Excellent source of: magnesium, iron
Good source of: folate
Low in saturated fat
Low in cholesterol
Very high source of fibre

Cottage Cheese with Fresh Fruit

This basic recipe for fresh fruit and cottage cheese makes for a breakfast that provides protein, fibre, and very little fat—a great combination to energize your day!

1 cup	cottage cheese	250 ml
3/4 cup	sliced strawberries	175 ml
3/4 cup	blueberries	175 ml
1	apple, diced	1

In a mixing bowl, combine cottage cheese, strawberries, blueberries, and apple. Toss to combine.

Serve immediately, or cover and refrigerate overnight.

Serves 2.

Per serving: 168 cal, 15 g pro, 2 g total fat (1 g saturated fat), 25 g carb, 4 g fibre, 5 mg chol, 474 mg sodium

Excellent source of: vitamin C
Good source of: vitamin K
Low in fat
Low in saturated fat
Low in cholesterol
High source of fibre

Orange Ginger Smoothie

Fresh ginger gives this smoothie a refreshing and delicious taste—my taste-testers couldn't seem to get enough of it! I often use jarred minced ginger-root as a convenient alternative to preparing fresh gingerroot, especially first thing in the morning!

Tip: When fresh berries are plentiful in the summer, freeze 1-cup (250 ml) portions in a freezer bag to use year-round in smoothies and baked goods.

1 cup	orange juice	250 ml
1 cup	low-fat (1% MF or less) milk or soymilk	250 ml
1 tsp	minced gingerroot	5 ml
1 cup	mixed fresh or frozen berries	250 ml

In a blender, combine orange juice, milk, gingerroot, and berries. Purée until smooth.

Serve cold.

Serves 2.

Per 1 1/2 cup (375 ml) serving: 148 cal, 6 g pro, 2 g total fat (1 g saturated fat), 30 g carb, 2 g fibre, 6 mg chol, 60 mg sodium

Excellent source of: vitamin D, vitamin C, folate
Good source of: calcium, potassium
Low in sodium
Low in fat
Low in saturated fat
Low in cholesterol

Rainbow Egg White Omelet

This omelet looks as good as it tastes. It uses egg whites instead of whole eggs, so it's low in fat and cholesterol-free. While it makes an excellent breakfast, it can double as a quick dinner when you're short on time.

1 tsp	canola oil	5 ml
1/4 cup	chopped red onion	50 ml
1	clove garlic, chopped	1
1/4 cup	shredded carrot	50 ml
1/4 cup	chopped red pepper	50 ml
2 cups	chopped spinach	500 ml
6	egg whites	6
2 tbsp	chopped chives	25 ml
	freshly ground black pepper, to taste	

Heat oil in a medium skillet over medium heat. Add onion and sauté until soft, about 3 or 4 minutes. Add garlic and carrots; sauté for another 2 minutes. Add red pepper and spinach; continue to sauté.

Meanwhile, in a small bowl, whisk egg whites, chives, and pepper until frothy; add to skillet and reduce heat to low. Cover and cook for about 6 to 8 minutes or until eggs are set.

Once omelet is set and firm, carefully fold in half.

Serves 2.

Per serving: 91 cal, 11 g pro, 3 g total fat (0 g saturated fat), 6 g carb, 1 g fibre, 0 mg chol, 171 mg sodium

Excellent source of: vitamin A, vitamin C, vitamin K
Low in fat
Low in saturated fat
Low in cholesterol

Strawberry Almond Oat Bran Cereal

Make your own instant oatbran with this quick and easy recipe. Combine the dry ingredients in advance and store the mix in a re-sealable container. In the morning, just add water, honey, and strawberries, and you're on your way to a healthy breakfast that will help keep your LDL cholesterol in check.

Tip: Try using blueberries and walnuts in place of the strawberries and almonds for an equally delicious and nutritious breakfast.

1 cup	water	250 ml
1/2 cup	oat bran	125 ml
1 tbsp	honey	15 ml
1 tbsp	sliced almonds	15 ml
1/2 cup	sliced strawberries	125 ml
1/2 tsp	cinnamon	2 ml

In a medium saucepan, bring water to a boil.

Add oat bran; simmer for 2 minutes, stirring constantly until oat bran is a smooth consistency.

Remove from heat; stir in honey, almonds, strawberries, and cinnamon.

Serve immediately.

Serves 2.

Per 3/4 cup (175 ml) serving: 153 cal, 6 g pro, 6 g total fat (1 g saturated fat), 31 g carb, 5 g fibre, 0 mg chol, 7 mg sodium

Excellent source of: vitamin C, magnesium
Good source of: iron
Low in sodium
Low in saturated fat
Low in cholesterol
High source of fibre

Heart Healthy Salads and Dressings

Chickpea and Black Bean Salad with Flaxseed Dressing

This easy-to-make salad is a sure-fire crowd pleaser at barbecues and picnics. Flavours intensify after sitting in the fridge overnight, so I suggest making it in advance if you have time. Thanks to the heart healthy legumes, this salad serves up 6 grams of fibre per serving and plenty of magnesium.

1	19 oz/540 ml can chickpeas, drained and rinsed	1
1	19 oz/540 ml can black beans, drained and rinsed	1
1	12 oz/341 ml can corn, drained	1
2	cloves garlic, chopped	2
1 tbsp	flaxseed oil	15 ml
1 tbsp	extra-virgin olive oil	15 ml
2 tbsp	seasoned rice vinegar	25 ml
3 tbsp	white wine vinegar	40 ml
1 tsp	honey	5 ml
	freshly ground black pepper, to taste	

In a large bowl, toss chickpeas, black beans, corn, and garlic.

Meanwhile, in a small bowl, whisk together flaxseed oil, olive oil, vinegars, honey, and pepper. Toss with chickpea mixture.

Serves 10.

Per 1/2 cup (125 ml) serving: 164 cal, 7 g pro, 4 g total fat (1 g saturated fat), 27 g carb, 6 g fibre, 0 mg chol, 179 mg sodium

Good source of: magnesium
Low in saturated fat
Low in cholesterol
Very high source of fibre

Crunchy Spinach and Sprouts Salad

This versatile whole-grain salad can change with the seasons. In place of the pear, add seasonal fruit such as apples or strawberries. Try making this salad with a variety of sprouts found in produce stores such as broccoli, sunflower, or lentil sprouts.

Tip: To cook quinoa, use 2 parts water to 1 part quinoa. For example, bring 2 cups of water to a boil, add 1 cup of quinoa and stir to combine. Reduce heat; cover and simmer for 12 minutes or until all of the moisture is absorbed. Remove from heat and fluff with a fork.

Tip: Pale yellow quinoa is the most widely available variety; however, some specialty food stores carry a dark reddish-brown variety. Make your own mix by combining equal parts yellow and brown quinoa—they take the same amount of time to cook and you'll end up with a more colourful dish.

8 cups	spinach (about 1 lb/454 g)	2 L
1 cup	sprouts, such as bean, lentil, or broccoli	250 ml
1 cup	cooked quinoa	250 ml
1	pear, cored and diced	1
1/2 cup	slivered almonds	125 ml
1/4 cup	dried cranberries	50 ml

In a large mixing bowl, toss spinach, sprouts, quinoa, pear, almonds, and cranberries.

Drizzle with Avocado Lime Dressing (page 266) just before serving.

Serves 6.

Per 1 1/2 cup (375 ml) serving without dressing: 142 cal, 6 g pro, 5 g total fat (0 g saturated fat), 21 g carb, 4 g fibre, 0 mg chol, 36 mg sodium

Per 1 1/2 cup (375 ml) serving with 2 tbsp (25 ml) dressing: 240 cal, 6 g pro, 15 g total fat (2 g saturated fat), 25 g carb, 6 g fibre, 0 mg chol, 40 mg sodium

(with dressing)
Excellent source of: vitamin A, vitamin K, magnesium, potassium
Good source of: iron, vitamin C
Low in sodium
Low in saturated fat
Low in cholesterol
Very high source of fibre

Fig and Roasted Walnut Salad

Dried figs, red onion, and roasted walnut pieces give this salad plenty of flavour and texture. The walnuts make this salad a great source of alpha-linolenic acid (ALA) while the figs boost its magnesium content.

1/4 cup	walnut pieces	50 ml
12	dried figs, cut into eighths	12
8 cups	spinach (about 1 lb/454 g)	2 L
1/2 cup	sliced red onion	125 ml
1/4 cup	crumbled feta cheese	50 ml

Preheat oven to 350°F (180°C).

Place walnut pieces on a baking sheet and bake for 5 to 7 minutes or until nuts are golden brown and fragrant. Remove from heat and cool.

In a large salad bowl, toss figs, spinach, onion, feta cheese, and roasted walnuts.

Drizzle with Honey Balsamic Dressing (page 268), or another reduced-fat dressing.

Serves 6.

Per 1 1/2 cup (375 ml) serving without dressing: 131 cal, 5 g pro, 8 g total fat (1 g saturated fat), 14 g carb, 3 g fibre, 6 mg chol, 102 mg sodium

Per 1 1/2 cup (375 ml) serving with 1 tbsp (15 ml) Honey Balsamic Dressing: 205 cal, 5 g pro, 14 g total fat (2 g saturated fat), 18 g carb, 3 g fibre, 6 mg chol, 119 mg sodium

(with dressing)
Excellent source of: vitamin A, vitamin K, magnesium
Good source of: potassium
Low in sodium
Low in saturated fat
Low in cholesterol

Mango Cashew Salad

This refreshing salad bursting with beta carotene requires no oil at all! Be sure to use mangos that are slightly firm so they hold their shape when you mix the salad.

2	mangos, peeled and cubed	2
1/2 cup	thinly sliced red onion	125 ml
1/4 cup	thinly sliced red bell pepper	50 ml
16	cashews	16
1/2 cup	chopped cilantro	125 ml
2 tbsp	freshly squeezed lime juice	25 ml
1/8 tsp	red pepper flakes	0.5 ml

In a large bowl, toss mango, red onion, bell pepper, cashews, and cilantro.

Add lime juice and pepper flakes; toss to coat.

Serves 4.

Per 3/4 cup (175 ml) serving: 166 cal, 3 g pro, 7 g total fat (1 g saturated fat), 26 g carb, 3 g fibre, 0 mg chol, 6 mg sodium

Excellent source of: vitamin A, vitamin C
Good source of: vitamin K, magnesium
Low in sodium
Low in saturated fat
Low in cholesterol

Mixed Berry Salad

This simple antioxidant-rich salad is at its best when local berries are available and plentiful. In addition to phytochemicals, this salad also serves up a hefty dose of vitamin C and potassium.

2 cups	sliced strawberries	500 ml
1 cup	blueberries	250 ml
1 cup	blackberries	250 ml
1 tbsp	lemon zest	15 ml
2 tbsp	finely chopped mint	25 ml
1 cup	low-fat (1% MF or less) plain yogurt	250 ml

In a large bowl, toss strawberries, blueberries, blackberries, lemon zest, mint, and yogurt. Serve immediately.

Serves 4.

Per 1 cup (250 ml) serving: 94 cal, 4 g pro, 1 g total fat (0 g saturated fat), 20 g carb, 5 g fibre, 1 mg chol, 45 mg sodium

Excellent source of: vitamin C
Good source of: vitamin K, potassium
Low in sodium
Low in fat
Low in saturated fat
Low in cholesterol
High source of fibre

Quinoa Tabbouleh

Tabbouleh is a Middle Eastern salad traditionally made with bulgur, a cracked wheat. I've changed things up and substituted quinoa, a whole grain that's high in protein. The result is a scrumptious high-fibre salad that's very low in sodium and, of course, contains no saturated fat!

Tip: See quinoa cooking instructions under Crunchy Spinach and Sprouts Salad (page 257).

4 cups	cooked quinoa	1 L
1 1/2 cups	diced cucumber	375 ml
3/4 cup	chopped parsley	175 ml
1/4 cup	chopped mint	50 ml
1 cup	chopped tomato	250 ml
2	green onions, chopped	2
1/4 cup	freshly squeezed lemon juice	50 ml
1 tbsp	extra-virgin olive oil	15 ml
3	cloves garlic, chopped	3

In a large bowl, toss quinoa, cucumber, parsley, mint, tomato, green onion, lemon juice, olive oil, and garlic.

Cover and refrigerate for at least 2 hours before serving.

Serves 6.

Per 1 cup (250 ml) serving: 191 cal, 6 g pro, 5 g total fat (0 g saturated fat), 32 g carb, 5 g fibre, 0 mg chol, 15 mg sodium

Excellent source of: vitamin K, magnesium
Good source of: iron, potassium
Low in sodium
Low in saturated fat
Low in cholesterol
High source of fibre

Roasted Beet Salad

Beets are an excellent source of anthocyanins, antioxidants that can help keep your heart healthy. This colourful salad takes a little longer to prepare than most of the salad recipes in this book, but the end result is well worth the time and effort.

4	medium-sized beets	4
1/2 cup	chopped red onion	125 ml
2 tbsp	seasoned rice vinegar	25 ml
1/2 tbsp	Dijon mustard	7 ml
1 tsp	extra-virgin olive oil	5 ml
2	green onions, finely sliced	2
1 tsp	orange zest	5 ml

Preheat oven to 375°F (190°C).

Trim beets and cut into quarters.

Place beets in a glass baking dish; cover with 1/2 cup (125 ml) water. Cover baking dish with foil; bake for 50 to 60 minutes or until beets are tender. (Keep an eye on the beets while they are baking; if the bottom of the dish dries out, add another 1/2 cup/125 ml of water.)

Remove from heat and cool.

When beets are cool enough to handle, peel and dice them.

In a large bowl, combine diced beets, red onion, rice vinegar, mustard, olive oil, green onions, and orange zest. Toss to coat.

Serves 4.

Per 3/4 cup (175 ml) serving: 60 cal, 2 pro, 1 g total fat (0 g saturated fat), 11 g carb, 2 g fibre, 0 mg chol, 121 mg sodium

Good source of: vitamin K
Low in sodium
Low in fat
Low in saturated fat
Low in cholesterol

Warm Spinach and Mushroom Salad with Goat Cheese

Low in sodium and saturated fat and packed with potassium, this decadent-tasting salad is ready in less than 20 minutes. The recipe suggests serving it warm, but it tastes just as good cold, so consider making extra for the next day's lunch.

2 tsp	canola oil	10 ml
1 cup	sliced red onion	250 ml
4 cups	sliced button mushrooms	1 L
1	clove garlic, minced	1
1 tbsp	balsamic vinegar	15 ml
8 cups	spinach (about 1 lb/454 g)	2 L
1/2 cup	crumbled goat cheese	125 ml
	freshly ground black pepper, to taste	

Heat oil in a skillet over medium heat.

Add onion; sauté about 5 to 6 minutes or until soft. Add mushrooms; sauté about 8 to 10 minutes or until soft and the pan begins to dry out. Add garlic; sauté for another minute.

Remove from heat. Add balsamic vinegar and scrape the bottom of the pan clean.

Meanwhile, place spinach in a large bowl. Spoon warm mushroom and onion mixture over spinach; toss to combine.

Sprinkle with goat cheese, season with pepper, and serve immediately.

Serves 4.

Per 2 cup (500 ml) serving: 87 cal, 5 g pro, 5 g total fat (2 g saturated fat), 7 g carb, 2 g fibre, 6 mg chol, 91 mg sodium

Excellent source of: vitamin A, vitamin K
Good source of: vitamin C, magnesium, iron, potassium
Low in sodium
Low in saturated fat
Low in cholesterol

Wild Rice and Black Bean Salad with Cilantro Lime Dressing

The combination of wild rice, black beans, corn, lime juice, and cilantro makes an incredibly flavourful Mexican-inspired salad that's low in sodium and saturated fat. Make the salad a few hours before you plan to serve it to allow the flavours to blend.

1 1/2 cups	cooked wild rice	375 ml
1 cup	black beans, rinsed and drained	250 ml
1 cup	corn kernels	250 ml
1/4 cup	freshly squeezed lime juice	50 ml
1/2 cup	chopped cilantro	125 ml
1/4 cup	thinly sliced green onion	50 ml
1/4 tsp	red chili flakes, or to taste	1 ml
2	cloves garlic, finely chopped	2

In a large bowl, toss rice, beans, corn, lime juice, cilantro, green onion, red pepper flakes, and garlic.

Cover and refrigerate for at least 2 hours before serving.

Serves 6.

Per 2/3 cup (150 ml) serving: 99 cal, 5 g pro, 1 g total fat (0 g saturated fat), 21 g carb, 3 g fibre, 0 mg chol, 51 mg sodium

Good source of: vitamin K
Low in sodium
Low in fat
Low in saturated fat
Low in cholesterol

Avocado Lime Dressing

Chipotle chili pepper gives a subtle smoky flavour to this creamy salad dressing, which is loaded with an omega-3 fatty acid called alpha-linolenic acid (ALA) thanks to the flaxseed oil. Not only a great dressing for a fresh salad, it's also a tasty dip for raw vegetables.

Tip: Depending on the size of avocado, the dressing might be quite thick. For a thinner consistency, add another tablespoon of lime juice and purée again.

1	ripe avocado, skin and pit removed	1
2 tbsp	flaxseed oil	25 ml
2	cloves garlic, chopped	2
3 tbsp	freshly squeezed lime juice	40 ml
2 tbsp	water	25 ml
1/4 tsp	dried chipotle chili pepper	1 ml

In a blender, combine avocado, flaxseed oil, garlic, lime juice, water, and chipotle chili pepper. Purée until smooth.

Serves 6.

Per 2 tbsp (25 ml) serving: 98 cal, 1 g pro, 10 g total fat (1 g saturated fat), 4 g carb, 2 g fibre, 0 mg chol, 4 mg sodium

Good source of: vitamin K
Low in sodium
Low in saturated fat
Low in cholesterol

Ginger Poppy Dressing

This flavourful low-fat dressing works well with a fresh spinach or chopped fruit salad.

1/2 cup	low-fat (1% MF or less) plain yogurt	125 ml
2 tsp	orange juice concentrate	10 ml
2 tsp	minced gingerroot	10 ml
1/4 tsp	poppy seeds	1 ml

In a small bowl, whisk together yogurt, orange juice concentrate, gingerroot, and poppy seeds.

Serves 4.

Per 2 tbsp (25 ml) serving: 22 cal, 2 g pro, 0 g total fat (0 g saturated fat), 4 g carb, 0 g fibre, 1 mg chol, 22 mg sodium

Low in sodium
Low in fat
Low in saturated fat
Low in cholesterol

Honey Balsamic Dressing

A triple-duty recipe! Try this delicious salad dressing, rich in monounsaturated fat and alpha-linolenic acid (ALA), as a marinade for meat and vegetables, or as a topping for baked potatoes.

Tip: Cut calories in a vinaigrette recipe by using less pungent vinegar, such as balsamic or white wine. That way you'll need less oil.

2 tbsp	extra-virgin olive oil	25 ml
1 tbsp	flaxseed oil	15 ml
3 tbsp	balsamic vinegar	40 ml
1 tbsp	honey	15 ml
1/2 tbsp	Dijon mustard	7 ml
1	clove garlic, minced	1

In a small bowl, whisk together olive oil, flaxseed oil, vinegar, honey, mustard, and garlic.

Store in an airtight container in the fridge until ready to serve.

Serves 6.

Per 1 tbsp (15 ml) serving: 74 cal, 0 g pro, 7 g total fat (1 g saturated fat), 4 g carb, 0 g fibre, 0 mg chol, 17 mg sodium

Low in sodium
Low in saturated fat
Low in cholesterol

Heart Healthy Soups

Carrot Ginger Soup

Psyllium (pronounced silly-um) comes from the crushed seeds of a plant most commonly grown in India. It's an excellent source of soluble fibre—the type that lowers elevated blood cholesterol. While psyllium is commonly added to breakfast cereals (for example, Kellogg's All-Bran Buds and Nature's Path Smart Bran) and baked goods, I've added it to this soup to help you sneak extra fibre into your meal. You'll find psyllium sold in drug stores as FibreSure (by the makers of Metamucil), which can be added to foods and beverages without changing taste or texture.

1 tbsp	canola oil	15 ml
1 cup	chopped onion	250 ml
4 cups	chopped carrot	1 L
2 cups	diced potato	500 ml
1 tbsp	minced gingerroot	15 ml
4 cups	water	1 L
1 cup	orange juice	250 ml
1/2 tsp	cinnamon	2 ml
1/2 tsp	ground cumin	2 ml
1/8 tsp	salt	0.5 ml
1 tbsp	psyllium, optional	15 ml

Heat oil in a large saucepan over medium heat. Add onion; sauté for about 4 to 5 minutes or until soft.

Add carrot, potato, gingerroot, water, orange juice, cinnamon, cumin, and salt.

Cover and simmer for 35 minutes.

Remove from heat. Purée with a hand blender to desired consistency.

Add psyllium just before serving to thicken soup.

Serves 8.

Per 1 cup (250 ml) serving: 94 cal, 2 g pro, 2 g total fat (0 g saturated fat), 18 g carb, 3 g fibre, 0 mg chol, 84 mg sodium

Excellent source of: vitamin A
Good source of: vitamin C, potassium
Low in sodium
Low in fat
Low in saturated fat
Low in cholesterol

Chicken Barley Soup

This stick-to-your-ribs soup (thanks to the soluble fibre–rich barley!) is the perfect choice for a cool autumn or winter day. The recipe calls for the whole-grain version of barley, called hulled barley or pot barley, which is available in most grocery and natural food stores.

Tip: Look for a reduced-sodium chicken bouillon product such as Knorr's OXO 25% Less Salt.

3 tbsp	canola oil	40 ml
1 cup	diced onion	250 ml
1 cup	diced celery	250 ml
2 cups	diced carrot	500 ml
3	cloves garlic, chopped	3
8 cups	water	2 L
1/2 cup	hulled barley	125 ml
4	4.5 g reduced-sodium chicken bouillon sachets	4
1/2 tsp	freshly ground black pepper	2 ml
1 tbsp	balsamic vinegar	15 ml
12 oz	cooked chicken breast, diced	350 g

Heat oil in a large saucepan, over medium heat. Add onion, celery, and carrot; sauté for about 10 minutes or until soft. Add garlic; sauté for another minute.

Add water, barley, chicken bouillon, pepper, and balsamic vinegar.

Cover and simmer for 45 to 50 minutes or until barley is soft and cooked through.

Add diced chicken; continue to simmer until heated through.

Serve warm.

Serves 6.

Per 1 1/2 cup (375 ml) serving: 237 cal, 20 g pro, 9 g total fat (1 g saturated fat), 20 g carb, 4 g fibre, 42 mg chol, 432 mg sodium

Excellent source of: vitamin A
Good source of: vitamin K, magnesium, potassium
Low in saturated fat
High source of fibre

Curried Lentil Soup

High in fibre and an excellent source of vitamin A and iron, this heart healthy soup has a creamy, thick texture after the lentils are puréed. A hearty meal in a bowl.

2 tbsp	canola oil	25 ml
1 cup	chopped onion	250 ml
1 cup	chopped celery	250 ml
2 cups	chopped carrot	500 ml
3	cloves garlic, chopped	3
8 cups	water	2 L
1 tsp	salt	5 ml
1 cup	dried brown lentils	250 ml
1 tbsp	curry powder	15 ml
1 tbsp	freshly squeezed lime juice	15 ml
1 tsp	minced gingerroot	5 ml
	chopped cilantro, to garnish	

Heat oil in a large saucepan over medium heat. Add onions, celery, and carrot; sauté for about 8 to 10 minutes or until soft. Add garlic; sauté for another minute.

Add water, salt, lentils, curry powder, lime juice, and gingerroot.

Cover and simmer for 45 minutes or until lentils are soft.

Remove from heat. Purée with a hand blender to desired consistency.

Garnish with cilantro.

Serves 6.

Per 1 1/2 cup (375 ml) serving: 182 cal, 10 g pro, 5 g total fat (0 g saturated fat), 26 g carb, 5 g fibre, 0 mg chol, 433 mg sodium

Excellent source of: vitamin A, iron
Good source of: vitamin K, magnesium, potassium
Low in saturated fat
Low in cholesterol
High source of fibre

Gazpacho

Gazpacho is a cold Spanish-style tomato soup loaded with vitamin C. It's very refreshing and meant for those summer days when it's too hot to cook and fresh local tomatoes are readily available. This soup gets better the longer it sits, so if you have time, make it the day before you plan to serve it.

4 cups	chopped tomato	1 L
2 cups	diced cucumber	500 ml
1 cup	chopped red onion	250 ml
2 cups	chopped red bell pepper	500 ml
1 tbsp	freshly squeezed lime juice	15 ml
1 tbsp	extra-virgin olive oil	15 ml
3	cloves garlic, minced	3
3 tbsp	red wine vinegar	40 ml
1 tbsp	finely chopped jalapeno pepper, optional	15 ml
	freshly ground black pepper, to taste	

In a large mixing bowl, combine all ingredients. Remove and reserve about 2 cups (500 ml) of mixture.

Purée ingredients in bowl with a hand blender until smooth. Add reserved solid ingredients; stir to combine.

Serve cold.

Serves 4.

Per 1 1/2 cup (375 ml) serving: 137 cal, 4 g pro, 5 g total fat (1 g saturated fat), 25 g carb, 5 g fibre, 0 mg chol, 25 mg sodium

Excellent source of: vitamin A, vitamin C, vitamin K, potassium
Good source of: folate, magnesium
Low in sodium
Low in saturated fat
Low in cholesterol
High source of fibre

Hot and Sour Soup

This low-sodium soup is quick to make—it's ready in less than 25 minutes! And you might want to double the recipe because it won't last long. My taste-testers liked it so much they wanted seconds and thirds.

Tip: What's the difference between unseasoned and seasoned rice vinegar? Seasoned rice vinegar has added sugar and salt. In fact, some brands of seasoned rice vinegar have up to 530 mg sodium per tablespoon—that's a fair bit! This recipe calls for a rice vinegar that's lower in sodium, so look for one with 60 mg or less per tablespoon.

Tip: Look for a reduced-sodium beef bouillon product such as Knorr's OXO 25% Less Salt.

1 tbsp	canola oil	15 ml
1 cup	finely chopped onion	250 ml
6 cups	water	1.5 L
2	4.5 g reduced-sodium beef bouillon sachets	2
1 cup	sliced button mushrooms	250 ml
1 cup	extra-firm tofu, cubed (about 1/3 block of tofu)	250 ml
2 tbsp	low-sodium seasoned rice vinegar	25 ml
2 tbsp	balsamic vinegar	25 ml
1 tbsp	chopped gingerroot	15 ml
1 tsp	sesame oil	5 ml
	freshly ground black pepper, to taste	
2 cups	kale, deveined and chopped	500 ml
2	green onions, chopped	2
1/8 tsp	red pepper flakes	0.5 ml

Heat oil in a large saucepan over medium heat. Add onions; sauté for about 4 to 5 minutes or until soft.

Add water, beef bouillon, mushrooms, tofu, rice vinegar, balsamic vinegar, gingerroot, sesame oil, pepper, kale, green onions, and red pepper flakes.

Cover and simmer for 15 to 20 minutes.

Serves 6.

Per 1 1/4 cup (300 ml) serving: 82 cal, 4 g pro, 5 g total fat (1 g saturated fat), 6 g carb, 1 g fibre, 0 mg chol, 209 mg sodium

Excellent source of: vitamin K
Good source of: calcium, iron
Low in saturated fat
Low in cholesterol

Miso Soup

A traditional Japanese soup made with miso paste, or fermented soybeans, this light, low-calorie soup is meant to complement a meal.

Tip: You can find miso paste in the Asian section of most major grocery stores or specialty food stores. Once opened, miso should be refrigerated. It's available in a variety of different colours and flavours, all of which work well in this recipe.

6 cups	water	1.5 L
1/4 cup	miso paste	50 ml
1/2 pkg	12 oz/350 g pkg extra-firm tofu, cut into 1/4-inch/0.5 cm cubes	1/2 pkg
1 cup	thinly sliced mushrooms	250 ml
1/4 cup	sliced green onions	50 ml

In a large saucepan, combine water, miso paste, tofu, mushrooms, and green onions. Cover and simmer for 5 minutes.

Remove from heat. Serve warm.

Serves 6.

Per 1 cup (250 ml) serving: 47 cal, 4 g pro, 2 g total fat (0 g saturated fat), 4 g carb, 1 g fibre, 0 mg chol, 435 mg sodium

Low in fat
Low in saturated fat
Low in cholesterol

Roasted Parsnip and Pear Soup

Parsnips are a white root vegetable related to carrots. While they lack their cousin's beta carotene, they're a good source of other heart healthy nutrients, including vitamin C, folate, and potassium. This recipe pairs the nutty flavour of parsnips with the sweetness of pears.

1 lb	parsnips (about 6 medium), cut into 1-inch/2.5 cm pieces	454 g
1	medium onion, quartered	1
2 tbsp	canola oil	25 ml
6 cups	water	1.5 L
2	pears, peeled, cored, and diced	2
1 tsp	salt	5 ml

Preheat oven to 375°F (190°C).

In a large bowl, toss parsnips, onion, and oil. Place on a baking sheet; bake for 30 minutes or until parsnips are cooked through and beginning to brown.

In a large saucepan, combine water, pears, salt, and roasted parsnips and onion.

Cover and simmer for 20 to 30 minutes or until pears are soft.

Remove from heat. Purée with a hand blender to smooth consistency.

Serve warm.

Serves 6.

Per 1 1/3 cup (325 ml) serving: 113 cal, 1 g pro, 4 g total fat (0 g saturated fat), 20 g carb, 4 g fibre, 0 mg chol, 301 mg sodium

Low in saturated fat
Low in cholesterol
High source of fibre

Spicy Black Bean Soup

This spicy, fibre-rich soup is a crowd-pleaser. And guests will love the fact that it's lower in sodium than store-bought varieties.

Tip: Look for a reduced-sodium beef bouillon product such as Knorr's OXO 25% Less Salt.

1 tbsp	canola oil	15 ml
1 cup	chopped onion	250 ml
3	cloves garlic, chopped	3
1 cup	chopped carrot	250 ml
8 cups	water	2 L
2	4.5 g reduced-sodium beef bouillon sachets	2
2	19 oz/540 ml cans black beans, drained and rinsed	2
1	28 oz/796 ml can no added salt diced tomatoes	1
1 tsp	ground cumin	5 ml
1	chopped jalapeno pepper, or to taste	1
2 tbsp	freshly squeezed lime juice	25 ml
1 cup	corn kernels	250 ml
1/2 cup	chopped cilantro	125 ml
3	green onions, chopped	3

Heat oil in a large saucepan over medium heat. Add onions; sauté for about 4 to 5 minutes or until soft. Add garlic; sauté another minute.

Add carrot, water, beef bouillon, beans, tomatoes, cumin, jalapeno pepper, and lime juice.

Cover and simmer for 30 minutes. Remove from heat.

Purée with a hand blender until beans are somewhat blended but still chunky.

Add corn, cilantro, and green onions; mix to combine.

Serve warm.

Serves 8.

Per 1 1/2 cup (375 ml) serving: 189 cal, 9 g pro, 3 g total fat (0 g saturated fat), 34 g carb, 8 g fibre, 0 mg chol, 396 mg sodium

Excellent source of: vitamin A
Good source of: vitamin K
Low in fat
Low in saturated fat
Low in cholesterol
Very high source of fibre

Squash and Apple Soup

This tasty and easy-to-make soup freezes well. The recipe calls for apples but you can use pears instead for a slightly different flavour. With only 80 calories and less than 200 milligrams of sodium per serving, this soup is definitely a heart healthy choice.

2 tbsp	canola oil	25 ml
2 cups	chopped onion	500 ml
6 cups	water	1.5 L
4 cups	cubed butternut squash	1 L
2	apples, peeled, cored, and chopped	2
1 tbsp	minced gingerroot	15 ml
1/2 tsp	salt	2 ml

Heat oil in a large pan over medium heat. Add onions; sauté for about 4 to 5 minutes or until soft.

Add water, squash, apples, gingerroot, and salt.

Cover and simmer for 30 minutes or until squash is tender.

Purée with a hand blender until smooth, or to desired consistency.

Serves 8.

Per 1 cup (250 ml) serving: 80 cal, 1 g pro, 4 g total fat (0 g saturated fat), 13 g carb, 2 g fibre, 0 mg chol, 152 mg sodium

Excellent source of: vitamin A
Low in saturated fat
Low in cholesterol

White Bean and Vegetable Soup

Serve this soup, chock full of soluble fibre and vitamin C, with a green salad and whole-grain crackers. If you want to nudge the sodium content down, use only 2 instead of 3 tablespoons of soy sauce.

1 tbsp	canola oil	15 ml
1 cup	chopped onion	250 ml
2 cups	chopped carrot	500 ml
1 cup	chopped celery	250 ml
1	red bell pepper, diced	1
3	cloves garlic, chopped	3
6 cups	water	1.5 L
	freshly ground black pepper, to taste	
1	19 oz/540 ml can white kidney beans, drained and rinsed	1
1 tbsp	balsamic vinegar	15 ml
3 tbsp	sodium-reduced soy sauce	40 ml
1 cup	chopped spinach	250 ml

Heat oil in a large saucepan over medium heat. Add onions; sauté for about 4 to 5 minutes or until soft.

Add carrot, celery, bell pepper, garlic, water, pepper, beans, balsamic vinegar, and soy sauce.

Cover and simmer for 30 minutes.

Remove from heat; add chopped spinach and stir until combined and spinach is wilted.

Serves 6.

Per 1 1/2 cup (375 ml) serving: 141 cal, 7 g pro, 3 g total fat (0 g saturated fat), 24 g carb, 8 g fibre, 0 mg chol, 597 mg sodium

Excellent source of: vitamin A, vitamin C
Good source of: vitamin K, magnesium, potassium
Low in fat
Low in saturated fat
Low in cholesterol
Very high source of fibre

Heart Healthy Side Dishes (Vegetables and Grains)

Caramelized Onions

The secret to this recipe is cooking the onions very slowly. Low heat allows the natural sugars to brown and caramelize, giving the onions a slightly sweet flavour. This is one of those recipes that's so tasty you'll want to double, or even triple, it! Enjoy these onions on their own, on a pizza, or in a sandwich.

2 tsp	canola oil	10 ml
3 cups	chopped onions	750 ml

Heat oil in a skillet over low heat.

Add onions; slowly sauté, stirring periodically, for about 40 to 45 minutes or until onions are golden brown.

Serves 4.

Per 1/4 cup (50 ml) serving: 66 cal, 1 g pro, 2 g total fat (0 g saturated fat), 11 g carb, 2 g fibre, 0 mg chol, 3 mg sodium

Low in sodium
Low in fat
Low in saturated fat
Low in cholesterol

Green Beans with Toasted Almonds

This side dish is simple, yet delicious. The almonds add a crunchy texture, while the nutmeg gives a slightly nutty flavour. Best of all, this dish is low in sodium and high in fibre.

6 cups	green beans, trimmed	1.5 L
1/4 cup	sliced or slivered almonds, toasted	50 ml
1/2 tsp	nutmeg	2 ml

In a medium pot, bring 1 cup (250 ml) of water to a boil. Add beans; steam for 5 to 7 minutes or until beans are bright green, but still slightly crunchy.

Remove from heat; drain.

In a medium bowl, toss cooked beans with almonds and sprinkle with nutmeg.

Serves 4.

Per 1 1/2 cup (375 ml) serving: 90 cal, 4 g pro, 4 g total fat (0 g saturated fat), 13 g carb, 6 g fibre, 0 mg chol, 12 mg sodium

Excellent source of: vitamin K
Good source of: vitamin C, magnesium, potassium
Low in sodium
Low in saturated fat
Low in cholesterol
Very high source of fibre

Grilled Balsamic Portobello Mushrooms

Portobello mushrooms have a meaty texture, making them a great alternative to a steak or beef burger. If you have guests who are vegetarian, they'll definitely enjoy these cholesterol- and saturated fat–free grilled mushrooms. In fact, you might want to barbecue extra, since meat eaters will enjoy them just as much.

4	portobello mushrooms, washed and trimmed	4
1 tsp	extra-virgin olive oil	5 ml
1 tbsp	balsamic vinegar	15 ml
	freshly cracked pepper, to taste	

Preheat grill over medium heat.

In a bowl, toss mushrooms with olive oil, vinegar, and pepper.

Place mushrooms on grill; cook for 4 to 5 minutes, turning once or twice, or until cooked through.

Serves 4.

Per mushroom: 37 cal, 3 g pro, 1g total fat (0 g saturated fat), 5 g carb, 2 g fibre, 0 mg chol, 6 mg sodium

Good source of: potassium
Low in sodium
Low in fat
Low in saturated fat
Low in cholesterol

Grilled Corn on the Cob with Cajun and Lime Rub

Mouth-watering corn on the cob without butter or salt? Absolutely! Fresh lime juice and a spicy Cajun rub turn corn on the cob into a heart healthy side dish you'll want to make again and again.

1 tbsp	paprika	15 ml
1/2 tbsp	garlic powder	7 ml
1 tsp	freshly ground black pepper	5 ml
1/8 tsp	cayenne pepper	0.5 ml
1	lime, cut into quarters	1
4	corn on the cob, husked	4

In a small bowl, combine paprika, garlic powder, and peppers.

Bring a pot of water to a boil. Add corn; boil for 3 to 4 minutes.

Remove from heat.

Serve each cob with a slice of lime. Sprinkle with Cajun seasoning.

Serves 4.

Per cob of corn with seasoning: 94 cal, 3 g pro, 1 g total fat (0 g saturated fat), 22 g carb, 3 g fibre, 0 mg chol, 14 mg sodium

Low in sodium
Low in fat
Low in saturated fat
Low in cholesterol

Grilled Eggplant with Ginger Dressing

These eggplant slices are delicious served as a side dish or rolled up with a toothpick and served as hors d'oeuvres.

1	large eggplant	1
2 tbsp	seasoned rice vinegar	25 ml
1/2 tsp	sesame oil	2 ml
1/2 tsp	minced gingerroot	2 ml
1	clove garlic, minced	1
1/2 tsp	sodium-reduced soy sauce	2 ml

Preheat grill over medium heat.

Cut eggplant lengthwise into 1/4-inch (.5 cm) slices; place in a shallow dish. Sprinkle with rice vinegar, sesame oil, gingerroot, garlic, and soy sauce; toss to coat. Set aside for 10 to 15 minutes.

Remove eggplant from marinade. Reserve any remaining marinade.

Place eggplant on grill. Cook for about 4 to 5 minutes or until eggplant is soft and begins to brown.

Remove from heat. Serve warm, drizzled with reserved marinade.

Serves 4.

Per serving: 42 cal, 2 g pro, 1 g total fat (0 g saturated fat), 9 g carb, 5 g fibre, 0 mg chol, 55 mg sodium

Low in sodium
Low in fat
Low in saturated fat
Low in cholesterol
High source of fibre

Orange Baked Squash

It's hard to beat winter squash for beta carotene, an antioxidant thought to guard against heart disease. Orange juice, added in the scooped-out hollow of the squash before baking, gently steams the vegetable and infuses a delicate citrus flavour.

1	acorn squash	1
2 tbsp	orange juice	25 ml
1/2 tsp	cinnamon	2 ml
1/4 tsp	nutmeg	1 ml
1 tsp	brown sugar	5 ml

Preheat oven to 375°F (190°C).

Cut squash in half lengthwise; scoop out seeds. Place in a casserole dish.

In a small bowl, combine orange juice, cinnamon, nutmeg, and sugar.

Pour equal amount of orange juice mixture into the hollow of each squash half.

Cover with foil; bake for 50 to 60 minutes or until squash is tender. Remove squash from oven once or twice during cooking to baste with the orange juice mixture.

Serves 4.

Per 1/4 squash: 53 cal, 1 g pro, 0 g total fat (0 g saturated fat), 14 g carb, 2 g fibre, 0 mg chol, 4 mg sodium

Good source of: potassium
Low in sodium
Low in fat
Low in saturated fat
Low in cholesterol

Roasted Squash with Ginger Orange Glaze

If you don't have time to peel and chop a whole squash, consider buying pre-chopped winter squash available in the produce section of grocery stores. And there's no need to worry you'll get less beta carotene. Pre-chopped squash has just as much of this heart healthy antioxidant as whole squash you'd chop and use immediately at home.

4 cups	diced butternut squash	1 L
2 tsp	canola oil	10 ml
1 tbsp	freshly squeezed orange juice	15 ml
1 tbsp	minced gingerroot	15 ml

Preheat oven to 375°F (190°C).

In a large bowl, toss squash with oil.

Place on a baking sheet; bake for 35 to 40 minutes or until squash is tender.

Remove from oven; toss with orange juice and ginger.

Serve warm.

Serves 4.

Per 1 cup (250 ml) serving: 61 cal, 1 g pro, 2 g total fat (0 g saturated fat), 10 g carb, 1 g fibre, 0 mg chol, 4 mg sodium

Excellent source of: vitamin A
Good source of: vitamin C
Low in sodium
Low in fat
Low in saturated fat
Low in cholesterol

Roasted Vegetables

Roasted vegetables are a delicious and versatile way to increase your family's intake of veggies. Serve them on their own with grilled fish, add them to a sandwich, toss them in a salad, or use them for a pizza topping. One serving dishes up 7 grams of fibre—making a hefty contribution to your daily fibre requirement.

2 cups	thinly sliced sweet potato, cut into 1/4-inch/0.5 cm pieces	500 ml
1 cup	thinly sliced parsnip, cut into 1/4-inch/0.5 cm coins	250 ml
1 cup	chopped artichoke, from fresh or frozen	250 ml
1	small onion, quartered	1
1 1/2 cups	thinly sliced carrot, cut into 1/4-inch/0.5 cm coins	375 ml
3	cloves garlic, chopped into large pieces	3
2 tbsp	extra-virgin olive oil	25 ml
2 tbsp	balsamic vinegar	25 ml
4	sprigs of fresh thyme	4
	freshly ground black pepper, to taste	

Preheat oven to 375°F (190°C).

Combine sweet potato, parsnip, artichoke, onion, and carrot on a baking sheet.

Toss with garlic, olive oil, balsamic vinegar, thyme, and pepper.

Bake for 40 to 50 minutes or until vegetables are tender.

Serves 4.

Per 1 cup (250 ml) serving: 203 cal, 5 g pro, 7 g total fat (1 g saturated fat), 34 g carb, 7 g fibre, 0 mg chol, 93 mg sodium

Excellent source of: potassium
Good source of: vitamin A, vitamin C, vitamin K, magnesium
Low in sodium
Low in saturated fat
Low in cholesterol
Very high source of fibre

Sautéed Cherry Tomatoes with Garlic and Fresh Basil

This side dish takes less than 5 minutes to cook and is delicious eaten warm or cold. For the best flavour, be sure to use fresh, locally grown cherry tomatoes when in season.

2 tbsp	extra-virgin olive oil	25 ml
4 cups	cherry tomatoes	1 L
2	cloves garlic, roughly chopped	2
1/4 cup	fresh basil, roughly chopped	50 ml
2 tbsp	pine nuts	25 ml
	freshly ground black pepper, to taste	

Heat olive oil in a skillet over medium heat. Add tomatoes; sauté for about 3 to 4 minutes or until warm. Add garlic; sauté for another minute.

Remove from heat; stir in basil and pine nuts.

Serve warm.

Serves 4.

Per 1 cup (250 ml) serving: 95 cal, 1 g pro, 10 g total fat (1 g saturated fat), 2 g carb, 1 g fibre, 0 mg chol, 2 mg sodium

Good source of: vitamin K
Low in sodium
Low in saturated fat
Low in cholesterol

Spicy Sesame Swiss Chard

Swiss chard has big green leaves and stalks that may be green, red, or yellow in colour. It's a versatile vegetable that can be added to soups, stir-fries, and casseroles, or steamed and enjoyed on its own.

2 tsp	sesame oil	10 ml
1	clove garlic, chopped	1
8 cups	Swiss chard, washed and trimmed	2 L
1/8 tsp	red pepper flakes, or to taste	0.5 ml
2 tsp	toasted sesame seeds	10 ml

Heat sesame oil in a skillet over medium heat. Add garlic; sauté for 1 minute. Add Swiss chard; cover and sauté for 6 to 8 minutes or until chard is wilted and soft.

Remove from heat. Sprinkle with pepper flakes and sesame seeds.

Serves 4.

Per serving: 32 cal, 1 g pro, 3 g total fat (0 g saturated fat), 1 g carb, 0 g fibre, 0 mg chol, 23 mg sodium

Excellent source of: vitamin K
Low in sodium
Low in saturated fat
Low in cholesterol

Heart Healthy Pasta and Stir-Fries

Beef Stroganoff

This tasty, heart healthy version of beef stroganoff uses no added sodium canned tomatoes, fat-free sour cream, and whole-wheat pasta, making it low in cholesterol and sodium and high in fibre—not to mention packed with potassium.

Tip: The sauce for this pasta can easily be prepared in a slow cooker. Brown the onions, mushrooms, and beef as called for in the recipe, but simmer the sauce in a slow cooker on low for 3 to 4 hours or until the beef is cooked through and falls apart when pierced with a fork.

1 tbsp	canola oil	15 ml
2 cups	sliced onions	500 ml
4 cups	sliced mushrooms	1 L
18 oz	lean stewing beef, cut into 1-inch/2.5 cm pieces	510 g
2 tbsp	whole-wheat flour	25 ml
1	28 oz/796 ml can no added salt diced tomatoes	1
1/8 tsp	freshly ground black pepper	0.5 ml
1 tsp	Worcestershire sauce	5 ml
1/2 cup	fat-free sour cream	125 ml
4 cups	cooked whole-wheat pasta, such as fettuccini	1 L

Heat oil in a skillet over medium heat. Add onions; sauté about 4 to 5 minutes or until soft.

Add mushrooms; continue to sauté about 8 to 10 minutes or until most of the moisture is out of the mushrooms. Remove onion and mushroom mixture from skillet into a large saucepan.

Meanwhile, dredge beef in flour. Add flour-coated beef to the skillet and cook about 6 to 8 minutes or until beef begins to brown. Place browned beef into saucepan with mushrooms and onions.

Add tomatoes, pepper, and Worcestershire sauce to the saucepan. Cover and simmer about 1 1/2 to 2 hours or until beef is cooked through and begins to fall apart.

Meanwhile, cook pasta according to package directions.

Toss cooked sauce with pasta.

Serve warm, garnished with a dollop of sour cream.

Serves 6.

Per 1 1/2 cup (375 ml) serving: 358 cal, 27 g pro, 11 g total fat (4 g saturated fat), 39 g carb, 5 g fibre, 48 mg chol, 86 mg sodium

Excellent source of: potassium
Good source of: vitamin D, magnesium, iron
Low in sodium
High source of fibre

Chicken Mango Stir-Fry

Fresh mango and strips of red pepper add colour to this tasty stir-fry, not to mention a considerable amount of vitamin C, potassium, and beta carotene.

1 tbsp	sesame oil	15 ml
12 oz	skinless boneless chicken breast, cut into 1-inch/2.5 cm strips	350 g
3	cloves garlic, chopped	3
1 tbsp	minced gingerroot	15 ml
2 cups	broccoli florets	500 ml
1	red pepper, sliced	1
1	mango, peeled and diced	1
2 tbsp	orange juice	25 ml
1/8 tsp	red pepper flakes	0.5 ml
2 tbsp	cashews	25 ml
2 cups	cooked brown rice	500 ml

Heat sesame oil in a skillet over medium heat. Add chicken; sauté until chicken begins to brown and is cooked through.

Add garlic and gingerroot; continue to sauté for another minute.

Add broccoli; sauté for 4 to 5 minutes.

Add red pepper, mango, orange juice, red pepper flakes, and cashews; sauté for another 2 to 3 minutes or until heated through.

Serve warm over rice.

Serves 4.

Per 1 1/2 cup (375 ml) serving: 398 cal, 33 g pro, 10 g total fat (2 g saturated fat), 46 g carb, 6 g fibre, 63 mg chol, 91 mg sodium

Excellent source of: vitamin A, vitamin C, vitamin K, magnesium, potassium

Good source of: iron
Low in sodium
Low in saturated fat
Very high source of fibre

Grilled Chicken and Mixed Vegetable Pasta

This colourful pasta is loaded with flavour and just as good whether eaten warm or cold. The best part: It's low in sodium and saturated fat and packed with fibre.

3 tbsp	olive oil	40 ml
3	cloves garlic, chopped	3
2 cups	broccoli florets	500 ml
1 cup	asparagus tips	250 ml
1 cup	shredded carrot	250 ml
2 cups	halved cherry tomatoes	500 ml
12 oz	sliced grilled chicken breast	350 g
1 cup	shredded spinach	250 ml
1/4 cup	chopped basil	50 ml
1/4 tsp	red pepper flakes	1 ml
	freshly ground black pepper, to taste	
2 cups	cooked whole-wheat pasta	500 ml

Heat olive oil in a large skillet over medium heat. Add garlic; sauté for 1 minute.

Add broccoli and asparagus; continue to sauté for 4 to 5 minutes.

Add carrot, cherry tomatoes, chicken breast, and spinach; sauté until heated through and spinach begins to wilt.

Remove from heat; toss with basil, red pepper flakes, pepper, and cooked pasta.

Serve warm.

Serves 4.

Per 2 cup (500 ml) serving: 379 cal, 34 g pro, 14 g total fat (2 g saturated fat), 31 g carb, 7 g fibre, 71 mg chol, 124 mg sodium

Excellent source of: vitamin A, vitamin C, vitamin K, magnesium, iron, potassium
Low in sodium
Low in saturated fat
Very high source of fibre

Honey Garlic Shrimp Stir-Fry

The honey garlic sauce for this stir fry is downright delicious. This dish is a little bit higher in sodium than most of the recipes in this book, so make sure your other meals during the day are lower in sodium. And no need to worry about shrimp! As you'll recall from Chapter 3, cholesterol in foods has little or no impact on most people's blood cholesterol level. So enjoy!

1/4 cup	honey	50 ml
4	cloves garlic, minced	4
1/4 cup	sodium-reduced soy sauce	50 ml
12 oz	cooked shrimp, peeled and deveined	350 g
1 tbsp	canola oil	15 ml
4 cups	snow peas, trimmed	1 L
1	227 ml can water chestnuts, drained	1
1	red pepper, cut into strips	1
1 tbsp	cornstarch	15 ml
3 tbsp	water	40 ml
2 cups	cooked brown rice	500 ml

In a shallow dish, combine honey, garlic, and soy sauce. Add shrimp; cover and refrigerate for at least 2 hours, or overnight.

Heat oil in a skillet over medium heat. Add snow peas, water chestnuts, and red pepper; sauté for 1 to 2 minutes or until heated through.

Add shrimp and honey garlic sauce; continue to sauté for another 2 to 3 minutes or until heated through.

Meanwhile, in a small bowl, whisk together cornstarch and water.

Add cornstarch mixture to skillet; continue to sauté, while stirring, for about 2 minutes or until sauce thickens.

Serve warm over rice.

Serves 4.

Per 2 cup (500 ml) serving: 378 cal, 26 g pro, 6 g total fat (1 g saturated fat), 57 g carb, 5 g fibre, 164 mg chol, 728 mg sodium

Excellent source of: vitamin A, vitamin C, vitamin K, magnesium, iron, potassium
Low in saturated fat
High source of fibre

Lemon Sesame Chicken Stir-Fry

This colourful stir-fry is an excellent way to boost your intake of heart healthy vegetables. Low in saturated fat, this meal is an excellent source of vitamins A and C, potassium, and dietary fibre.

1 tbsp	sesame oil	15 ml
2	cloves garlic, minced	2
1 tbsp	minced gingerroot	15 ml
2 cups	broccoli florets	500 ml
2 cups	chopped cauliflower	500 ml
1 cup	chopped red pepper	250 ml
16 oz	roasted skinless, boneless chicken breast, diced	480 g
2 tbsp	sodium-reduced soy sauce	25 ml
3 tbsp	lemon juice	40 ml
1 tbsp	sesame seeds	15 ml
1/4 cup	cilantro to garnish	50 ml
2 cups	cooked brown rice	500 ml

Heat sesame oil in a skillet over medium heat. Add garlic and gingerroot; sauté for 1 minute.

Add broccoli, cauliflower, and red pepper; sauté for 4 to 5 minutes.

Add chicken, soy sauce, and lemon juice; heat through.

Sprinkle with sesame seeds and garnish with cilantro. Serve with rice.

Serves 4.

Per 2 cup (500 ml) serving: 473 cal, 47 g pro, 9 g total fat (2 g saturated fat), 56 g carb, 12 g fibre, 84 mg chol, 449 mg sodium

Excellent source of: vitamin A, vitamin C, vitamin K, iron, potassium
Good source of: calcium
Low in saturated fat
Very high source of fibre

Pasta Salad with Tuna, Capers, and Lemon

This citrus-flavoured pasta is excellent for a picnic or as part of a healthy brown bag lunch. It's a source of heart healthy omega-3 fats and it's low in saturated fat and sodium.

2	170 g cans low-sodium water-packed tuna, drained	2
2 tbsp	extra-virgin olive oil	25 ml
3 tbsp	freshly squeezed lemon juice	40 ml
2 tbsp	capers	25 ml
2	cloves garlic, minced	2
	freshly ground black pepper, to taste	
4 cups	cooked whole-wheat pasta (such as penne)	1 L
2	green onions, sliced	2

In a large bowl, toss tuna, olive oil, lemon juice, capers, garlic, pepper, pasta, and green onions.

Serve cold.

Serves 6.

Per 1 cup (250 ml) serving: 227 cal, 20 g pro, 6 g total fat (1 g saturated fat), 26 g carb, 3 g fibre, 17 mg chol, 92 mg sodium

Good source of: vitamin K, magnesium, iron
Low in sodium
Low in saturated fat
Low in cholesterol

Pasta with Salmon and Snap Peas

Fresh garlic, black olives, basil, and white wine give plenty of flavour to this pasta salad. And thanks to the salmon, this dish is a great source of vitamin D! If you have leftover cooked salmon, consider using that in place of the canned salmon.

1 tbsp	extra-virgin olive oil	15 ml
2 tbsp	finely chopped onion	25 ml
1	cloves garlic, chopped	1
1 cup	chopped tomatoes	250 ml
2 tbsp	chopped black olives	25 ml
2 tbsp	dry white wine	25 ml
1 cup	snap peas	250 ml
2	213 g cans low-sodium salmon, drained	2
1/2 cup	chopped basil	125 ml
	zest of 1 lemon	
4 cups	cooked whole-wheat pasta, such as penne	1 L

In a large bowl, toss olive oil, onion, garlic, tomatoes, olives, wine, snap peas, salmon, basil, lemon zest, and pasta.

Serve cold.

Serves 6.

Per 1 cup (250 ml) serving: 264 cal, 21 g pro, 7 g total fat (2 g saturated fat), 29 g carb, 4 g fibre, 28 mg chol, 84 mg sodium

Excellent source of: vitamin D, vitamin K, magnesium
Good source of: vitamin C, calcium, iron, potassium
Low in sodium
Low in saturated fat
High source of fibre

Roasted Vegetable Pasta

Loaded with flavour, this whole-grain pasta dish is low in sodium and saturated fat and a very high source of fibre. It's delicious eaten warm or cold.

2 tbsp	extra-virgin olive oil	25 ml
2	cloves garlic, chopped	2
pinch	red pepper flakes, to taste	pinch
2 cups	cooked whole-wheat pasta, such as spaghetti	500 ml
4 cups	roasted vegetables (page 290)	1 L

Heat olive oil in a skillet over medium heat.

Add garlic and pepper flakes; sauté for 1 minute.

Add cooked pasta and roasted vegetables; toss to coat. Sauté until heated through.

Serves 4.

Per 1 1/2 cup (375 ml) serving: 350 cal, 8 g pro, 14 g total fat (2 g saturated fat), 52 g carb, 9 g fibre, 0 mg chol, 95 mg sodium

Excellent source of: vitamin K, magnesium, potassium
Good source of: vitamin A, vitamin C, iron
Low in sodium
Low in saturated fat
Low in cholesterol
Very high source of fibre

Sweet and Sour Tofu Stir-Fry

Slightly sweet and slightly sour, this tasty stir-fry is a great way to entice your family to try tofu. You can substitute cooked whole-grain or whole-wheat noodles for the brown rice.

1/2 cup	100% pure pineapple juice	125 ml
1/2 cup	white vinegar	125 ml
1/4 cup	honey	50 ml
2 tbsp	sodium-reduced soy sauce	25 ml
1	12 oz/350 g pkg extra-firm tofu, cut into cubes	1
1 tbsp	canola oil	15 ml
1	clove garlic, chopped	1
2	carrots, sliced	2
1	green pepper, cut into strips	1
1	red pepper, cut into strips	1
1 tbsp	cornstarch	15 ml
3 tbsp	water	40 ml
2 cups	cooked brown rice	500 ml

In a shallow dish, combine pineapple juice, vinegar, honey, soy sauce, and tofu. Cover and refrigerate sauce for at least 2 hours.

Heat oil in a skillet over medium heat. Add garlic; sauté for 1 minute.

Add carrots; sauté for 3 to 4 minutes. Add peppers and sauté for another minute.

Add tofu and sauce; sauté until heated through.

Meanwhile, in a small bowl whisk together cornstarch and water. Add to skillet; sauté while stirring until sauce thickens.

Serve warm over rice.

Serves 4.

Per 2 cup (500 ml) serving: 340 cal, 11 g pro, 9 g total fat (1 g saturated fat), 59 g carb, 5 g fibre, 0 mg chol, 306 mg sodium

Excellent source of: vitamin A, vitamin C, calcium, iron
Good source of: vitamin K, magnesium, potassium
Low in saturated fat
Low in cholesterol
High source of fibre

Tempeh Stir-Fry with Orange Garlic Sauce

Tempeh, (pronounced tem-pay) is a fermented soy product that's similar to tofu because it's so versatile. It can be cubed, chopped, or crumbled and tends to take on the flavour of the ingredients it's cooked with—in this case, a delicious orange garlic sauce. Tempeh is sold refrigerated or frozen at most major grocery stores and natural food stores.

1 tsp	sesame oil	5 ml
1	85 oz/250 g block tempeh	1
1/2 cup	freshly squeezed orange juice	125 ml
1	clove garlic, chopped	1
1 tbsp	sodium-reduced soy sauce	15 ml
2 cups	bok choy, chopped	500 ml
2 cups	shredded carrot	500 ml
1 cup	cauliflower, chopped	250 ml
1 tbsp	cornstarch	15 ml
3 tbsp	water	40 ml
2 cups	cooked brown rice	500 ml

Heat sesame oil in a skillet over medium heat. Add tempeh; sauté for 3 to 4 minutes.

Add orange juice, garlic, and soy sauce; continue to sauté for another minute.

Add bok choy, carrot, and cauliflower; sauté for 4 to 5 minutes or until bok choy is wilted.

Meanwhile, in a small bowl, whisk together cornstarch and water.

Add cornstarch mixture to skillet; simmer for 2 to 3 minutes or until sauce thickens slightly.

Serve warm over rice.

Serves 4.

Per 1 1/2 cup (375 ml) serving: 298 cal, 16 g pro, 9 g total fat (2 g saturated fat), 41 g carb, 4 g fibre, 0 mg chol, 208 mg sodium

Excellent source of: vitamin A, vitamin C, vitamin K, magnesium, potassium
Good source of: calcium, iron
Low in saturated fat
Low in cholesterol
High source of fibre

Heart Healthy Meatless Main Dishes

Almond-Crusted Tofu

This tofu tastes better the longer it marinates. If you have time, let it sit in the marinade overnight. Breading and frying makes the tofu crispy. This dish is great with veggies and a whole-grain side dish, or in a whole-grain pita pocket sandwich.

Tip: If you don't have a food processor, blend the almond and oat mixture in a cleaned coffee grinder. To clean a coffee grinder, place a small piece of bread in the grinder and grind away—it'll quickly loosen and pick up any loose bits of coffee.

Tip: See tip on rice vinegar under Hot and Sour Soup (page 275).

Tofu:

1/2 cup	rice vinegar	125 ml
1 tbsp	honey	15 ml
2 tbsp	orange juice concentrate	25 ml
2 tbsp	minced gingerroot	25 ml
1	12 oz/350 g pkg extra-firm tofu, cut into 16 slices	1

Coating:

1/4 cup	sliced almonds	50 ml
1/4 cup	rolled oats	50 ml
1 tsp	lemon zest	5 ml
1 tsp	paprika	5 ml
1 tbsp	canola oil	15 ml

In a shallow dish, combine rice vinegar, honey, orange juice concentrate, and gingerroot. Stir to combine. Place tofu in marinade; cover and refrigerate for at least 2 hours (overnight if possible).

Meanwhile, in a food processor, blend almonds, oats, lemon rind, and paprika.

Heat oil in a skillet over medium heat.

Place almond mixture on a plate. Remove tofu from marinade; dredge in almond mixture. Place coated tofu in the skillet and cook for 2 to 3 minutes per side or until tofu is brown and slightly crispy.

Serve warm.

Serves 4.

Per 4 slices: 215 cal, 10 g pro, 13 g total fat (1 g saturated fat), 18 g carb, 2 g fibre, 0 mg chol, 128 mg sodium

Excellent source of: calcium, magnesium, iron
Low in sodium
Low in saturated fat
Low in cholesterol

Asparagus and Red Pepper Frittata with Goat Cheese

This colourful frittata uses egg whites instead of whole eggs, so it's very low in saturated fat and virtually cholesterol-free. This dish makes for a delicious breakfast, lunch, or dinner.

2 tsp	canola oil	10 ml
1/2 cup	chopped red onion	125 ml
1 cup	asparagus spears, cut into 1-inch/2.5 cm pieces	250 ml
1	clove garlic, chopped	1
1 cup	chopped red bell pepper	250 ml
6	egg whites	6
1/4 cup	crumbled goat cheese	50 ml

Preheat oven to 375°F (190°C).

In an ovenproof skillet, heat oil over medium heat. Add onions; sauté about 4 to 5 minutes or until soft. Add asparagus spears; sauté another 4 to 5 minutes.

Add garlic and red pepper; sauté 1 minute.

Meanwhile in a mixing bowl, whisk egg whites until frothy and white.

Add egg whites and goat cheese to skillet; stir for 30 seconds.

Place skillet in oven and bake for 10 to 12 minutes or until eggs are set.

Serves 4.

Per serving: 90 cal, 8 g pro, 4 g total fat (1 g saturated fat), 7 g carb, 2 g fibre, 3 mg chol, 102 mg sodium

Excellent source of: vitamin A, vitamin C, vitamin K
Low in sodium
Low in saturated fat
Low in cholesterol

Chickpea Goulash

Goulash is a traditional Hungarian dish made from beef, onions, red peppers, and paprika. This heart healthy version uses fibre-rich chickpeas in place of the beef and calls for extra veggies. The end result: a hearty meal that's very low in saturated fat and very high in fibre!

1 tbsp	canola oil	15 ml
2 cups	chopped onion	500 ml
3	cloves garlic, chopped	3
2 cups	chopped celery, cut into 1-inch/2.5 cm pieces	500 ml
3 cups	chopped carrots, cut into 1-inch/2.5 cm pieces	750 ml
2 cups	diced potatoes (about 2 medium)	500 ml
1	19 oz/540 ml can chickpeas, drained and rinsed	1
1 cup	chopped red pepper	250 ml
2 tbsp	paprika	25 ml
2 cups	water	500 ml
1/4 cup	white vinegar	50 ml
2 tbsp	tomato paste	25 ml
1/2 tsp	freshly ground black pepper	2 ml
1 tbsp	Worcestershire sauce	15 ml

Heat oil in a large saucepan over medium heat. Add onions; sauté about 4 to 5 minutes or until soft. Add garlic; sauté for another minute.

Add celery, carrots, potatoes, chickpeas, red pepper, paprika, water, vinegar, tomato paste, pepper, and Worcestershire sauce. Cover and simmer for 1 hour.

Serve warm.

Serves 4.

Per 1 1/2 cup (375 ml) serving: 361 cal, 12 g pro, 6 g total fat (1 g saturated fat), 70 g carb, 13 g fibre, 0 mg chol, 557 mg sodium

Excellent source of: vitamin A, vitamin C, vitamin K, magnesium, iron, potassium
Low in saturated fat
Low in cholesterol
Very high source of fibre

Chipotle Chili

This recipe uses dried chipotle chili pepper powder, which gives it a rich, smoky flavour. You can find it in the spice section of your local grocery store or gourmet food shop. Be sure to save some of this chili for leftovers—it's even tastier after sitting in the fridge for a day.

1 tbsp	canola oil	15 ml
1 cup	chopped onion	250 ml
3	cloves garlic, chopped	3
1 1/2 cup	chopped green pepper (about 1 large)	375 ml
1	28 oz/796 ml can no added salt diced tomatoes	1
1	19 oz/540 ml can kidney beans, drained and rinsed	1
1	19 oz/540 ml can chickpeas, drained and rinsed	1
1	12 oz/341 ml can corn, drained	1
1	14 oz/398 ml can baked beans in tomato sauce	1
2 tbsp	molasses	25 ml
2 tbsp	white vinegar	25 ml
1 tbsp	cocoa powder	15 ml
1/4 tsp	dried chipotle chili pepper powder	1 ml

Heat oil in a large saucepan over medium heat. Add onions; sauté about 4 to 5 minutes or until soft. Add garlic and green pepper; sauté another minute.

Add tomatoes, kidney beans, chickpeas, corn, baked beans, molasses, vinegar, cocoa powder, and chipotle chili pepper. Cover and simmer for 30 minutes.

Serves 8.

Per 1 cup (250 ml) serving: 287 cal, 12 g pro, 4 g total fat (1 g saturated fat), 54 g carb, 13 g fibre, 4 mg chol, 694 mg sodium

Excellent source of: magnesium, iron, potassium
Good source of: vitamin C
Low in saturated fat
Low in cholesterol
Very high source of fibre

Honey Garlic Soy Meatballs

Textured vegetable protein, also known as TVP, is a meat alternative made from soybeans. It's high in protein and virtually free of cholesterol-raising saturated fat. You can purchase it dried or hydrated, such as Yves Veggie Cuisine Ground Round. Hydrated versions are refrigerated in the produce section of major grocery stores.

Tip: The trick to this recipe is getting your hands dirty. Use your hands to thoroughly combine the textured vegetable protein, oats, and breadcrumbs—the meatballs will hold their shape much better if ingredients are well mixed.

12 oz	hydrated textured vegetable protein	350 g
1/2 cup	finely chopped onion	125 ml
1	clove garlic, minced	1
1/3 cup	rolled oats	75 ml
1/3 cup	whole-wheat breadcrumbs	75 ml
2 tbsp	ground flaxseed	25 ml
1/4 cup	honey	50 ml
2 tbsp	sodium-reduced soy sauce	25 ml
3	cloves garlic, minced	3
1/4 cup	water	50 ml

Preheat oven to 350°F (180°C).

In a mixing bowl, combine textured vegetable protein, onion, garlic, oats, breadcrumbs, and flaxseed. Mix to combine well. Form into 16 1 1/2-inch (3.75 cm) balls.

Place in a small casserole dish.

Meanwhile, in a small bowl, combine honey, soy sauce, garlic, and water. Pour over soy meatballs in casserole dish.

Bake for 30 to 35 minutes or until meatballs are cooked through and begin to brown. If meatballs begin to burn, add 1/4 cup (50 ml) of water to the casserole dish.

Serves 4.

Per 4 meatballs: 220 cal, 18 g pro, 3 g total fat (0 g saturated fat), 35 g carb, 5 g fibre, 0 mg chol, 688 mg sodium

Good source of: potassium
Low in fat
Low in saturated fat
Low in cholesterol
High source of fibre

Refried Bean Baked Tortilla

These fibre-rich baked tortillas are delicious and a cinch to make. I suggest baking the tortillas until the edges start to brown and get crispy, but be careful not to burn them. These make great leftovers too!

2	10-inch/25 cm whole-grain tortilla shells	2
1 cup	low-fat refried beans	250 ml
1/2 cup	sliced red bell pepper	125 ml
1/2	jalapeno, finely chopped (or to taste)	1/2
1/4 cup	sliced green onions	50 ml
1/4 cup	chopped cilantro	50 ml
1 tsp	freshly squeezed lime juice	5 ml
1/2 cup	low-fat cheddar style cheese (4% MF or less)	125 ml

Preheat oven to 350°F (180°C).

Lay tortilla shells flat on a baking sheet.

Divide refried beans over each shell. Top with bell pepper, jalapeno, green onions, cilantro, lime juice, and cheese.

Bake for 10 to 12 minutes or until cheese begins to melt and the tortilla is heated through. Place under broiler for an additional minute to brown cheese.

Remove from oven and serve immediately.

Serves 2.

Per tortilla: 348 cal, 15 g pro, 8 g total fat (2 g saturated fat), 56 g carb, 12 g fibre, 10 mg chol, 880 mg sodium

Excellent source of: vitamin A, vitamin C, vitamin K
Good source of: magnesium, iron, potassium
Low in saturated fat
Low in cholesterol
Very high source of fibre

Roasted Vegetable Sandwich

For extra flavour, consider using seasoned goat cheese, such as herbed or peppercorn, in this recipe.

1/2 cup	goat cheese (at room temperature)	125 ml
8	thinly sliced pieces of whole-grain rye bread	8
2 cups	roasted vegetables (page 290)	500 ml
1 cup	baby spinach leaves	250 ml

Using a food processor, or the back of a fork, mash the goat cheese until it is a soft and spreadable. Set aside.

Lightly toast the bread.

Divide the goat cheese among the slices of bread, and spread thinly.

Divide the roasted vegetables onto 4 slices of bread. Top with spinach leaves and a slice of bread.

Serves 4.

Per sandwich: 300 cal, 10 g pro, 8 g total fat (3 g saturated fat), 48 g carb, 7 g fibre, 6 mg chol, 514 mg sodium

Excellent source of: magnesium, potassium
Good source of: folate, vitamin K, iron
Low in cholesterol
Very high source of fibre

Slow Cooker Stewed Lentils

Using a slow cooker is a great way to cook meals with little effort. Because they cook slowly, these stewed lentils are infused with a delicious curry flavour. Even better, they're packed with fibre, folate, and potassium.

2 cups	diced onion	500 ml
2 cups	diced celery	500 ml
2	cloves garlic, minced	2
2 cups	diced sweet potato	500 ml
2 cups	diced carrot	500 ml
1	28 oz/796 ml can no added salt diced tomatoes	1
1 cup	dried brown lentils, washed and drained	250 ml
3 cups	water	750 ml
3 tbsp	lime juice	40 ml
1 tsp	salt	5 ml
1 tbsp	curry powder	15 ml
1/2 cup	chopped cilantro	125 ml

In a slow cooker, combine onion, celery, garlic, sweet potato, carrot, tomatoes, brown lentils, water, lime juice, salt, and curry powder.

Cover and simmer on high for 3 to 4 hours or until lentils are soft.

Garnish with cilantro just before serving.

Serves 8.

Per 1 cup (250 ml) serving: 169 cal, 9 g pro, 1 g total fat (0 g saturated fat), 33 g carb, 6 g fibre, 0 mg chol, 335 mg sodium

Excellent source of: vitamin A, folate, potassium
Good source of: vitamin K, magnesium, iron
Low in fat
Low in saturated fat
Low in cholesterol
Very high source of fibre

Spicy Baked Tofu Bites

These spicy tofu bites are excellent served with steamed veggies and brown rice or quinoa. They also make a great high-protein snack that even kids will enjoy!

3 tbsp	sodium-reduced soy sauce	40 ml
3 tbsp	white wine vinegar	40 ml
1 tbsp	honey	15 ml
2	cloves garlic, chopped	2
1 tsp	sesame oil	5 ml
1/4 tsp	red pepper flakes	1 ml
1	12 oz/350 g pkg extra-firm tofu, cut into 1-inch/2.5 cm cubes	1

In a shallow dish, combine soy sauce, vinegar, honey, garlic, sesame oil, and red pepper flakes. Add tofu; cover and marinate in the fridge for a couple of hours or overnight.

Preheat oven to 350°F (180°C).

Remove tofu from marinade and place on a baking sheet. Drizzle with marinade.

Bake for 15 to 20 minutes or until brown and slightly crispy.

Serves 4.

Per serving: 103 cal, 8 g pro, 5 g total fat (1 g saturated fat), 8 g carb, 1 g fibre, 0 mg chol, 408 mg sodium

Excellent source of: calcium, iron
Low in saturated fat
Low in cholesterol

Thai Tofu Cutlets

Serve these low-calorie vegetarian cutlets with roasted vegetables, or use them in a veggie sandwich or burger.

1/4 cup	lime juice (about 2 limes)	50 ml
2 tbsp	sodium-reduced soy sauce	25 ml
1	clove garlic, minced	1
1 tsp	minced gingerroot	5 ml
1 tsp	honey	5 ml
1/4 tsp	red pepper flakes	1 ml
1	12 oz/350 g pkg extra-firm tofu, cut into 16 slices	1
1/4 cup	chopped cilantro	50 ml

In a shallow dish, combine lime juice, soy sauce, garlic, gingerroot, honey, and red pepper flakes. Add tofu; cover and marinate in the fridge for a couple of hours or overnight.

Pour marinade and tofu cutlets into a skillet and heat over medium heat. Cover and simmer for 4 to 5 minutes or until tofu is warmed through.

Remove from heat and serve warm.

Serves 4.

Per 4 slices: 82 cal, 8 g pro, 4 g total fat (1 g saturated fat), 6 g carb, 1 g fibre, 0 mg chol, 275mg sodium

Excellent source of: calcium, iron
Low in saturated fat
Low in cholesterol

Heart Healthy Fish and Seafood

Grilled Salmon with Sesame Cilantro Pesto

This heart healthy salmon recipe is an Asian twist on traditional pesto: Sesame oil and cilantro are used instead of olive oil and basil. If you don't have limes on hand, freshly squeezed lemon juice works well, too.

1 cup	cilantro	250 ml
1 cup	chopped spinach	250 ml
1/2 cup	mint	125 ml
1 tbsp	minced gingerroot	15 ml
1 tsp	sesame oil	5 ml
3 tbsp	freshly squeezed lime juice	40 ml
2	cloves garlic	2
4	4 oz/120 g salmon fillets	4

Preheat grill over medium heat.

In a food processor, mince cilantro, spinach, mint, gingerroot, sesame oil, lime juice, and garlic.

Coat salmon in pesto mixture. Place salmon fillets on grill and cook for 5 to 7 minutes per side or until fish flakes easily when tested with a fork.

Serves 4.

Per fillet: 177 cal, 23 g pro, 8 g total fat (1 g saturated fat), 2 g carb, 0 g fibre, 62 mg chol, 53 mg sodium

Excellent source of: vitamin D, potassium
Good source of: vitamin K
Low in sodium
Low in saturated fat

Lemon Pepper Salmon Dip

This creamy dip is excellent with cut raw vegetables or whole-grain crackers. It also makes a tasty sandwich spread that's low in saturated fat.

Tip: To store fresh dill, absorb any excess moisture with a towel and place the dill in a re-sealable freezer bag in the crisper of the fridge. Do not wash the dill before storing because moisture will cause the leaves to deteriorate.

1	8 oz / 226 g pkg light cream cheese	1
1	213 g can low-sodium salmon, drained	1
1 tbsp	prepared horseradish	15 ml
2 tbsp	fresh dill	25 ml
1 tbsp	freshly squeezed lemon juice	15 ml
1	green onion, chopped	1
2 tbsp	low-fat (1% MF or less) milk	25 ml

In a mixing bowl, beat cream cheese with an electric mixer until smooth. Add salmon, horseradish, dill, lemon juice, green onion, and milk. Mix until combined.

Cover and refrigerate until ready to serve.

Serves 12.

Per 2 tbsp (25 ml) serving: 69 cal, 6 g pro, 5 g total fat (2 g saturated fat), 1 g carb, 0 g fibre, 19 mg chol, 149 mg sodium

Good source of: vitamin D
Low in saturated fat
Low in cholesterol

Lemon Thyme Grilled Trout

Trout is a great alternative to salmon. It's just as flavourful and an excellent source of heart healthy omega-3 fatty acids. Rainbow and lake trout both work well for this recipe. If you eat fish at least twice per week, consider growing your own lemon thyme, a citrus-flavoured variety that's especially good with fish and seafood.

1/4 cup	fresh thyme	50 ml
2 tbsp	lemon juice	25 ml
1 tsp	honey	5 ml
4	slices lemon	4
4	4 oz/120 g trout fillets	4

In a small bowl, combine thyme, lemon juice, and honey.

Place trout fillets in a skillet and drizzle with lemon mixture. Top each fillet with a lemon slice. Cover and steam for 8 to 10 minutes or until fish flakes easily when tested with a fork.

Serves 4.

Per fillet: 142 cal, 23 g pro, 4 g total fat (1 g saturated fat), 3 g carb, 0 g fibre, 64 mg chol, 31 mg sodium

Excellent source of: potassium
Good source of: magnesium, iron
Low in sodium
Low in saturated fat

Mussels Steamed in a White Wine Sauce

It doesn't take long at all to cook mussels; however, properly preparing them can be time-consuming. Clean the mussels well and discard any that are chipped, broken or cracked, or that don't close when you're rinsing them (read the tip below for more details).

Tip: To ensure you are serving mussels that are safe and free of sand, follow these simple steps:

1. Buy mussels from a reputable fishmonger and avoid mussels that are chipped, broken, or cracked. Ask for a bag of ice from the fish counter so you can keep them cool until you can get them home and in the fridge.

2. To clean mussels, dump them in a large bowl or sink of cold water. Some mussels will have a fibrous web of vegetation, called a "beard." This can be removed with a firm tug. Scrub the mussels and remove any barnacles. Tap any mussels that are open; if they do not close, they are dead and should be discarded.

3. Rinse mussels a few times before cooking to ensure all sand and grit is removed.

4. Any mussels that are closed after cooking are dead and should be thrown away.

2 tsp	canola oil	10 ml
1/2 cup	onion, finely chopped	125 ml
1	clove garlic, chopped	1
1 cup	dry white wine	250 ml
1/4 cup	finely chopped parsley	50 ml
2 lbs	mussels, scrubbed and de-bearded	900 g

Heat oil in a large saucepan over medium heat. Add onions; sauté for 4 to 5 minutes or until onions begin to turn golden yellow. Add garlic; sauté for another minute.

Add wine and parsley. Bring to a simmer.

Add mussels; cover and steam for 2 to 3 minutes or until the mussels open. Serve immediately.

Serves 4.

Per serving: 265 cal, 27 g pro, 7 g total fat (1 g saturated fat), 11 g carb, 0 g fibre, 64 mg chol, 653 mg sodium

Excellent source of: magnesium, iron, potassium
Good source of: vitamin C
Low in saturated fat

Pepper-Crusted Salmon

Salmon is a heart healthy food because it's packed with omega-3 fatty acids. Use a good quality pepper mill to coarsely grind the fresh pepper for this recipe—it will make a big difference.

2 tbsp	maple syrup	25 ml
2 tbsp	sodium-reduced soy sauce	25 ml
2	cloves garlic, chopped	2
1/4 cup	fresh coarsely ground pepper	50 ml
1 tsp	canola oil	5 ml
4	4 oz/120 g salmon fillets	4

In a shallow dish, combine maple syrup, soy sauce, and garlic. Place salmon fillets, skin side up in marinade. Cover and refrigerate for at least 2 hours (overnight if possible).

Place ground pepper on a plate. Remove salmon from marinade and firmly press each fillet (skin side up) into pepper.

Meanwhile, heat oil in a skillet over medium heat. Place salmon in the skillet, starting with skin side up, and cook for 4 to 5 minutes per side or until fish flakes easily when tested with a fork.

Serves 4.

Per fillet: 207 cal, 23 g pro, 9 g total fat (1 g saturated fat), 9 g carb, 2 g fibre, 62 mg chol, 320 mg sodium

Excellent source of: vitamin D, potassium
Good source of: magnesium, iron
Low in saturated fat

Seared Tuna Sandwich with Caramelized Onions

This delicious sandwich is a good source of omega-3 fats as well as magnesium and potassium, two minerals that help keep blood pressure in check. The caramelized onions add a touch of sweetness. For a quick version of this recipe, use a can of water-packed light tuna in place of the tuna steaks.

Tip: If you're short of time, skip the caramelized onions and use a handful or so of chopped red onion. Fresh sprouts also work very well in this recipe.

2 tsp	canola oil	10 ml
4	4 oz/120 g tuna steaks	4
4	slices tomato	4
1/2	avocado, sliced	1/2
1 cup	spinach	250 ml
1 cup	caramelized onions (page 283)	250 ml
4	whole-grain rolls	4
	freshly cracked pepper, to taste	

Heat oil in a skillet over medium-high heat. Add tuna steaks and cook 2 to 3 minutes per side or to desired degree of doneness.

Remove fish from pan.

Divide tomato slices, mashed avocado, spinach, and caramelized onions among whole-grain rolls. Add tuna steak to each roll; season with pepper. Serve warm.

Serves 4.

Per roll with tuna steak and condiments: 363 cal, 30 g pro, 15 g total fat (3 g saturated fat), 28 g carb, 3 g fibre, 43 mg chol, 187 mg sodium

Excellent source of: vitamin A, vitamin D, vitamin K, magnesium, potassium
Good source of: iron

Smoked Salmon Sandwich with Capers and Red Onions

I suggest using a whole-grain rye or pumpernickel bread for this sandwich. Not only does it pair well with the smoked salmon, it's also a low-glycemic bread. You'll feel satisfied and energized for hours after this meal!

Tip: Wondering how to store an avocado that is already cut? Leave the unused portion of the avocado in its skin, and gently rub the flesh side of the avocado with lemon juice. Firmly press the avocado, flesh side down, into the bottom of a resealable container—it'll keep for a couple of days without turning brown.

4	slices dark rye bread	4
3 oz	thinly sliced smoked salmon (about 4 slices)	85 g
1/2	avocado, sliced	1/2
1/2 cup	sliced red onion	125 ml
1 tbsp	capers	15 ml
1	small tomato, sliced	1
1 cup	spinach	250 ml
1/4 cup	cilantro, chopped	50 ml
	freshly ground black pepper, to taste	

Evenly divide salmon, avocado, red onion, capers, tomato, spinach, and cilantro between the 2 sandwiches.

Serves 2.

Per sandwich: 286 cal, 15 g pro, 12 g total fat (2 g saturated fat), 30 g carb, 7 g fibre, 31 mg chol, 675 mg sodium

Excellent source of: vitamin K
Good source of: vitamin C, folate, magnesium, potassium
Low in saturated fat
Very high source of fibre

Sole with Tomatoes and Olives

This Mediterranean-inspired dish is very low in saturated fat and cholesterol. It's delicious served over a bed of whole-grain brown rice or quinoa.

1 tbsp	extra-virgin olive oil	15 ml
1/2 cup	chopped onion	125 ml
3	cloves garlic, chopped	3
1	tomato, coarsely chopped	1
1/4 cup	finely chopped black olives	50 ml
1/4 cup	white wine	50 ml
1 tbsp	capers, optional	15 ml
1/4 cup	finely chopped basil	50 ml
1 tsp	lemon zest	5 ml
	freshly ground pepper, to taste	
4	4 oz/120 g sole fillets	4

Heat olive oil in a skillet over medium heat. Add onions; sauté for 4 to 5 minutes or until onions are soft. Add garlic; sauté for another minute.

Add tomatoes, olives, wine, capers, basil, lemon zest, and pepper. Bring to a simmer.

Add sole fillets; cover and simmer for 10 to 12 minutes or until fish flakes easily when tested with a fork.

Serves 4.

Per fillet: 170 cal, 22 g pro, 6 g total fat (1 g saturated fat), 5 g carb, 1 g fibre, 54 mg chol, 209 mg sodium

Excellent source of: vitamin D, vitamin K
Good source of: magnesium, potassium
Low in saturated fat

Tilapia in a Tomato Fennel Sauce

Tilapia is an extremely versatile white fish that has a delicate taste and tends to take on the flavour of the ingredients it's cooked with. This recipe is low in saturated fat and sodium. Serve the fish with steamed brown rice or whole-wheat couscous.

1 tsp	canola oil	5 ml
2	cloves garlic, chopped	2
1 cup	no added salt crushed tomatoes	250 ml
2 tbsp	lemon juice	25 ml
1 tbsp	lemon zest	15 ml
1 tbsp	capers	15 ml
1/4 cup	chopped parsley	50 ml
1 tsp	fennel seeds	5 ml
4	4 oz/120 g tilapia fillets	4

Heat oil in a skillet over medium heat. Add garlic; sauté for 1 to 2 minutes. Add tomatoes, lemon juice, lemon zest, capers, parsley, and fennel seeds. Bring to a simmer.

Gently lay tilapia fillets in tomato sauce. Cover and simmer for 8 to 10 minutes or until fish flakes easily when tested with a fork.

Serves 4.

Per fillet: 145 cal, 24 g pro, 3 g total fat (1 g saturated fat), 6 g carb, 2 g fibre, 56 mg chol, 142 mg sodium

Good source of: potassium
Low in fat
Low in saturated fat

Tuna Bruschetta

Any variety of fresh tomato works well in this recipe. If you have access to locally grown heirloom tomatoes, which come in a variety of colours including red, purple, yellow, and pink, consider using them to add a splash of colour.

2 cups	tomatoes, seeded and diced (about 3 large)	500 ml
1 tbsp	olive oil	15 ml
1/2 cup	chopped basil	125 ml
1	clove garlic, chopped	1
1	170 g can low-sodium water-packed flaked tuna	1
1	whole-grain baguette, halved lengthwise	1

Preheat broiler.

In a mixing bowl, combine tomatoes, olive oil, basil, and garlic. Cover and refrigerate for 2 hours. Remove from fridge; drain any excess liquid. Add flaked tuna to tomato mixture.

Place baguette halves on a baking sheet. Spread the tomato and tuna mixture over each half. Grill for 4 to 5 minutes or until baguette begins to brown around the edges. Remove from heat. Serve immediately.

Serves 4.

Per serving: 281 cal, 18 g pro, 6 g total fat (1 g saturated fat), 39 g carb, 4 g fibre, 13 mg chol, 421 mg sodium

Excellent source of: folate, vitamin K
Good source of: vitamin C, magnesium, iron, potassium
Low in saturated fat
Low in cholesterol
High source of fibre

Heart Healthy Poultry and Meat

Grilled Honey Tarragon Turkey Breasts

If you can't find turkey breasts, chicken breasts work just as well in this recipe. Regular Dijon mustard can be substituted for the grainy mustard.

1/2 cup	grainy Dijon mustard	125 ml
1/4 cup	lemon juice	50 ml
2 tbsp	finely chopped fresh tarragon	25 ml
	ground black pepper, to taste	
4	4 oz/120 g skinless, boneless turkey breasts	4

In a shallow casserole dish, combine mustard, lemon juice, tarragon, and pepper. Add turkey breasts; toss to coat.

Meanwhile, preheat grill.

Place turkey breasts on grill; brush with remaining marinade. Grill for 16 to 20 minutes or until cooked through.

Serve warm.

Serves 4.

Per turkey breast: 159 cal, 27 g pro, 4 g total fat (1 g saturated fat), 3 g carb, 0 g fibre, 57 mg chol, 478 mg sodium

Good source of: vitamin D, potassium
Low in saturated fat

Honey Garlic Pork Chops

If you have time, let the pork chops marinate overnight in the fridge. They pair well with grilled vegetables such as red peppers, asparagus, and portobello mushrooms.

3 tbsp	tomato paste	40 ml
1 tbsp	sodium-reduced soy sauce	15 ml
2 tbsp	honey	25 ml
1 tsp	white vinegar	5 ml
4	cloves garlic, minced	4
1/4 tsp	red pepper flakes	1 ml
4	4 oz/120 g boneless centre cut loin chops	4

Preheat grill over medium heat.

In a shallow dish, combine tomato paste, soy sauce, honey, vinegar, garlic, and red pepper flakes.

Brush marinade over pork; place on grill. Grill for 3 to 4 minutes per side or until cooked through.

Serves 4.

Per pork chop: 194 cal, 26 g pro, 4 g total fat (1 g saturated fat), 13 g carb, 1 g fibre, 77 mg chol, 221 mg sodium

Excellent source of: potassium
Low in saturated fat

Lemon Chicken

Want to have a quick week-night dinner ready to go? Then this is the recipe for you. Combine the chicken and tangy marinade in a re-sealable freezer bag and pop it in the freezer. For dinner in a hurry, thaw the bag in the microwave and grill the chicken. You'll have a delicious meal with very little effort!

1/4 cup	freshly squeezed lemon juice	50 ml
1/2 tbsp	granulated sugar	7 ml
1/2 tbsp	sodium-reduced soy sauce	7 ml
3	cloves garlic, minced	3
1 tsp	canola oil	5 ml
	zest of 1 lemon	
	freshly ground black pepper, to taste	
4	4 oz/120 g skinless, boneless chicken breasts	4

In a shallow dish, combine lemon juice, sugar, soy sauce, garlic, oil, lemon zest, and pepper. Add chicken; toss to coat. Cover and refrigerate for 1 to 2 hours.

Preheat grill.

Place chicken breasts on grill. Grill for 18 to 20 minutes or until cooked through.

Serves 4.

Per chicken breast: 148 cal, 25 g pro, 3 g total fat (1 g saturated fat), 4 g carb, 0 g fibre, 64 mg chol, 125 mg sodium

Low in sodium
Low in fat
Low in saturated fat

Moroccan Turkey Meat Loaf

This is a low in saturated fat twist on traditional meat loaf made with ground beef. This low-calorie version uses lean ground turkey and is infused with a variety of Moroccan-style spices. Serve with whole-grain couscous.

1/2 cup	finely diced onion	125 ml
1	clove garlic, chopped	1
1 tsp	chopped fresh gingerroot	5 ml
1.25 lb	lean ground turkey	570 g
1 tsp	cinnamon	5 ml
1/2 tsp	ground cumin	2 ml
1 tbsp	tomato paste	15 ml
1/2 cup	rolled oats	125 ml
1/4 cup	sliced almonds	50 ml

Preheat oven to 375°F (190°C).

In a mixing bowl, combine onion, garlic, gingerroot, turkey, cinnamon, cumin, tomato paste, and oats. Mix well.

Grease a 9 x 5 inch (2 L) loaf pan. Firmly press turkey mixture into loaf pan. Top with sliced almonds.

Bake uncovered for 60 to 70 minutes or until loaf begins to brown and pull away from sides of pan.

Preheat broiler. Place loaf under broiler for about 4 to 5 minutes or until almonds begin to brown.

Serves 8.

Per 1-inch (2.5 cm) slice: 157 cal, 17 g pro, 7 g total fat (2 g saturated fat), 6 g carb, 1 g fibre, 46 mg chol, 46 mg sodium

Low in sodium
Low in saturated fat

Mustard-Glazed Chicken

This quick and simple chicken dish is loaded with flavour and is low in saturated fat. I suggest baking the chicken breasts rather than grilling them because the honey tends to burn on the grill.

4 tbsp	whole-grain mustard	60 ml
2 tbsp	honey	25 ml
2 tsp	sodium-reduced soy sauce	10 ml
1 tbsp	canola oil	15 ml
4	4 oz/120 g skinless, boneless chicken breasts	4

Preheat oven to 375°F (190°C).

In a casserole dish, combine mustard, honey, soy sauce, and oil. Add chicken; toss to coat.

Bake for 20 to 25 minutes or until chicken is cooked through.

Serves 4.

Per chicken breast: 202 cal, 26 g pro, 6 g total fat (1 g saturated fat), 10 g carb, 0 g fibre, 64 mg chol, 351 mg sodium

Low in saturated fat

Pork Loin Chops with Apple Chutney

Many people think pork chops are a high-fat meat. Not so! This recipe derives less than 30% of its calories from fat and less than 10% from saturated fat. And it tastes great, too. The apple chutney adds just the right touch of spice to the pork chops, making it simply delicious.

4	apples, peeled and grated	4
1 tbsp	apple cider vinegar	15 ml
1/8 tsp	cayenne pepper	0.5 ml
1/2 tsp	ground cloves	2 ml
1 tsp	cinnamon	5 ml
1 tsp	cumin seeds	5 ml
1/2 tbsp	olive oil	7 ml
1 tsp	ground cumin	5 ml
6	4 oz/120 g boneless centre cut loin chops	6

In a small saucepan, combine apples, vinegar, cayenne pepper, cloves, cinnamon, and cumin seeds. Cover and simmer for 15 to 20 minutes or until apple is soft and chutney is fragrant.

Meanwhile, preheat broiler.

In a small bowl, combine olive oil and cumin. Rub over loin chops and place on a baking sheet.

Place under broiler; cook for 3 to 4 minutes per side or until chops are cooked through.

Remove from heat. Serve with warm apple chutney.

Serves 6.

Per pork chop with apple chutney: 200 cal, 26 g pro, 6 g total fat (2 g saturated fat), 12 g carb, 1 g fibre, 77 mg chol, 76 mg sodium

Good source of: potassium
Low in sodium
Low in saturated fat

Roasted Chicken Breasts with Curry Sauce

Nothing boring about this low-fat recipe! I'm sure you'll enjoy this spiced-up version of skinless chicken breasts.

Tip: This dish pairs well with steamed brown rice or quinoa and a spinach salad.

1 tbsp	canola oil	15 ml
1/2 cup	chopped onions	125 ml
1 cup	chopped tomatoes	250 ml
1 tsp	turmeric	5 ml
1 tsp	ground coriander	5 ml
1 tsp	ground cumin	5 ml
1/2 tsp	chili powder	2 ml
4	4 oz/120 g skinless, boneless chicken breasts, cubed	4
1/4 cup	chopped cilantro	50 ml

Preheat oven to 375°F (190°C).

Combine all ingredients except cilantro in a casserole dish. Toss to coat chicken.

Bake for 18 to 20 minutes or until chicken is cooked through.

Garnish with cilantro.

Serves 4.

Per chicken breast: 240 cal, 36 g pro, 8 g total fat (1 g saturated fat), 5 g carb, 1 g fibre, 95 mg chol, 93 mg sodium

Excellent source of: vitamin K
Good source of: magnesium, iron, potassium
Low in sodium
Low in saturated fat

Slow Cooker Beef and Vegetable Stew

This stick-to-your ribs stew is low in sodium and cholesterol and a great source of fibre. It freezes well, so be sure to make extra for a quick weekday meal or brown bag lunch.

Tip: If you don't have a slow cooker, simmer all the ingredients in a large saucepan on the stovetop for 2 to 3 hours or until beef is tender.

2 tsp	canola oil	10 ml
1 lb	lean stewing beef, cut into 1-inch (2.5 cm) pieces	454 g
1 1/2 cups	chopped onions	375 ml
4	cloves garlic, chopped	4
2 tbsp	flour	25 ml
1 cup	water	250 ml
2 cups	chopped carrot	500 ml
1 cup	chopped parsnip, optional	250 ml
2 cups	chopped celery	500 ml
2 cups	diced potato	500 ml
1 cup	diced sweet potato	250 ml
1 cup	diced eggplant	250 ml
1/8 tsp	salt	0.5 ml
1/2 cup	dry red wine	125 ml
2 cups	water	500 ml
2	bay leaves	2
	freshly ground black pepper	

Heat oil in a large skillet over medium-high heat. Add stewing beef; sauté about 5 to 7 minutes or until the meat begins to brown.

Add onions to the frying pan with the beef; sauté over medium heat for 4 to 5 minutes or until onions are soft. Add garlic; sauté for another minute.

Sprinkle skillet with flour; sauté for another 30 seconds. Remove from heat.

Add first amount of water to the skillet, scraping the bottom of the pan with a spatula to loosen any brown bits. Pour beef, onion, garlic, and flour mixture into a slow cooker.

Add carrot, parsnip, celery, potato, sweet potato, eggplant, salt, red wine, second amount of water, and bay leaves to the slow cooker. Season to taste with black pepper.

Cover slow cooker and simmer on low for 4 to 6 hours or until beef is tender and shreds easily when pierced with a fork.

Serve warm.

Serves 8.

Per 1 cup (250 ml) serving: 213 cal, 15 g pro, 6 g total fat (2 g saturated fat), 23 g carb, 4 g fibre, 31 mg chol, 112 mg sodium

Excellent source of: vitamin A, potassium
Good source of: magnesium
Low in sodium
High source of fibre

Slow Cooker Citrus Chicken with Potatoes

This citrusy stew is delicious served with steamed brown rice or quinoa. In addition to being low in saturated fat and sodium, it's a great source of heart healthy nutrients such as vitamin C, magnesium, and potassium.

4	4 oz/120 g skinless, boneless chicken breasts	4
1	large onion, quartered	1
12	baby red potatoes	12
1	large sweet potato, peeled and diced	1
4	cloves garlic, peeled	4
	zest of 1 lemon	
3 tbsp	freshly squeezed lemon juice	40 ml
1/2 cup	dry white wine	125 ml
4	sprigs fresh thyme	4

Place chicken in bottom of slow cooker. Layer on top onions, potatoes, garlic, lemon zest, lemon juice, wine, and thyme. Cover and simmer on high for 3 to 4 hours or until chicken is cooked through and vegetables are tender.

Serves 4.

Per 1 1/2 cup (375 ml) serving: 291 cal, 28 g pro, 2 g total fat (1 g saturated fat), 35 g carb, 4 g fibre, 64 mg chol, 70 mg sodium

Excellent source of: vitamin C, magnesium, potassium
Good source of: iron
Low in sodium
Low in fat
Low in saturated fat
High source of fibre

Turkey Burgers

Who would have guessed you could sneak cholesterol-lowering soluble fibre into burgers? I've added rolled oats, ground flaxseed, and diced apple to these turkey burgers to make them heart healthy.

1.3 lb	lean ground turkey, or chicken	570 g
1/2 cup	rolled oats	125 ml
2 tbsp	ground flaxseed	25 ml
1/2 cup	oat bran	125 ml
1	egg	1
1/4 cup	sliced green onion	50 ml
1 tbsp	Dijon mustard	15 ml
1	apple, peeled and diced	1
1 tbsp	freshly squeezed lemon juice	15 ml
3	cloves garlic, minced	3
1/2 cup	low-fat salsa	125 ml
1/2 tsp	red pepper flakes, optional	2 ml
	freshly ground black pepper, to taste	
8	whole-grain rolls	8

Preheat oven to 375°F (190°C).

In a large bowl, combine ground turkey, rolled oats, flaxseed, oat bran, egg, green onion, mustard, apple, lemon juice, garlic, salsa, pepper flakes, and pepper. Mix well.

Form mixture into 8 small patties and place on a baking sheet.

Bake for 30 minutes, turning once after 20 minutes.

Serve patties on whole-grain rolls with fresh vegetables, such as tomato slices and shredded spinach.

Serves 8.

Per patty and whole-grain roll: 259 cal, 22 g pro, 8 g total fat (2 g saturated fat), 27 g carb, 2 g fibre, 67 mg chol, 316 mg sodium

Excellent source of: magnesium
Good source of: iron, potassium
Low in saturated fat

Heart Healthy Quick Breads and Muffins

Apple Blueberry Bran Muffins

If you're looking for a low-fat muffin that delivers the goodness of whole grain, this recipe is a must-try! While it calls for apples and blueberries, consider substituting other fresh fruit, such as peaches and strawberries.

2 cups	whole-wheat flour	500 ml
1 1/2 cup	oat bran	375 ml
1/4 cup	ground flaxseed	50 ml
2 tsp	baking powder	10 ml
1 tsp	baking soda	5 ml
1/4 tsp	salt	1 ml
1 tsp	cinnamon	5 ml
1/2 tsp	ground cloves	2 ml
1/2 tsp	nutmeg	2 ml
1 cup	unsweetened applesauce	250 ml
1/2 cup	low-fat (1% MF or less) milk or soymilk	125 ml
1 cup	diced apple (about 1 small apple)	250 ml
3/4 cup	brown sugar	175 ml
2 tbsp	canola oil	25 ml
2	eggs	2
1 tsp	orange zest	5 ml
1/2 cup	blueberries, fresh or frozen	125 ml

Preheat oven to 375°F (190°C).

In a large mixing bowl, combine flour, oat bran, flaxseed, baking powder, baking soda, salt, cinnamon, cloves, and nutmeg.

In a separate bowl, combine applesauce, milk, apple, sugar, oil, eggs, orange zest, and blueberries.

Add wet ingredients to dry ingredients; mix just enough to combine.

Pour batter into 16 lined muffin tins.

Bake for 25 minutes or until cooked through (when a knife inserted in the centre comes out clean).

Serves 16.

Per muffin: 167 cal, 5 g pro, 4 g total fat (1 g saturated fat), 33 g carb, 4 g fibre, 27 mg chol, 165 mg sodium

Good source of: magnesium
Low in saturated fat
High source of fibre

Carrot Walnut Bread

This delicious bread is a great way to increase your intake of alpha linolenic acid, an omega-3 fatty acid in walnuts that's linked with protection from heart disease. The recipe also calls for whole-wheat flour and oats, making it a great source of fibre.

1 cup	whole-wheat flour	250 ml
1/4 cup	all-purpose flour	50 ml
1/2 cup	rolled oats	125 ml
1 tsp	baking soda	5 ml
1 tsp	baking powder	5 ml
1/2 tsp	salt	2 ml
1 tsp	cinnamon	5 ml
1/2 tsp	nutmeg	2 ml
1	egg	1
2 tbsp	canola oil	25 ml
1/3 cup	brown sugar	75 ml
1/2 cup	low-fat (1% MF or less) milk or soymilk	125 ml
1 cup	shredded carrot	250 ml
1/4 cup	walnut pieces	50 ml
1/2 tsp	lemon zest	2 ml

Preheat oven to 375°F (190°C).

Grease and flour a 9 x 5 inch (2 L) loaf pan.

In a large mixing bowl, combine whole-wheat and all-purpose flour, oats, baking soda, baking powder, salt, cinnamon, and nutmeg.

In a separate bowl, whisk together egg, oil, and brown sugar. Add milk, carrots, walnuts, and lemon zest; stir to combine.

Add wet ingredients to dry ingredients; mix just enough to combine.

Pour batter into loaf pan.

Bake for 30 to 35 minutes or until cooked through (when a knife inserted in the centre comes out clean).

Serves 9.

Per 1-inch (2.5 cm) slice: 225 cal, 7 g pro, 9 g total fat (1 g saturated fat), 32 g carb, 4 g fibre, mg 25 chol, 314 mg sodium

Excellent source of: vitamin A
Good source of: magnesium
Low in saturated fat
High source of fibre

Chocolate Zucchini Muffins

Yes, chocolate is heart healthy! The cocoa beans used to make cocoa powder are an excellent source of antioxidants that studies suggest help keep blood pressure in check. These low-fat chocolaty muffins freeze well.

2 1/2 cups	whole-wheat flour	625 ml
1/2 cup	oat bran	125 ml
3 tbsp	ground flaxseed	40 ml
1/3 cup	unsweetened cocoa powder	75 ml
2 1/2 tsp	baking powder	12 ml
1 1/2 tsp	baking soda	7 ml
1/4 tsp	salt	1 ml
1 tsp	cinnamon	5 ml
2 tsp	psyllium	10 ml
2 cups	shredded zucchini	500 ml
2/3 cup	low-fat (1% MF or less) milk or soymilk	150 ml
4	egg whites	4
2 tbsp	canola oil	25 ml
1/2 cup	granulated sugar	125 ml
1 tsp	vanilla extract	5 ml
1 tbsp	orange zest	15 ml

Preheat oven to 375°F (190°C).

In a large mixing bowl, combine flour, oat bran, flaxseed, cocoa, baking powder, baking soda, salt, and cinnamon.

In a separate bowl, combine psyllium, zucchini, milk, egg whites, oil, sugar, vanilla, and orange zest.

Add wet ingredients to dry ingredients; mix just enough to combine.

Pour batter into 16 lined muffin tins.

Bake for 25 minutes or until cooked through (when a knife inserted in the centre comes out clean).

Serves 16.

Per muffin: 133 cal, 5 g pro, 3 g total fat (0 g saturated fat), 25 g carb, 4 g fibre, 1 mg chol, 213 mg sodium

Good source of: magnesium
Low in saturated fat
Low in cholesterol
High source of fibre

Cinnamon Orange Loaf

No doubt you've heard the adage: "beans, beans, they're good for your heart ..." Legumes are an excellent source of vegetarian protein and fibre. That's why I've added them to this delicious quick bread. Might seem strange but, I think you'll be pleasantly surprised once you try a slice. None of my taste testers could detect the secret ingredient!

1 1/2 cup	whole-wheat flour	375 ml
1 tsp	baking soda	5 ml
1/2 tsp	baking powder	2 ml
1/4 tsp	salt	1 ml
2 tsp	cinnamon	10 ml
2	eggs	2
1/4 cup	packed brown sugar	50 ml
1 cup	romano beans, rinsed and mashed	250 ml
2 tbsp	canola oil	25 ml
1 tsp	vanilla extract	5 ml
1 tbsp	orange juice concentrate	15 ml
1/2 cup	low-fat (1% MF or less) milk or soymilk	125 ml

Preheat oven to 375°F (190°C).

Grease and flour a 9 x 5 inch (2 L) loaf pan.

In a large mixing bowl, combine flour, baking soda, baking powder, salt, and cinnamon.

In a separate bowl, beat together eggs, sugar, beans, oil, vanilla, orange juice concentrate, and milk.

Add wet ingredients to dry ingredients; mix just enough to combine.

Pour batter into loaf pan.

Bake for 35 to 40 minutes or until cooked through (when a knife inserted in the centre comes out clean).

Serves 9.

Per 1-inch (2.5 cm) slice: 214 cal, 9 g pro, 5 g total fat (1 g saturated fat), 35 g carb, 6 g fibre, 49 mg chol, 231 mg sodium

Good source of: vitamin K, iron, potassium
Low in saturated fat
Very high source of fibre

Easy Beer Bread

Beer isn't just for drinking anymore! This simple recipe uses beer and the result is a dense bread that tastes great with soup or chili, or as toast. The type of beer you choose will change the flavour and colour of the bread, so try a few different kinds to see what you prefer. Light and dark beer work equally well.

Bread:

1 1/2 cups	all-purpose flour	375 ml
1 1/2 cups	whole-wheat flour	375 ml
1 tsp	salt	5 ml
5 tsp	baking powder	25 ml
3 tbsp	granulated sugar	40 ml
12 oz	beer	375 ml

Topping:

2 tsp	olive oil	10 ml
1 tsp	dried rosemary	5 ml
1/2 tsp	coarse sea salt	2 ml

Preheat oven to 375°F (190°C).

Grease and flour a 9 x 5 inch (2 L) loaf pan.

In a large mixing bowl, combine flours, salt, baking powder, and sugar. Add beer, and quickly mix until just combined.

In a small mixing bowl, combine olive oil, rosemary, and salt.

Add batter to loaf pan and drizzle with olive oil mixture.

Bake for 45 to 60 minutes or until bread is cooked through (when a knife inserted in the centre comes out clean).

Let the bread cool for at least 15 minutes before serving.

Serves 12.

Per 3/4-inch (2 cm) slice: 139 cal, 4 g pro, 1 g total fat (0 g saturated fat), 27 g carb, 2 g fibre, 0 mg chol, 387 mg sodium

Low in fat
Low in saturated fat
Low in cholesterol

Jalapeno Cornmeal Muffins

These muffins are a cinch to make! They're a great snack to enjoy on their own or extra-delicious paired with my mouth-watering Chipotle Chili (page 312).

Tip: Chopping a fresh jalapeno can cause mild skin irritation. Consider wearing gloves while chopping, or be sure to wash your hands very well to remove any oil.

1	egg	1
1 cup	low-fat (1% MF or less) milk or soymilk	250 ml
2 tbsp	canola oil	25 ml
3/4 cup	cornmeal	175 ml
1 1/2 cup	whole-wheat flour	375 ml
4 tsp	baking powder	20 ml
1/2 tsp	salt	2 ml
2 tsp	minced jalapeno	10 ml
1/2 tsp	chili powder	2 ml
1 tbsp	lime juice	15 ml
1 tbsp	granulated sugar	15 ml

Preheat oven to 425°F (220°C).

In a large mixing bowl, whisk together egg, milk, and oil.

Add cornmeal, flour, baking powder, salt, jalapeno, chili powder, lime juice, and sugar. Mix just enough to combine. Note: Batter will be very thick.

Pour batter into 12 lined muffin tins.

Bake for 13 to 15 minutes or until cooked through (when a knife inserted in the centre comes out clean).

Serves 12.

Per muffin: 119 cal, 4 g pro, 4 g total fat (1 g saturated fat), 19 g carb, 2 g fibre, 19 mg chol, 229 mg sodium

Low in saturated fat
Low in cholesterol

Lemon Poppy Seed Loaf

The combination of lemon and poppy seeds in a quick bread is a favourite of mine. Here's my heart healthy, whole-grain version that's low in saturated fat and cholesterol and high in fibre.

1 1/2 cups	whole-wheat flour	375 ml
1/2 cup	rolled oats	125 ml
1/2 tsp	baking soda	2 ml
2 tsp	baking powder	10 ml
1/4 tsp	salt	1 ml
1 tbsp	poppy seeds	15 ml
1/2 cup	low-fat (1% MF or less) plain yogurt	125 ml
1	egg	1
1/2 cup	granulated sugar	125 ml
3 tbsp	canola oil	40 ml
1/4 cup	freshly squeezed lemon juice	50 ml
1 tbsp	lemon zest	15 ml

Preheat oven to 375°F (190°C).

Grease and flour a 9 x 5 inch (2 L) loaf pan.

In a large mixing bowl, combine flour, oats, baking soda, baking powder, salt, and poppy seeds.

In a separate bowl, combine yogurt, egg, sugar, oil, lemon juice, and lemon zest.

Add wet ingredients to dry ingredients; mix just enough to combine.

Pour batter into loaf pan.

Bake for 35 to 40 minutes or until cooked through (when a knife inserted in the centre comes out clean).

Serves 9.

Per 1-inch (2.5 cm) slice: 223 cal, 6 g pro, 7 g total fat (1 g saturated fat), 36 g carb, 4 g fibre, 24 mg chol, 220 mg sodium

Good source of: magnesium
Low in saturated fat
High source of fibre

Marbled Chocolate Banana Bread

If you have bananas that are starting to turn brown, peel them and pop them into a re-sealable freezer bag and then into the freezer. They're ready to use when you want to make this recipe—just mash the frozen bananas with the back of a fork.

1 3/4 cups	whole-wheat flour	425 ml
1 1/2 tsp	baking powder	7 ml
1/2 tsp	baking soda	2 ml
1/2 cup	granulated sugar	125 ml
1/4 cup	canola oil	50 ml
2	eggs	2
1 cup	mashed banana (about 2 medium)	250 ml
2 tbsp	cocoa powder	25 ml
1 tbsp	ground flaxseed	15 ml

Preheat oven to 350°F (180°C).

Grease and flour a 9 x 5 inch (2 L) loaf pan.

In a large mixing bowl, combine flour, baking powder, baking soda, and sugar.

In a separate bowl, whisk together oil, eggs, and mashed banana.

Add banana mixture to flour mixture; mix until just combined. Remove 1/4 cup (50 ml) of the batter and set aside.

Pour the batter into the prepared loaf pan.

Mix the reserved 1/4 cup (50 ml) batter with the cocoa powder. Drizzle over the batter in the pan, and then drag a knife through the batter to create the marble effect.

Sprinkle loaf with flaxseed.

Bake for 40 to 45 minutes or until cooked through (when a knife inserted in the centre comes out clean).

Serves 12.

Per 3/4-inch (2 cm) slice: 165 cal, 4 g pro, 6 g total fat (1 g saturated fat), 26 g carb, 3 g fibre, 36 mg chol, 100 mg sodium

Good source of: vitamin K
Low in sodium
Low in saturated fat

Pumpkin Quinoa Muffins

Quinoa (pronounced keen-wa) is an ancient grain from South America that's high in protein. It can be used in place of rice in many recipes. Quinoa is easy to cook and can be eaten warm or cold. Thanks to psyllium, flaxseed, and whole-wheat flour, these heart healthy muffins deliver 4 grams of fibre each!

Tip: Quinoa is usually available in a pale yellow colour; however, some specialty food stores carry a dark reddish-brown variety. Either one works well in this recipe, but consider making your own mix by combining equal parts yellow and brown quinoa.

2 1/2 cups	whole-wheat flour	625 ml
1 tbsp	ground flaxseed	15 ml
2 tsp	cinnamon	10 ml
1 tsp	ground cloves	5 ml
2 tsp	baking powder	10 ml
1/2 tsp	baking soda	2 ml
1/4 tsp	salt	1 ml
1/3 cup	quinoa, uncooked	75 ml
1 cup	pure pumpkin purée	250 ml
2/3 cup	low-fat (1% MF or less) milk or soymilk	150 ml
1/4 cup	canola oil	50 ml
2	eggs	2
1/2 cup	brown sugar	125 ml
1/4 cup	granulated sugar	50 ml
1/4 cup	psyllium	50 ml

Preheat oven to 375°F (190°C).

In a large mixing bowl, combine flour, flaxseed, cinnamon, cloves, baking powder, baking soda, salt, and quinoa.

In a separate bowl, combine pumpkin purée, milk, oil, eggs, and sugars.

Add wet ingredients to dry ingredients; mix just enough to combine.

Pour batter into 16 lined muffin tins. Sprinkle psyllium on top of muffins.

Bake for 20 to 25 minutes or until cooked through (when a knife inserted in the centre comes out clean).

Serves 16.

Per muffin: 171 cal, 4 g pro, 5 g total fat (1 g saturated fat), 29 g carb, 4 g fibre, 27 mg chol, 131 mg sodium

Excellent source of: vitamin A
Good source of: magnesium
Low in sodium
Low in saturated fat
High source of fibre

Strawberry Rhubarb Muffins

If you're lucky enough to have a patch of rhubarb in your backyard, this is a great way to use up the famously tart vegetable. If you're buying rhubarb for this recipe, clean and chop what you don't use and store it in the freezer to make these homemade muffins year-round.

1 1/2 cups	whole-wheat flour	375 ml
1/2 cup	oat bran	125 ml
2 tsp	baking powder	10 ml
1/2 tsp	baking soda	2 ml
1 tsp	cinnamon	5 ml
1 cup	sliced rhubarb, cut into 1/2-inch/1 cm pieces	250 ml
1 cup	sliced strawberries	250 ml
3/4 cup	low-fat (1% MF or less) milk or soymilk	175 ml
1	egg	1
1/3 cup	granulated sugar	75 ml
1/4 cup	canola oil	50 ml
1 tsp	vanilla extract	5 ml

Preheat oven to 375°F (190°C).

In a large mixing bowl, combine flour, oat bran, baking powder, baking soda, and cinnamon.

In a separate bowl, combine rhubarb, strawberries, milk, egg, sugar, oil, and vanilla.

Add wet ingredients to dry ingredients; mix just enough to combine.

Pour batter into 12 lined muffin tins.

Bake for 30 minutes or until cooked through (when a knife inserted in the centre comes out clean).

Serves 12.

Per muffin: 144 cal, 4 g pro, 6 g total fat (1 g saturated fat), 22 g carb, 3 fibre, 19 mg chol, 116 mg sodium

Good source of: vitamin K
Low in sodium
Low in saturated fat
Low in cholesterol

Heart Healthy Desserts

Apple Raspberry Crisp with Maple Oat Topping

I've revamped my traditional apple crisp recipe by using whole-wheat flour and oat bran to make it heart healthy—as a result it's a great source of fibre. This recipe is delicious made with a variety of seasonal fruit. Try locally grown peaches or pears in place of apples, and blueberries or strawberries in place of raspberries.

Tip: Double the recipe for the crumble topping and freeze half in a re-sealable freezer bag. When you want to make this recipe, all you have to do is slice the fruit and add the topping directly from the freezer.

1/2 cup	whole-wheat flour	125 ml
3/4 cup	rolled oats	175 ml
1/2 cup	oat bran	125 ml
1 tsp	cinnamon	5 ml
1 tsp	ground cloves	5 ml
1 tsp	vanilla extract	5 ml
3 tbsp	maple syrup	40 ml
2 tbsp	canola oil	25 ml
8 cups	peeled and sliced apples	2 L
1 cup	raspberries	250 ml

Preheat oven to 375°F (190°C).

In a large bowl, combine flour, oats, oat bran, cinnamon, cloves, vanilla, maple syrup, and oil. Mix until crumbly.

In an 8 x 8 inch (2 L) glass baking dish, combine apples and raspberries. Sprinkle crumble mixture over fruit.

Bake for 40 to 50 minutes or until fruit is soft and the top begins to brown.

Serves 6.

Per serving: 235 cal, 5 g pro, 7 g total fat (1 g saturated fat), 45 g carb, 7 g fibre, 0 mg chol, 3 mg sodium

Good source of: vitamin K, magnesium
Low in sodium
Low in saturated fat
Low in cholesterol
Very high source of fibre

Broiled Grapefruit with Ginger Glaze

With only three ingredients, dessert recipes don't get much simpler—or healthier—than this one! This dessert is low in calories and fat, cholesterol-free, and a great source of heart healthy vitamin C. Garnish the grapefruit with a fresh sprig of mint to add colour and refreshing flavour.

Tip: To ensure the grapefruit sits level on the baking sheet, trim the bottom of each fruit to create a flat surface.

2	red grapefruits, halved	2
1/4 cup	brown sugar	50 ml
2 tsp	minced gingerroot	10 ml

Preheat broiler.

With a sharp knife, cut grapefruits in half. Run knife around each section to loosen flesh from membranes.

In a small bowl, combine sugar and gingerroot to form a paste.

Place grapefruit halves cut-side up on a baking sheet.

Divide and spread sugar mixture over cut-side of each grapefruit half.

Place grapefruit under broiler for 2 to 4 minutes or until sugar topping begins to bubble.

Serves 4.

Per 1/2 grapefruit: 104 cal, 1 g pro, 0 g total fat (0 g saturated fat), 27 g carb, 2 g fibre, 0 mg chol, 6 mg sodium

Excellent source of: vitamin C
Low in sodium
Low in fat
Low in saturated fat
Low in cholesterol

Chocolate Cake with Crystallized Ginger

This decadent chocolate cake is delicious served on its own or topped with fresh antioxidant-packed blueberries and strawberries.

Tip: Crystallized ginger is ginger that's been dried and preserved in a sugar coating. It's slightly chewy, spicy, and sweet. You can find it in the bulk section of most major grocery stores or at your local bulk food store.

1 cup	all-purpose flour	250 ml
1 1/2 tsp	baking powder	7 ml
3 tbsp	cocoa	40 ml
3 tbsp	finely chopped crystallized ginger	40 ml
1/8 tsp	salt	0.5 ml
2	eggs	2
2/3 cup	granulated sugar	150 ml
5 tbsp	water	65 ml
1 tsp	vanilla extract	5 ml

Preheat oven to 350°F (180°C).

Lightly grease and flour a 9-inch (23 cm) round cake pan.

In a small bowl, combine flour, baking powder, cocoa, ginger, and salt. Set aside.

In a large mixing bowl, beat eggs for 2 minutes using an electric mixer. Gradually add sugar; continue beating for 3 to 4 minutes or until pale yellow and fluffy.

Add water and vanilla; mix to combine. Add dry ingredients; continue to beat with an electric mixer for another minute.

Pour batter into prepared cake pan and bake for 25 to 30 minutes or until a knife inserted in the centre comes out clean.

Serves 8.

Per 1/8 cake slice: 164 cal, 4 g pro, 2 g total fat (1 g saturated fat), 35 g carb, 1 g fibre, 54 mg chol, 122 mg sodium

Good source of: iron
Low in sodium
Low in fat
Low in saturated fat

Chocolate Fruit Fondue

Chocolate fondue recipes usually call for heavy cream, a source of cholesterol-raising saturated fat. This version skips the cream, making it slightly thicker but considerably lower in saturated fat. While the recipe calls for regular semi-sweet or unsweetened chocolate, you can also use plain or flavoured specialty dark chocolate bars such as orange, mint, espresso, or green tea. Buy dark chocolate with 70% cocoa solids: the higher the cocoa solids, the greater the concentration of antioxidants that might help keep blood pressure in check.

Tip: A double boiler is two saucepans that stack on top of each other. The bottom saucepan is filled with simmering water, while the top saucepan is filled with food that is cooked, or in this case melted, by the heat from below. If you don't have a double boiler, make your own: In a small saucepan, bring 1 to 2 inches (2.5 to 5 cm) of water to a boil, then place a stainless steel bowl over the mouth of the saucepan to hold the chocolate.

1 cup	chopped dark chocolate (about 5 oz/140 g)	250 ml
4 cups	mixed fruit, cut into 1-inch/2.5 cm chunks (such as strawberries, mango, apples, banana, kiwi, or pineapple)	1 L

Using a double boiler (see tip), and stirring constantly, melt chocolate until warm and smooth.

Remove from heat; pour into a heat-resistant bowl. Serve immediately with fresh fruit for dipping.

Serves 4.

Per serving: 302 cal, 5 g pro, 18 g total fat (10 g saturated fat), 44 g carb, 4 g fibre, 0 mg chol, 4 mg sodium

Excellent source of: vitamin C, potassium
Good source of: iron
Low in sodium
Low in cholesterol
High source of fibre

Cinnamon Pecan Baked Apples

Baked apples conjure up thoughts of cool autumn days; however, these apples can be enjoyed year-round. Choose an apple variety that will hold its shape when cooked, such as Spy or Idared.

4	apples, cored	4
1/4 cup	brown sugar	50 ml
1 tbsp	chopped pecans	15 ml
1 tsp	cinnamon	5 ml
1 tbsp	dried cranberries	15 ml
1/2 tsp	vanilla extract	2 ml

Preheat oven to 375°F (190°C).

Using an apple corer, remove most of the apple core, leaving about 1/2 inch (1 cm) at the bottom.

In a small bowl, combine sugar, pecans, cinnamon, cranberries, and vanilla.

Place the apples in a glass baking dish.

Place equal portions of sugar mixture in the hollow centre of each apple.

Cover the bottom of the dish with 1/4 inch (.5 cm) of water.

Bake for 40 to 50 minutes or until apples are soft, but still hold their shape.

Serves 4.

Per apple: 166 cal, 1 g pro, 3 g total fat (0 g saturated fat), 37 g carb, 3 g fibre, 0 mg chol, 6 mg sodium

Low in sodium
Low in fat
Low in saturated fat
Low in cholesterol

Dessert Crepes

These delicious crepes, inspired by a recent trip to France, make an attractive dessert and can even double as a hearty breakfast. Use a heavy cast-iron frying pan if you have one—it will help the crepes cook evenly and they won't burn as easily.

Tip: Berries, grated dark chocolate, and icing sugar taste great on these crepes. But use your imagination to change them up a bit—try a sprinkle of brown sugar and fresh lemon juice, or locally grown blueberries and maple syrup.

Crepes:

1 cup	low-fat (1% MF or less) milk or soymilk	250 ml
2	eggs	2
1 tsp	vanilla extract	5 ml
1 cup	all-purpose flour	250 ml
1 tsp	baking powder	5 ml
1/8 tsp	salt	0.5 ml
1 tsp	canola oil	5 ml

Topping:

1 cup	mixed berries	250 ml
1 tbsp	grated dark chocolate	15 ml
2 tbsp	icing sugar	25 ml

In a mixing bowl, whisk together milk, eggs, and vanilla.

In a separate mixing bowl, combine flour, baking powder, and salt.

Meanwhile, heat oil in a heavy frying pan over medium-high heat.

Add flour mixture to egg mixture; briskly whisk until just combined.

Pour a quarter of batter into the hot frying pan; quickly tilt the pan in a circle to spread batter across the bottom of the pan in a very thin layer.

When small air bubbles begin to appear on the top of crepe, flip it and continue to cook until it begins to brown. Remove from pan and repeat with remaining batter.

When crepes are cooked, place equal portion of berries down the centre of each crepe. Gently roll up crepes; sprinkle with grated chocolate and icing sugar.

Serve warm.

Serves 4.

Per crepe with 1/4 cup (50 ml) berries, grated chocolate, and icing sugar: 237 cal, 9 g pro, 6 g total fat (2 g saturated fat), 37 g carb, 2 g fibre, 111 mg chol, 220 mg sodium

Excellent source of: folate
Good source of: vitamin C, vitamin K, iron
Low in saturated fat

Ginger Flax Cookies

To enjoy freshly baked cookies any day of the week, portion 1/2-inch (1 cm) balls of dough onto a baking sheet and place them in the freezer. Once frozen, transfer them into a re-sealable freezer bag and put them back in the freezer. When you want home-baked cookies, place a few frozen balls on a baking sheet and pop them in the oven.

2/3 cup	brown sugar	150 ml
1/4 cup	canola oil	50 ml
1/4 cup	molasses	50 ml
2	eggs	2
2 tsp	minced gingerroot	10 ml
2 cups	whole-wheat flour	500 ml
1/2 cup	wheat germ	125 ml
2 tbsp	whole flaxseed	25 ml
1/4 cup	oat bran	50 ml
2 tsp	baking soda	10 ml
2 tsp	cinnamon	10 ml

Preheat oven to 350°F (180°C).

In a large mixing bowl, beat sugar, oil, molasses, eggs, and ginger until light and fluffy.

In a separate bowl, combine flour, wheat germ, flaxseed, oat bran, baking soda, and cinnamon.

Add flour mixture to egg mixture; mix just enough to combine.

Shape dough into 36 1/2-inch (1 cm) balls; place on a baking sheet lightly coated with cooking spray. Bake for 12 minutes or until lightly brown.

Remove from pan; let cool on a wire rack before serving.

Serves 18 (makes 36 cookies).

Per 2 cookies: 143 cal, 4 g pro, 5 g total fat (1 g saturated fat), 24 g carb, 3 g fibre, 24 mg chol, 134 mg sodium

Good source of: magnesium
Low in sodium
Low in saturated fat

Orange Fig Granola Bars

These bars take a little bit longer to make than most of the other recipes in this section, but they're well worth the effort. They make a great dessert or mid-day energy-boosting snack.

Tip: Use a clean pair of sharp kitchen scissors to quickly chop the dried figs.

Filling:

2 cups	dried figs (about 18), chopped (stems removed)	500 ml
3/4 cup	freshly squeezed orange juice	175 ml
1 tbsp	orange zest	15 ml

Crust:

1	egg	1
2 tbsp	canola oil	25 ml
1/2 cup	brown sugar	125 ml
3/4 cup	whole-wheat flour	175 ml
1 1/4 cups	rolled oats	300 ml
1/2 cup	oat bran	125 ml
2 tbsp	ground flaxseed	25 ml
2 tsp	ground cinnamon	10 ml

Filling:

In a saucepan, combine figs, orange juice, and orange zest. Bring to a boil; simmer for 5 minutes.

Remove from heat and let stand for an hour to allow figs to soften.

Transfer cooled mixture to a food processor; purée until smooth.

Preheat oven to 350°F (180°C).

Crust:

In a large mixing bowl, whisk together egg, oil, and sugar.

In a separate bowl, combine flour, oats, oat bran, flaxseed, and cinnamon.

Add egg mixture to flour mixture; mix until combined and crumbly.

Firmly press three-quarters of crumb mixture onto the bottom of an 8 x 8 (2 L) baking dish. (Using the back of a floured spatula works well.)
Spread puréed fig filling over crust.

Top with remaining quarter of crumb mixture and press firmly.

Bake for 35 to 40 minutes or until top begins to brown.

Serves 18.

Per 2 1/2 x 1 1/2 inch (6.5 x 4 cm) bar: 126 cal, 3 g pro, 3 g total fat (0 g saturated fat), 25 g carb, 3 g fibre, 12 mg chol, 8 mg sodium

Low in sodium
Low in fat
Low in saturated fat
Low in cholesterol

Pomegranate Poached Pears with Fresh Raspberries

While any type of pear will work in this recipe, I suggest using ones that are slightly firm. The antioxidant-rich pomegranate juice and red wine give the pears a beautiful deep red colour that's sure to impress guests. Serve this dessert on light-coloured dishes for a dramatic effect.

2 cups	pomegranate juice	500 ml
1/2 cup	red wine	125 ml
1	1-inch (2.5 cm) piece cinnamon stick	1
1	1-inch (2.5 cm) piece vanilla bean	1
4	whole cloves	4
4	pears, cored, peeled and halved	4
1/2 cup	fresh raspberries	125 ml
1 tbsp	orange zest	15 ml
4	mint sprigs	4

In a medium saucepan, bring pomegranate juice, wine, cinnamon stick, vanilla bean, and cloves to a boil.

Add pears; cover and simmer for 20 to 40 minutes or until pears are soft when pierced with a fork. (Cooking time will depend on the ripeness of the pears. Keep an eye on them while they're simmering so they don't overcook.)

Remove from heat; let cool slightly.

Portion pears out into 8 dishes; garnish with fresh raspberries, orange zest, and mint. Serve warm.

Serves 8.

Per 1/2 pear: 104 cal, 1 g pro, g total fat (0 g saturated fat), 24 g carb, 3 g fibre, 0 mg chol, 4 mg sodium

Low in sodium
Low in fat
Low in saturated fat
Low in cholesterol

Pumpkin Ginger Pie

This pumpkin pie is simply irresistible. My taste-testers agreed it was the best they'd ever had! Traditional pumpkin pie, often made with cream and topped with whipped cream, can deliver a whopping 400 calories per serving! My version is made with low-fat milk and ground flaxseed for a guilt-free dessert that's half the calories and very low in saturated fat.

Tip: Jarred minced gingerroot works especially well in this recipe.

Tip: Use an 8- or 9-inch (20 or 23 cm) pie plate to firmly press the graham crumb mixture onto the bottom of the 10-inch (25 cm) pie plate—it works like a charm.

Crust:

1 1/2 cups	honey graham crumbs	375 ml
3 tbsp	canola oil	40 ml
1/4 cup	granulated sugar	50 ml
1 tsp	minced gingerroot	5 ml

Filling:

2	eggs	2
1 cup	pure pumpkin purée	250 ml
1 cup	low-fat (1% MF or less) milk or soymilk	250 ml
3/4 cup	brown sugar	175 ml
2 tsp	cinnamon	10 ml
1 tbsp	minced gingerroot	15 ml
1/2 tsp	ground cloves	2 ml
1/2 tsp	nutmeg	2 ml
1 tbsp	ground flaxseed	15 ml

Preheat oven to 375°F (190°C).

In a mixing bowl, combine graham crumbs, oil, granulated sugar, and ginger-root. Press firmly into a 10-inch (25 cm) pie plate. Bake for 6 to 8 minutes or until it begins to brown.

Reduce oven temperature to 350°F (180°C).

In a mixing bowl, combine eggs, pumpkin purée, milk, brown sugar, cinnamon, gingerroot, cloves, nutmeg, and flaxseed. Whisk until smooth.

Pour pumpkin mixture into pre-baked crust. Bake for 40 minutes or until filling is firm.

Serves 10.

Per 1/10 slice: 196 cal, 3 g pro, 7 g total fat (1 g saturated fat), 31 g carb, 2 g fibre, 46 mg chol, 162 mg sodium

Excellent source of: vitamin A
Good source of: vitamin K
Low in saturated fat

Appendix

Internet resources for consumers

ABOUT HEART DISEASE

Heart and Stroke Foundation of Canada

www.heartandstroke.ca

The association's comprehensive website provides plenty of health information about heart disease and stroke, including risk assessment, cholesterol, blood pressure, diet and nutrition, and healthy living. The website also offers many recipes and nutrition columns written by the Heart and Stroke Foundation's registered dietitians. Kids, parents, and teachers can visit the website's "kids/teens zone" for health information geared to youth.

American Heart Association

www.americanheart.org

Although written for Americans, this website offers a wealth of resources for individuals, caregivers, and health professionals about cardiovascular disease. You'll find information on heart attack, high blood pressure, high cholesterol, and diabetes as well as plenty of nutrition, weight control, and exercise tips to prevent heart disease.

CardioSmart

www.cardiosmart.org

This website of the American College of Cardiology provides extensive consumer information about various aspects of cardiovascular disease. Here, you'll learn about risk factors, tests, and treatments related to heart disease as well as ways to reduce your risk for the disease. You'll also find answers to commonly asked questions written by cardiologists.

Mayo Clinic

www.mayoclinic.com

Various disease centres provide information for preventing and managing heart disease and its many risk factors, including high blood pressure, hypertension, and diabetes. Topics covered include heart disease basics, treating heart disease, and living with heart disease. The website's healthy living centres offer tips on diet, nutrition, weight loss, fitness, and smoking cessation.

National Heart Lung and Blood Institute

www.nhbli.nih.gov

This U.S.–based institute provides leadership for a national program in diseases of the heart, blood vessels, lungs, and blood. The organization's website disseminates information for individuals, patients, and health professionals on heart disease, heart attack, high blood pressure, obesity, and physical activity. You can download fact sheets, booklets, and recipes that help you live a heart healthy lifestyle.

Canadian Cardiac Rehabilitation Foundation

www.cardiacrehabilitation.ca

Cardiac rehabilitation is a comprehensive, multidisciplinary approach to the prevention, stabilization, and possible reversal of cardiovascular disease. This national foundation supports community cardiac rehabilitation programs across Canada, funds research that investigates better methods of cardiac rehabilitation, encourages secondary prevention of heart disease, and educates those with heart disease to live a productive lifestyle. Visit the website to learn about cardiac rehabilitation—including nutrition and exercise—and to find cardiac rehab centres across Canada.

ABOUT DIET AND NUTRITION

Canadian Council of Food and Nutrition

www.ccfn.ca

This multi-sectorial, science-based organization on food and nutrition policy and education is dedicated to providing leadership in promoting nutrition for the benefit of all Canadians. On the website, you can read Canadian nutrition news and publications prepared by the organization as well as access webcasts on topics such as trans fat, childhood obesity, and Canadian nutrition trends.

Dietitians of Canada

www.dietitians.ca

Dietitians of Canada is an association of food and nutrition professionals committed to the health and well-being of Canadians. Visit the website for fact sheets, tips, and answers to frequently asked questions about nutrition, or to assess your current food intake and activity level. The website also enables you to locate a private practice dietitian in your community.

HealthCastle.com—Simply Better Health

www.healthcastle.com

This is a comprehensive nutrition community run by registered dietitians on the Internet. The U.S.–based website's mission is to empower people to manage their health and prevent disease through healthy eating. Among the wealth of nutrition information, you'll find diet strategies for heart health, cholesterol management, weight control, and diabetes as well as tips for dining out and grocery shopping. I don't think there's a topic these registered dietitians have left uncovered!

Health Check

www.healthcheck.ca

Health Check™ is the Heart and Stroke Foundation's food information program. The not-for-profit program is open to food companies and restaurants that voluntarily submit products or menu items to be evaluated by registered dietitians. The website provides the nutrient criteria that foods must meet in order to carry the Health Check symbol. You'll also find resources for label reading, dining out, and healthy cooking.

Canada's Food Guide

www.hc-sc.gc.ca/fn-an/food-guide-aliment/index-eng.php

On Health Canada's website you'll learn about the most recent version of Canada's Food Guide, released in 2007. The guide outlines how many servings from each food group you need to eat based on your age and gender. Serving sizes are given for an extensive list of foods, including many ethnic foods. The food guide section of Health Canada's website also provides tips for menu planning, grocery shopping, label reading, eating out, and healthy snacking.

ABOUT DIABETES

The Canadian Diabetes Association
www.diabetes.ca
The association's website is a comprehensive source of facts about diabetes and pre-diabetes. You'll find nutrition, diet, and exercise information if you've been diagnosed with diabetes or if you're trying to prevent the disease. Through the website's online order desk, you can purchase one or more of the association's healthy living booklets, menu planning guides, and cookbooks.

ABOUT PHYSICAL ACTIVITY

Canada's Physical Activity Guide
www.phac-aspc.gc.ca/pau-uap/paguide/index.html
Here you'll find physical activity guides for children, teenagers, and adults that help you improve your health and prevent disease. Each guide is available in a one-page, easy-to-read format that's available to order on its own, or as a pull-out section in a handbook that gives you even more information on building physical activity into your daily life.

Canadian Centre for Activity and Aging
www.uwo.ca/actage
This website offers resources and tips to develop, encourage, and promote an active, healthy lifestyle for Canadian adults that will enhance the dignity of the aging process.

ABOUT SMOKING CESSATION

Health Canada: Quit Smoking
www.hc-sc.gc.ca/hl-vs/tobac-tabac/quit-cesser/index-eng.php
This section of Health Canada's website offers information for individuals trying to quit smoking and those who are helping a family member or friend quit, as well as tips for parents to keep their kids smoke-free. Tips

and strategies are also provided in a free, downloadable guide titled, *On the Road to Quitting—Guide to becoming a non-smoker.*

Quit Smoking Canada

www.quitsmoking.ca

This support network for individuals in the process of quitting smoking offers tips to help you quit, self-help booklets, and a free helpline (1-877-513-5333) that provides personalized support.

References

Chapter 1: What Is Heart Disease?

1. Heart Attack Warning Signals. The Heart and Stroke Foundation of Canada. March 2008. Available at: www.heartandstroke.com/site/c.ikIQLcMWJtE/b.3483917/k.BF6E/Heart_attack_warning_signals.htm#warningsignals.
2. Ridker, PM, M Cushman, MJ Stampfer, et al. Inflammation, aspirin, and the risk of cardiovascular disease in apparently healthy men. *N Engl J Med* 1997, 336(14):973–999.
3. Ridker, PM, JE Buring, J Shih, M Matias, and CH Hennekens. Prospective study of C-reactive protein and the risk of future cardiovascular events among apparently healthy women. *Circulation* 1998, 98(8):731–733.
4. Khaw, KT, N Wareham, S Bingham, R Luben, et al. Association of hemoglobin A1c with cardiovascular disease and mortality in adults: The European prospective investigation into cancer in Norfolk. *Ann Intern Med* 2004, 141(6):413–420.

Chapter 2: Are You at Risk for Heart Disease?

1. Yusuf, S, S Hawken, S Ounpuu, T Dans, et al. Effect of potentially modifiable risk factors associated with myocardial infarction in 52 countries (the INTER-HEART study): Case-control study. *Lancet* 2004, 364(9438):937–952.
2. Anand, SS, S Islam, A Rosengren, MG Franzosi, et al. Risk factors for myocardial infarction in women and men: Insights from the INTERHEART study. *Eur Heart J* 2008, 29(7):932–940.
3. The Heart and Stroke Foundation of Canada. Tipping the Scales of Progress: Heart Disease and Stroke in Canada 2006. Available at: ww2.heartandstroke.ca/Page.asp?PageID=33&ArticleID=5043&Src=news&From=SubCategory.
4. Shields, M. Measured Obesity: Overweight Canadian Children and Adolescents. Statistics Canada, 2005. Available at: wwwstatcan.ca/english/research/82-620-MIE/2005001/pdf/cobesity.pdf.
5. Rossouw, JE, GL Anderson, RL Prentice, AZ LaCroix, C Kooperberg, ML Stefanick, RD Jackson, SA Beresford, BV Howard, KC Johnson, JM Kotchen, J Ockene; Writing Group for the Women's Health Initiative Investigators. Risks and benefits of estrogen plus progestin in healthy post-menopausal women:

Principal results from the Women's Health Initiative randomized controlled trial. *JAMA* 2002, 288(3):321–333.

6. Hsia, J, RD Langer, JE Manson, L Kuller, KC Johnson, SL Hendrix, M Pettinger, SR Heckbert, N Greep, S Crawford, CB Eaton, JB Kostis, P Caralis, R Prentice; Women's Health Initiative Investigators. Conjugated equine estrogens and coronary heart disease: The Women's Health Initiative. *Arch Intern Med* 2006, 166(3):357–365.

7. Koon, KT, S Ounpuu, S Hawken, V Valentin, et al. Tobacco use and risk of myocardial infarction in 52 countries in the INTERHEART study: A case-control study. *Lancet* 2006, 368(9536):647–658.

8. Critchlet, J, and S Capewell. Smoking cessation for the secondary prevention of coronary heart disease. *Cochrane Database of Systematic Reviews* 2003, Issue 4. Art No: CD003041. DOI: 10.1002/14651858. CD003041.pub2.

9. Health Canada. Canadian Tobacco Use Monitoring Survey (CTUMS) 2007. Available at: www.hc-sc.gc.ca/hl-vs/tobac-tabac/research-recherche/stat/ctums-esutc_2007-eng.php.

10. Statistics. Heart and Stroke Foundation of Canada. Available at: www.heartandstroke.com/site/c.ikIQLcMWJtE/b.3483991/k.34A8/Statistics.htm.

11. Tu, K, C Zhongliang, and LL Lipscombe. Prevalence and incidence of hypertension from 1995 to 2005: A population-based study. *CMAJ* 2008, 178(11):1429–1435.

12. Statistics. Heart and Stroke Foundation of Canada. Available at: www.heartandstroke.com/site/c.ikIQLcMWJtE/b.3483991/k.34A8/Statistics.htm.

13. Canadian Fitness and Lifestyle Research Institute. 2004 Physical Activity and Sport Monitor. Available at: www.cflri.ca/eng/statistics/surveys/pam2004.php.

14. Shields, M. Measured Obesity: Overweight Canadian Children and Adolescents. Statistics Canada, 2005. Available at: www.statcan.ca/english/research/82-620-MIE/2005001/pdf/cobesity.pdf.

15. Public Health Agency of Canada. Diabetes in Canada. Health Canada, 2003. Available at: www.phac-aspc.gc.ca/publicat/dic-dac2/english/01cover_e.html. The prevalence and costs of diabetes. Canadian Diabetes Association, 2008. Available at: www.diabetes.ca/Files/prevalence-and-costs.pdf.

16. Knowler, WC, E Barrett-Connor, SE Fowler, RF Hamman, JM Lachin, EA Walker, DM Nathan. Diabetes Prevention Program Research Group. Reduction in the incidence of type 2 diabetes with lifestyle intervention or metformin. *N Engl J Med* 2002, 346(6):393–403.

17. Anand, SS, Q Yi, H Gerstein, E Lonn, R Jacobs, V Vuksan, K Teo, B Davis, P Montague, and S Yusuf. Study of Health Assessment and Risk in Ethnic Groups; Study of Health Assessment and Risk Evaluation in Aboriginal Peoples Investigators. Relationship of metabolic syndrome and fibrinolytic dysfunction to cardiovascular disease. *Circulation* 2003,108(4):420–425.

18. The IDF consensus worldwide definition of the metabolic syndrome, International Diabetes Federation, 2006. Table 1: The International Diabetes Federation definition (of the Metabolic Syndrome).

Chapter 3: Foods and Nutrients to Limit or Avoid

1. Hu, FB, MJ Stampfer, JE Manson, E Rimm, et al. Dietary fat intake and the risk of coronary heart disease in women. N Eng J Med 1997, 337(21):1491–1499.
2. Mensink, RP, PL Zock, A Kester, and MB Katan. Effects of dietary fatty acids and carbohydrates on the ratio of serum total to HDL cholesterol and on serum lipids and apolipoproteins: A meta-analysis of 60 controlled trials. Am J Clin Nutr 2003, 77(5):1146–1155.
3. Yu, S, J Derr, TD Etherton, and P Kris-Etherton. Plasma cholesterol-predictive equations demonstrate that stearic acid is neutral and monounsaturated fats are hypocholesterolemic. Am J Clin Nutr 1995, 61(5):1129–1139. Aro, A, M Jauhiainen, R Partanen, I Salminen and M Mutanen. Stearic acid, trans fatty acids, and diary fat: Effects on serum and lipoprotein lipids, apoplioproteins, lipoprotein(a), and lipid transfer proteins in healthy subjects. Am J Clin Nutr 1997, 65(5):1491–1426. Mitropoulos, KA, GJ Miller, JC Martin, BEA Reeves and J Cooper. Dietary fat induces changes in factor VII coagulant activity through effects on plasma free stearic acid concentration. Arterioscler Thromb 1994, 14(2):214–222. Furguson, J, N Mackay, and G McNichol. Effect of feeding fat on fibrinolysis, Stypven time, and platelet aggregation in Africans, Asians, and Europeans. J Clin Pathol 1970, 23(7):580–585.
4. Pietinen, P, A Ascherio, P Korhonen, AM Hartman, et al. Intake of fatty acids and risk of coronary heart disease in a cohort of Finnish men. The Alpha-Tocopherol, Beta-Carotene Cancer Prevention Study. Am J Epidemiol 1997, 145(10):876–887. Ascherio, A, EB Rimm, EL Giovannucci, D Spiegelman, et al. Dietary fat intake and risk of coronary heart diseae in men: Cohort follow-up study in the United States. BMJ 1996, 13(7049):84–90. Hu, FB, MJ Stampfer, JE Manson, E Rimm, et al. Dietary fat intake and the risk of coronary heart disease in women. N Eng J Med 1997, 337(21): 1491–499.
5. Motard-Bélanger, A, A Charest, G Grenier, P Paquin, et al. Study of the effect of trans fatty acids from ruminants on blood lipids and other risk factors for cardiovascular disease. Am J Clin Nutr 2008, 87(3):593–599.
6. Transforming the Food Supply. Report of the Trans Fat Task Force Submitted to the Minister of Health. Minister of Health, June 2006. Available at: www.hc-sc.gc.ca/fn-an/nutrition/gras-trans-fats/tf-ge/tf-gt_rep-rap-eng.php.
7. Herron, KL, IE Lofgren, M Sharman, JS Volek, and ML Fernandez. High intake of cholesterol results in less atherogenic low-density lipoprotein particles in men and women independent of response classification. Metabolism 2004, 53(6):823–830. Mutungi, G, J Ratliff, M Puglisi, M Torres-Gonzalez, et al. Dietary cholesterol from eggs increases plasma HDL cholesterol in overweight men consuming a carbohydrate-restricted diet. J Nutr 2008, 138(2):272–276.

Greene, CM, D Waters, RM Clark, JH Contois, and ML Fernandez. Plasma LDL and HDL characteristics and carotenoid content are positively influenced by egg consumption in an elderly population. *Nutr Metab* (Lond) 2006, 3(6):1–10. Goodrow, EF, TA Wilson, SC Houde, R Vishwanathan, et al. Consumption of one egg per day increases serum lutein and zeaxanthin concentrations in older adults without altering serum lipid and lipoprotein cholesterol concentrations. *J Nutr* 2006, 136(10):2519–2524.

8. Hu, FB, MJ Stampfer, EB Rimm, JE Manson, et al. A prospective study of egg consumption and risk of cardiovascular disease in men and women. *JAMA* 1999, 281(15):1387–1394.

9. Qureshi, AI, FK Suri, S Ahmed, A Nasar, AA Divani, and JF Kirmani. Regular egg consumption does not increase the risk of stroke and cardiovascular diseases. *Med Sci Monit* 2007, 13(1):CR1–8. Djoussé, L, and JM Gaziano. Egg consumption in relation to cardiovascular disease and mortality: The Physicians' Health Study. *Am J Clin Nutr* 2008, 87(4):964–969.

10. Archer, SL, K Liu, AR Dyer, KJ Ruth, et al. Relationship between changes in dietary sucrose and high density lipoprotein cholesterol: The CARDIA study. Coronary Artery Risk Development in Young Adults. *Ann Epidemiol* 1998, 8(7):433–438.

11. Barclay, AW, P Petocz, J McMillan-Price, VM Flood, et al. Glycemic index, glycemic load, and chronic disease risk: A meta-analysis of observational studies. *Am J Clin Nutr* 2008, 87(3):627–637.

12. Sacks, FM, LP Svetkey, WM Vollmer, LJ Appel, et al; DASH-Sodium Collaborative Research Group. Effects on blood pressure of reduced dietary sodium and the Dietary Approaches to Stop Hypertension (DASH) diet. DASH-Sodium Collaborative Research Group. *N Engl J Med* 2001, 344(1):3–10.

13. Cook, NR, JA Cutler, E Obarzanek, JE Buring, et al. Long-term effects of dietary sodium reduction on cardiovascular disease outcomes: Observational follow-up of the trials of hypertension prevention (TOHP). *BMJ* 2007; doi:10.1136/bmj.39147.604896.55.

14. Bulpitt, CJ. How many alcoholic drinks might benefit an older person with hypertension? *J Hypertens* 2005, 23(11):1947–1951.

Chapter 4: Heart Healthy Foods

Omega-3 fatty acids (Polyunsaturated fat)

1. Mozaffarian, D, and EB Rimm. Fish intake, contaminants, and human health: Evaluating the risks and the benefits. *JAMA* 2006, 296(15):1885–1899.

2. Marchioli, R, F Barzi, E Bomba, et al. Early protection against sudden death by n-3 polyunsaturated fatty acids after myocardial infarction. *Circulation* 2002, 105(16):1897–1903. Erkkilä, AT, NR Matthan, DM Herrington, and AH Lichtenstein. Higher plasma docosahexaenoic acid is associated with reduced progression of coronary atherosclerosis in women with CAD. *J Lipid Res* 2006, 47(12):2814–2819.

3. Hartweg J, R Perera, V Montori, S Dinneen, HA Neil, and AFarmer. Omega-3 polyunsaturated fatty acids (PUFA) for type 2 diabetes mellitus. *Cochrane Database Syst Rev* 2008. (1):CD003205.

4. Hill, AM, JD Buckley, KJ Murphy, and PR Howe. Combining fish-oil supplements with regular aerobic exercise improves body composition and cardiovascular disease risk factors. *Am J Clin Nutr* 2007, 85(5):1267–1274. Wang, C, WS Harris, M Chung, AH Lichtenstein, et al. n-3 Fatty acids from fish or fish-oil supplements, but not alpha-linolenic acid, benefit cardiovascular disease outcomes in primary- and secondary-prevention studies: A systematic review. *Am J Clin Nutr* 2006, 84(1):5–17.

5. Jenkins, DJ, AR Josse, J Beyene, P Dorian, et al. Fish-oil supplementation in patients with implantable cardioverter defibrillators: A meta-analysis. *CMAJ* 2008, 178(2):157–164.

6. Hu, FB, MJ Stampfer, JE Manson, EB Rimm, et al. Dietary intake of a-linolenic acid and risk of fatal ischemic heart disease among women. *Am J Clin Nutr* 1999, 69(5):890–897.

7. Albert, CM, O Kyungwon, W Whang, JE Manson, et al. Dietary a-linolenic acid intake and risk of sudden cardiac death and coronary heart disease. *Circulation* 2005, 112(21):3232–3238.

8. Oomen, CM, MC Ocké, EJ Feskens, FJ Kok, and D Kromhout. Alpha-Linolenic acid intake is not beneficially associated with 10-y risk of coronary artery disease incidence: The Zutphen Elderly Study. *Am J Clin Nutr* 2001, 74(4):457–463. Brouwer, IA, MB Katan, and PL Zock. Dietary alpha-linolenic acid is associated with reduced risk of fatal coronary heart disease, but increased prostate cancer risk: A meta-analysis. *J Nutr* 2004, 134(4):919–922. Pietinen, P, A Ascherio, P Korhonen, AM Hartman, et al. Intake of fatty acids and risk of coronary heart disease in a cohort of Finnish men. The Alpha-Tocopherol, Beta-Carotene Cancer Prevention Study. *Am J Epidemiol* 1997, 145(10):876–887. Mozaffarian, D, A Ascherio, FB Hu, MJ Stampfer, et al. Interplay between different polyunsaturated fatty acids and risk of coronary heart disease in men. *Circulation* 2005, 111(2):157–164.

9. Djoussé, L, DK Arnett, JJ Carr, JH Eckfeldt, PN Hopkins, MA Province, RC Ellison; Investigators of the NHLBI FHS. Dietary linolenic acid is inversely associated with calcified atherosclerotic plaque in the coronary arteries: The National Heart, Lung, and Blood Institute Family Heart Study. *Circulation* 2005, 111(22):2921–2926.

10. Christensen, JH, K Fabrin, K Borup, N Barber, and J Poulsen. Prostate tissue and leukocyte levels of n-3 polyunsaturated fatty acids in men with benign prostate hyperplasia or prostate cancer. *BJU Int* 2006, 97(2):270–273. Koralek, DO, U Peters, G Andriole, D Reding, et al. A prospective study of dietary alpha-linolenic acid and the risk of prostate cancer (United States). *Cancer Causes Control* 2006, 17(6):783–791.

Monounsaturated fats

11. Hu, FB, MD Stampfer, JE Manson, E Rimm, et al. Dietary fat intake and the risk of coronary heart disease in women. *N Eng J Med* 1997, 337(21):1491–1499.

12. Appel, LJ, FM Sacks, VJ Carey, E Obarzanek, JF Swain, ER Miller 3rd, PR Conlin, TP Erlinger, BA Rosner, NM Laranjo, J Charleston, P McCarron, LM Bishop; OmniHeart Collaborative Research Group. Effects of protein, monounsaturated fat, and carbohydrate intake on blood pressure and serum lipids: Results of the OmniHeart randomized trial. *JAMA* 2005, 294(19):2455–2464.

Whole grains

13. Mellen, PB, TF Walsh, and DM Herrington. Whole grain intake and cardiovascular disease: A meta-analysis. *Nutr Metab Cardiovasc Dis* 2007. Apr 19; [Epub ahead of print].

14. Erkkila, AT, DM Herrington, D Mozaffarian, et al. Cereal fiber and whole-grain intake are associated with reduced progression of coronary-artery atherosclerosis in post-menopausal women with coronary artery disease. *Am Heart J* 2005, 150(1):94–101.

15. Mozaffarian, D, SK Kumanyika, RN Lemaitre, et al. Cereal, fruit, and vegetable fiber intake and the risk of cardiovascular disease in elderly individuals. *JAMA* 2003, 289(13):1659–1666.

16. Katcher, HI, RS Legro, AR Kunselman, PJ Gillies, et al. The effects of a whole grain–enriched hypocaloric diet on cardiovascular risk factors in men and women with metabolic syndrome. *Am J Clin Nutr* 2008. 87(1):79–90.

17. Mellen, PB, AD Liese, JA Tooze, et al. Whole-grain intake and carotid artery atherosclerosis in a multiethnic cohort: The Insulin Resistance Atherosclerosis Study. *Am J Clin Nutr* 2007, 85(6):1495–1502.

18. Meyer, KA, LH Kushi, DR Jacobs, Jr, J Slavin, et al. Carbohydrates, dietary fiber, and incident type 2 diabetes in older women. *Am J Clin Nutr* 2000, 71(4):921–930. Liu, S, JE Manson, MJ Stampfer, FB Hu, et al. A prospective study of whole-grain intake and risk of type 2 diabetes mellitus in US women. *Am J Public Health* 2000, 90(9):1409–1415.

19. Brown, L, B Rosner, WW Willett, and FM Sacks. Cholesterol-lowering effects of dietary fiber: A meta-analysis. *Am J Clin Nutr* 1999, 69(1):30–42. Anderson, JW, LD Allgood, A Lawrence, LA Altringer, et al. Cholesterol-lowering effects of psyllium intake adjunctive to diet therapy in men and women with hypercholesterolemia: Meta-analysis of 8 controlled trials. *AM J Clin Nutr* 2000, 71(2):472–479. Keenan, JM, JB Wenz, S Myers, C Ripsan, and ZQ Huang. Randomized, controlled, crossover trial of oat bran in hypercholesterolemic subjects. *J Fam Prac* 1991, 33(6):60–608.

Legumes and soy

20. Bazzano, LA, J He, LG Ogden, et al. Legume consumption and risk of coronary heart disease in US men and women: NHANES I Epidemiologic Follow-up Study. *Arch Intern Med* 2001, 161(21):2573–2578.

21. Hu, FB, EB Rimm, MJ Stampfer, et al. Prospective study of major dietary patterns and risk of coronary heart disease in men. *Am J Clin Nutr* 2000, 72(4):912–921.

22. Anderson, JW, and AW Major. Pulses and lipaemia, short- and long-term effect: Potential in the prevention of cardiovascular disease. *Br J Nutr* 2002, 88 Suppl 3:S263–271.

23. Sacks, FM, LP Svetkey, WM Vollmer, LJ Appel, GA Bray, D Harsha, E Obarzanek, PR Conlin, ER Miller 3rd, DG Simons-Morton, N Karanja, PH Lin; DASH-Sodium Collaborative Research Group. Effects on blood pressure of reduced dietary sodium and the Dietary Approaches to Stop Hypertension (DASH) diet. DASH-Sodium Collaborative Research Group. *N Engl J Med* 2001, 344(1):3–10. Conlin, PR, D Chow, ER Miller 3rd, LP Svetkey, et al. The effect of dietary patterns on blood pressure control in hypertensive patients: Results from the Dietary Approaches to Stop Hypertension (DASH) trial. *Am J Hypertens* 2000, 13(9):949–955.

24. Villegas, R, YT Gao, G Yang, HL Li, et al. Legume and soy food intake and the incidence of type 2 diabetes in the Shanghai Women's Health Study. *Am J Clin Nutr* 2008, 87(1):162–167.

25. Anderson, JW, et al. Meta-analysis of the effects of soy protein intake or serum lipids. *N Engl J Med* 1995, 333(5):276–282. Washburn, S, et al. Effect of soy protein supplementation on serum lipoproteins, blood pressure, and menopausal symptoms in perimenopausal women. *Menopause* 1999, 6(1):7–13. Crouse, JR, et al. A randomized trial comparing the effect of casein with that of soy protein containing varying amounts of isoflavones on plasma concentrations of lipids and lipoproteins. *Arch Intern Med* 1999, 159(17):2070–2076.

26. Washburn, S, et al. Effect of soy protein supplementation on serum lipoproteins, blood pressure, and menopausal symptoms in perimenopausal women. *Menopause* 1999, 6(1):7–13. Schieber, MD, et al. Dietary soy isoflavones favorably influence lipids and bone turnover in healthy post-menopausal women. Abstract. Third International Symposium on the Role of Soy in Preventing and Treating Chronic Disease. October 1999. Wilcox, JN, and BF Blumenthal. Thrombotic mechanism in atherosclerosis: Potential impact of soy proteins. *J Nutr* 1995, 125(3 Suppl):631–638.

Nuts

27. Albert, CM, JM Gaziano, WC Willett, and JE Manson. Nut consumption and decreased risk of sudden cardiac death in the Physicians' Health Study. *Arch Intern Med* 2002, 162(12):1382–1387. Hu, FB, MJ Stampfer, JE Manson, EB Rimm, et al. Frequent nut consumption and risk of coronary heart disease in women: Prospective cohort study. *BMJ* 1998, 317(7169):1341–1345. Ellsworth, JL, LH Kushi, and AR Folsom. Frequent nut intake and risk of death from coronary heart disease and all causes in post-menopausal women: The Iowa Women's Health Study. *Nutr Metab Cardiovasc Dis* 2001, 11(6):372–377.

Fraser, GE, J Sabaté, WL Beeson, and TM Strahan. A possible protective effect of nut consumption on risk of coronary heart disease. The Adventist Health Study. *Arch Intern Med* 1992, 152(7):1416–24.

28. Jenkins, DJ, CW Kendall, A Marchie, TL Parker, et al. Dose response of almonds to coronary heart disease risk factors: Blood lipids, oxidized low-density lipoproteins, lipoprotein(a), homocysteine, and pulmonary nitric oxide: A randomized, controlled, crossover trial. *Circulation* 2002, 106(11):1327–1332.

29. Jiang, R, JE Manson, MJ Stampfer, et al. Nut and peanut butter consumption and risk of type 2 diabetes in women. *JAMA* 2002, 288(20):2554–2560.

30. Katan, MB, SM Grundy, P Jones, M Law, et al. Efficacy and safety of plant stanols and sterols in the management of blood cholesterol levels. *Mayo Clin Proc* 2003, 78(8): 965–978.

Fruit and vegetables

31. He, FJ, CA Nowson, M Lucas, and GA MacGregor. Increased consumption of fruit and vegetables is related to reduced risk of coronary heart disease: Meta-analysis of cohort studies. *J Human Hypertens* 2007, 21(9):717–728. Liu, S, JE Manson, IM Lee, SR Cole, et al. Fruit and vegetable intake and risk of cardio-vascular disease: The Women's Health Study. *Am J Clin Nutr* 2000, 72(4):922–928. Liu, S, IM Lee, U Ajani, SR Cole, JE Buring, and JE Manson; Physicians' Health Study. Intake of vegetables rich in carotenoids and risk of coronary heart disease in men: The Physicians' Health Study. *Int J Epidemiol* 2001, 30(1):130–135.

32. Dauchet, L, P Amouyel, and J Dallongeville. Fruit and vegetable consumption and risk of stroke: A meta-analysis of cohort studies. *Neurology* 2005, 65(8):1193–1197.

33. Appel, LJ, TJ Moore, E Obarzanek, WM Vollmer, et al. A clinical trial of the effects of dietary patterns on blood pressure. DASH Collaborative Research Group. *N Engl J Med* 1997, 17;336(16):1117–1124.

34. He, K, FB Hu, GA Colditz, JE Manson, et al. Changes in intake of fruits and vegetables in relation to risk of obesity and weight gain among middle-aged women. *Int J Obes Relat Metab Disord* 2004, 28(12):1569–1574.

35. Erlund, I, R Koli, G Alfthan, J Marniemi, et al. Favorable effects of berry consumption on platelet function, blood pressure and HDL cholesterol. *Am J Clin Nutr* 2008, 87(2):323–331.

36. Silaste, ML, G Alfthan, A Aro, YA Kesaniemi, and S Horkko. Tomato juice decreases LDL cholesterol levels and increases LDL resistance to oxidation. *Br J Nutr* 2007, 98(6):1251–1258.

37. Hung, HC, KJ Joshipura, R Jiang, et al. Fruit and vegetable intake and risk of major chronic disease. *J Natl Cancer Inst* 2004, 96(21):1577–1584. Joshipura, KJ, FB Hu, JE Mason, et al. The effect of fruit and vegetable intake on risk for coronary heart disease. Ann Intern Med 2001. 134(12):1106–1114.

Tea

38. Peters, U, C Poole, and L Arab. Does tea affect cardiovascular disease? A meta-analysis. *Am J Epidemiol* 2001, 154(6):495–503. Sesso, HD, JM Gaziano, S Liu, and JE Buring. Flavonoid intake and the risk of cardiovascular disease in women. *Am J Clin Nutr* 2003, 77(6):1400–1408. Geleijnse, JM, LJ Launer, DA Van der Kuip, et al. Inverse association of tea and flavonoid intakes with incident myocardial infarction: The Rotterdam Study. *Am J Clin Nutr* 2002, 75(5):880–886.

39. Mukamal, KJ, M Maclure, JE Muller, et al. Tea consumption and mortality after acute myocardial infarction. *Circulation* 2002, 105(21):2476–2481.

40. Shimazu, T, S Kuriyama, A Hozawa, K Ohmori, et al. Dietary patterns and cardiovascular disease mortality in Japan: A prospective cohort study. *Int J Epidemiol* 2007, 36(3):600–609. Kuriyama, S, T Shimazu, K Ohmori, N Kikuchi, N Nakaya, et al. Green tea consumption and mortality due to cardio-vascular disease, cancer, and all causes in Japan: The Ohsaki study. *JAMA* 2006, 296(10):1255–1265.

41. Duffy, SJ, JF Keaney Jr, M Holbrook, N Gokce, et al. Short- and long-term black tea consumption reverses endothelial dysfunction in patients with coronary artery disease. *Circulation* 2001, 104(2):151–156. Hodgson, JM, IB Puddey, V Burke, GF Watts, and LJ Beilin. Regular ingestion of black tea improves brachial artery vasodilator function. *Clin Sci* (Lond) 2002, 102(2):195–201.

42. Winkelmayer, WC, MJ Stampfer, WC Willett, and GC Curhan. Habitual caffeine intake and the risk of hypertension in women. *JAMA* 2005, 294(18):2330–2335.

Dark chocolate

43. Grassi, D, S Necozione, C Lippi, G Croce, et al. Cocoa reduces blood pressure and insulin resistance and improves endothelium-dependent vasodilation in hypertensives. *Hypertension* 2005, 46(2):398–405.

44. Taubery, D, R Roesen, C Lehmann, N Jung, and E Schomig. Effects of low habitual cocoa intake in blood pressure and bioactive nitric oxide: A randomized controlled trial. *JAMA* 2007, 298(1):49–60.

45. Wang-Polagruto, JF, AC Villablanca, JA PolagrutoA, L Lee, et al. Chronic consumption of flavonol-rich cocoa improves endothelial function and decreases vascular cell adhesion molecule in hypercholesterolemic post-menopausal women. *J Cardiovasc Pharmacol* 2006, 47 Suppl2:S177–186.

46. Farouque, HM, M Leung, SA Hope, M Baldi, et al. Acute and chronic effects of flavonol-rich cocoa on vascular subjects with coronary artery disease: A randomized double-blind placebo-controlled study. *Clin Sci* (Lond) 2006, 111(1):71–80.

Chapter 5: Heart Healthy Vitamins, Minerals, and Supplements

Antioxidants

1. The effect of vitamin E and beta carotene on the incidence of lung cancer and other cancers in male smokers. The Alpha-Tocopherol, Beta Carotene Cancer Prevention Study Group. *N Engl J Med* 1994, 330(15):1029–1035. Available at: www.ncbi.nlm.nih.gov/entrez/query.fcgi?cmd=Retrieve&db=pubmed&dopt= Abstract&list_uids=8127329. Omenn, GS, GE Goodman, MD Thornquist, et al. Risk factors for lung cancer and for intervention effects in CARET, the Beta-Carotene and Retinol Efficacy Trial. *J Natl Cancer Inst* 1996, 88(21):1550–1559.

2. Rimm, EB, MJ Stampfer, A Ascherio, E Giovannucci, et al. Vitamin E consumption and the risk of coronary heart disease in men. *N Engl J Med* 1993, 328(20):1450–1456. Stampfer, MJ, CH Hennekens, JE Manson, GA Colditz, et al. Vitamin E consumption and the risk of coronary disease in women. *N Engl J Med* 1993, 328(20):1444–1449.

3. Lee, IM, NR Cook, JM Gaziano, D Gordon, et al. Vitamin E in the primary prevention of cardiovascular disease and cancer: The Women's Health Study: A randomized controlled trial. *JAMA* 2005, 294(1):56–65.

4. Yusuf, S, G Dagenais, J Pogue, J Bosch, and P Sleight. Vitamin E supplementation and cardiovascular events in high-risk patients. The Heart Outcomes Prevention Evaluation Study Investigators. *N Engl J Med* 2000, 342(3):154–160. Gruppo Italiano per lo Studio della Sopravvivenza nell'Infarto miocardico. Dietary supplementation with n-3 polyunsaturated fatty acids and vitamin E after myocardial infarction: Results of the GISSI-Prevenzione trial. Gruppo Italiano per lo Studio della Sopravvivenza nell'Infarto miocardico. *Lancet* 1999, 354(9177):447–455. Lonn, E, J Bosch, S Yusuf, P Sheridan, J Pogue, JM Arnold, C Ross, A Arnold, P Sleight, J Probstfield, GR Dagenais; HOPE and HOPE-TOO Trial Investigators. Effects of long-term vitamin E supplementation on cardiovascular events and cancer: A randomized controlled trial. *JAMA* 2005, 293(11):1338–1347.

5. Miller 3rd, ER, R Pastor-Barriuso, D Dalal, RA Riemersma, et al. Meta-analysis: High-dosage vitamin E supplementation may increase all-cause mortality. *Ann Intern Med* 2005, 142(1):37–46.

B vitamins

6. Homocysteine Studies Collaboration. Homocysteine and risk of ischemic heart disease and stroke: A meta-analysis. *JAMA* 2002, 288(16):2015–2022.

7. Lonn, E, S Yusuf, MJ Arnold, P Sheridan, J Pogue, M Micks, MJ McQueen, J Probstfield, G Fodor, C Held, J Genest Jr; Heart Outcomes Prevention Evaluation (HOPE) 2 Investigators. Homocysteine lowering with folic acid and B vitamins in vascular disease. *N Engl J Med* 2006, 354(15):1567–1577.

8. Albert, CM, NR Cook, JM Gaziano, E Zaharris, et al. Effect of folic acid and B vitamins on risk of cardiovascular events and total mortality among women at high risk for cardiovascular disease: A randomized trial. *JAMA* 2008, 299(17):2027–2036.

9. Bazzano, LA, K Reynolds, KN Holder, J He. Effect of folic acid supplementation on risk of cardiovascular diseases: A meta-analysis of randomized controlled trials. *JAMA* 2006, 296(22):2720–2726.

10. Giovannucci, E, MJ Stampfer, GA Colditz, DJ Hunter, et al. Multivitamin use, folate, and colon cancer in the Nurses' Healthy Study. *Ann Intern Med* 1998, 129(7):517–524. Su, LJ, and L Arab. Nutritional status of folate and colon cancer risk: Evidence from NHANES I epidemiologic follow-up study. *Ann Epidemiol* 2001, 11(1):65–72.

11. Cole, BF, JA Baron, RS Sandler, RW Haile, DJ Ahnen, RS Bresalier, G McKeown-Eyssen, RW Summers, RI Rothstein, CA Burke, DC Snover, TR Church, JI Allen, DJ Robertson, GJ Beck, JH Bond, T Byers, JS Mandel, LA Mott, LH Pearson, EL Barry, JR Rees, N Marcon, F Saibil, PM Ueland, ER Greenberg; Polyp Prevention Study Group. Folic acid for the prevention of colorectal adenomas: A randomized clinical trial. *JAMA* 2007, 297(21):2351–2359.

Vitamin D

12. Giovannucci, E, Y Liu, BW Hollis, and EB Rimm. 25-hydroxyvitamin D and risk of myocardial infarction in men. *Arch Intern Med* 2008, 168(11):1174–1180.

13. Dobnig, H, S Pilz, H Scharnagl, W Renner, et al. Independent association of low serum 25-hydroxyvitamin D and 1,25-dihydroxyvitamin D levels with all-cause mortality and cardiovascular mortality. *Arch Intern Med* 2008, 168(12):1340–1349.

Magnesium

14. Lopez-Ridaura, R, WC Willett, EB Rimm, S Liu, et al. Magnesium intake and risk of type 2 diabetes in men and women. Diabetes Care 2004, 27(1):134–40. Meyer, KA, LH Kishi, DR Jacobs Jr., J Slavin, et al. Carbohydrates, dietary fiber, and incident type 2 diabetes in older women. *Am J Clin Nutr* 1999, 71(4):921–930. Song, V, JE Manson, JE Buring, and S Liu. Dietary magnesium intake in relation to plasma insulin levels and risk of type 2 diabetes in women. *Diabetes Care* 2003, 27(1):59–65. Larsson, SC and A Wolk. Magnesium intake and risk of type 2 diabetes: A meta-analysis. *J Intern Med* 2007, 262(2):208–214.

15. Rodriguez-Moran, M and F Guerrero-Romero. Oral magnesium supplementation improves insulin sensitivity and metabolic control in type 2 diabetic subjects. *Diabetes Care* 2003, 26(4):1147–1152.

16. Shechter, M, CN Bairey Merz, HG Stuehlinger, et al. Effects of oral magnesium therapy on exercise tolerance, exercise-induced chest pain, and quality of life in patients with coronary artery disease. *Am J Cardiol* 2003, 91(5): 517–521.

Coenzyme Q10

17. Tran, MT, TM Mitchell, DT Kennedy, and JT Giles. Role of coenzyme Q10 in chronic heart failure, angina, and hypertension. *Pharmacotherapy* 2001, 21(7):797–806.

18. Singh, RB, MA Niaz, SS Rastogi, PK Shukla, and AS Thakur. Effect of hydrosoluble coenzyme Q10 on blood pressures and insulin resistance in hypertensive patients with coronary artery disease. *J Hum Hypertens* 1999,13(3):203–208. Burke, BE, R Neuenschwander, and RD Olson. Randomized, double-blind, placebo-controlled trial of coenzyme Q10 in isolated systolic hypertension. *South Med J* 2001, 94(11):1112–1117.

19. Watts, GF, DA Playford, KD Croft, NC Ward, et al. Coenzyme Q(10) improves endothelial dysfunction of the brachial artery in Type II diabetes mellitus. *Diabetologia* 2002, 45(3):420–426.

Garlic

20. Gardner, CD, LD Lawson, E Block, et al. Effect of raw garlic vs. commercial garlic supplements on plasma lipid concentrations in adults with moderate hypercholesterolemia: A randomized clinical trial. *Arch Intern Med* 2007, 167(4):346–353.

21. Koscielny, J, D Klussendorf, R Latza, R Schmitt, et al. The antiatherosclerotic effect of *Allium sativum*. *Atherosclerosis* 1999,144(1):237–249.

22. Budoff, MJ, J Takasu, FR Flores, Y Niihara, et al. Inhibiting progression of coronary calcification using Aged Garlic Extract in patients receiving statin therapy: A preliminary study. *Prev Med* 2004; 39(5):985–991.

Chapter 6: Diet Plans to Help Prevent Heart Disease

1. Appel, LJ, TJ Moore, E Obarzanek, WM Vollmer, et al. A clinical trial of the effects of dietary patterns on blood pressure. DASH Collaborative Research Group. *N Engl J Med* 1997, 336(16):1117–1124.

2. Sacks, FM, LP Svetkey, WM Vollmer, LJ Appel, GA Bray, D Harsha, E Obarzanek, PR Conlin, ER Miller 3rd, DG Simons-Morton, N Karanja, PH Lin; DASH-Sodium Collaborative Research Group. Effects on blood pressure of reduced dietary sodium and the Dietary Approaches to Stop Hypertension (DASH) diet. DASH-Sodium Collaborative Research Group. *N Engl J Med* 2001, 344(1):3–10.

3. Obarzanek, E, FM Sacks, WM Vollmer, GA Bray, ER Miller 3rd, PH Lin, NM Karanja, MM Most-Windhauser, TJ Moore, JF Swain, CW Bales, MA Proschan; DASH Research Group. Effects on blood lipids of a blood pressure-lowering diet: The Dietary Approaches to Stop Hypertension (DASH) Trial. *Am J Clin Nutr* 2001, 74(1):80–89.

4. Azadbakht, L, P Mirmiran, A Esmaillzadeh, T Azizi, and F Azizi. Beneficial effects of a Dietary Approaches to Stop Hypertension eating plan on features of the metabolic syndrome. *Diabetes Care* 2005, 28(12):2823–2831.

5. Fung, TT, SE Chiuve, ML McCullough, KM Rexrode, G Logroscino, and FB Hu. Adherence to a DASH-style diet and risk of coronary heart disease and stroke in women. *Arch Intern Med* 2008, 168(7):713–720.

6. Appel, LJ, FM Sacks, VJ Carey, E Obarzanek, JF Swain, ER Miller 3rd, PR Conlin, TP Erlinger, BA Rosner, NM Laranjo, J Charleston, P McCarron, LM Bishop; OmniHeart Collaborative Research Group. Effects of protein, monounsaturated fat, and carbohydrate intake on blood pressure and serum lipids: Results of the OmniHeart randomized trial. *JAMA* 2005, 294(19):2455–2464.

7. Jenkins, DJ, CW Kendall, A Marchie, DA Faulkner, et al. Direct comparison of a dietary portfolio of cholesterol-lowering foods with a statin in hypercholesterolemic participants. *Am J Clin Nutr* 2005, 81(2):380–387.

8. Jenkins, DJ, CW Kendall, DA Faulkner, T Nguyen, et al. Assessment of the longer-term effects of a dietary portfolio of cholesterol-lowering foods in hypercholesterolemia. *Am J Clin Nutr* 2006, 83(3):582–591.

9. Jenkins, DJ, CW Kendall, DA Faulkner, T Kemp, et al. Long-term effects of a plant-based dietary portfolio of cholesterol-lowering foods on blood pressure. *Eur J Clin Nutr* 2008, 62(6):781–788. Jenkins, DJ, CW Kendall, A Marchie, DA Faulkner, et al. Direct comparison of dietary portfolio vs statin on C-reactive protein. *Eur J Clin Nutr* 2005, 59(7):851–860.

Chapter 9: Maintaining a Healthy Weight

1. Heart and Stroke Foundation of Canada. Overweight, Obesity, and Heart Disease and Stroke. Heart and Stroke Foundation of Canada Position Statement. Available at: www.heartandstroke.com/site/c.ikIQLcMWJtE/b.3799193/k.C2EF/Overweight_obesity_and_heart_disease_and_stroke.htm. Shields, Margot. Measured Obesity: Overweight Canadian children and adolescents. Statistics Canada, 2005. Available at: www.statcan.ca/english/research/82-620-MIE/2005001/pdf/cobesity.pdf

2. Bowman, TS, T Kurth, HD Sesso, JE Manson, and JM Gaziano. Eight-year change in body mass index and subsequent risk of cardiovascular disease among healthy non-smoking men. *Prev Med* 2007, 45(6):436–441.

3. Rimm, EB, MJ Stampfer, E Giovannucci, A Ascherio, et al. Body size and fat distribution as predictors of coronary heart disease among middle-aged and older U.S. men. *AM J Epidemiol* 1995, 141(12):1117–1127.

4. Lakka, HM, TA Lakka, J Tuomilehto, and JT Salonen. Abdominal obesity is associated with increased risk of acute coronary events in men. *Eur Heart J* 2002, 23(9):706–713. De Koning, L, AT Merchant, J Pogue, and SS Anand. Waist circumference and waist-to-hip ratio as predictors of cardiovascular events: Meta-regression of prospective studies. *Eur Heart J* 2007, 28(7):850–856. Canoy, D, SM Boekholdt, N Wareham, R Luben, et al. Body fat distribution and risk of coronary heart disease in men and women in the European Prospective Investigation into Cancer and Nutrition in Norfolk cohort: A population-based prospective study. *Circulation* 2007, 116(25):2933–2943.

5. Yusuf, S, S Hawken, S Ounpuu, L Bautista, MG Franzosi, P Commerford, CC Lang, Z Rumboldt, CL Onen, L Lisheng, S Tanomsup, P Wangai Jr, F Razak, AA Sharma, SS Anand; INTERHEART Study Investigators. Obesity and the risk of myocardial infarction in 27,000 participants from 52 countries: A case-control study. *Lancet* 2005, 366(9497):1640–1649.

6. JF Hollis, CM Gullion, VJ Stevens, PJ Brantley, LJ Appel, JD Ard, CM Champagne, A Dalcin, TP Erlinger, K Funk, D Laferriere, PH Lin, CM Loria, C Samuel-Hodge, WM Vollmer, LP Svetkey; Weight Loss Maintenance Trial Research Group. Weight loss during the intensive intervention phase of the weight-loss maintenance trial. *Am J Prev Med* 2008, 35(2):118–126.

7. McGuire, MT, et al. Behavioural strategies of individuals who have maintained long-term weight losses. *Obes Research* 1999, 7(4):334–341.

8. Ibid.

Chapter 10: Exercise for Preventing Heart Disease

1. Sesso, HD, RS Paffenbarger, and IM Lee. Physical activity and coronary heart disease in men. The Harvard Alumni Health Study. *Circulation* 2000, 102(9):975–980. Tanasescu, M, MF Leitzmann, EB Rimm, WC Willet, MJ Stampfer, and FB Hu. Exercise type and intensity in relation to coronary heart disease. *JAMA* 2002, 288(6):1994–2000.

2. Lee, IM, HD Sesso, and RS Paffenbarger. Physical activity and coronary heart disease in men. Does the duration of exercise episodes predict risk? *Circulation* 2000, 102(9):981–986. Tanasescu, M, MF Leitzmann, EB Rimm, WC Willet, MJ Stampfer, and FB Hu. Exercise type and intensity in relation to coronary heart disease. *JAMA* 2002, 288(6):1994–2000.

3. Tanasescu, M, MF Leitzmann, EB Rimm, WC Willet, MJ Stampfer, and FB Hu. Exercise type and intensity in relation to coronary heart disease. *JAMA* 2002, 288(6):1994–2000.

General index

abdominal obesity, 47
Accupril, 46
ACE inhibitors, 45–46
Adalat, 46
adrenal glands, 9
adrenaline, 9
aerobic exercise, 223–25
age
   and hypertension, 43
   and type 2 diabetes, 49
aging
   and cholesterol, 7
   as risk factor, 31–32
ALA fatty acid, 84, 88–90, 113
alcohol
   and cholesterol, 79
   daily intake, 38, 80
   and heart disease, 53, 79
   and high blood pressure, 58
   intake and hypertension, 44
   red wine, 79–80
   and triglycerides, 80
Aldactone, 45
alpha-linolenic acid. See ALA fatty acid
Altace, 46
Alzheimer's disease, 19
angina pectoris, 7–8
   and CRP levels, 18
   and heart attack, 4
   symptoms, 8
   treatment, 8
angioplasty, 11
angiotensin receptor blockers, 46
anthocyanins, 117
anticoagulants, 88
anti-inflammatories, 95, 115

antioxidants, 80, 113, 115, 117, 132–33, 136, 138. (*See also* beta carotene; vitamin C; vitamin E)
apo B cholesterol, 38
Apo-Hydro, 45
apolipoprotein B, 17–18
arginine, 113
arrhythmias, 12, 20, 85, 87–88
   and magnesium, 146
   prevention, 89
arteries, 6–7
aspirin, 11
atherosclerosis, 6–7, 123
   and ALA, 89
   and blood clots, 8
   in children, 138
   and garlic supplements, 153
   and homocysteine, 19
   and inflammation, 18
   risk ratio, 15–16
Avapro, 46

"bad" cholesterol. See LDL cholesterol
berries
   role in diet, 117–18
beta blockers, 11, 45
beta carotene, 117, 132, 134–35
bile acid, 40, 102
bioavailability, 149
blood cholesterol, xxii
   and DASH diet, 160
   and diet, 37–38
   and garlic, 152–53
   and genetics, 37–38
   high, 36–41
   and oils, 60

and saturated fat, 58
and soy, 108–10
blood clots, 8–9, 34, 53, 61, 79, 90, 95, 113, 117, 153
  drugs to treat, 11
  and liver, 19
  and smoking, 35
blood glucose, 20
blood lipids, 39–41
blood pressure, xxii. (*See also* hypertension)
  and caffeine, 124
  DASH diet and, 159–60
  effect of chocolate on, 126–27
  effect of legumes on, 105
  and garlic, 153
  and heredity, 77
  high, 30, 41–46, 58
  high, in youths, 31
  lowering, 94–95, 116
  and magnesium, 146
  measuring, 5
  normal, 76
  and nuts, 112
  and potassium, 77
  and sodium intake, 75, 76
blood sugar, 20–21, 58
  and diabetes, 48
  levels, and hypertension, 44
  lowering through exercise, 47
  and whole grains, 101
blood tests
  for heart disease, 13–21
blood thinners, 88, 151, 154
body fat, 206
body mass index (BMI), 206–8, 211
brain natriuretic peptide (BNP), 19–20
bread products
  purchasing, 186
breakfasts
  in restaurants, 202
  and weight loss, 213
breastfeeding
  ALA intake while, 90
butter, 59

caffeine, 124–25
calcium
  and hypertension, 46
  increasing, 181
  and vitamin D, 143
calcium channel blockers, 46
calories, 179
  children's requirements, 193
  daily requirements, 191
  reducing, 211–12
  in restaurant meals, 190–94
  in selected foods, 217
Canada's Food Guide, 96, 119, 176, 177
cancer, 34
  and alcohol intake, 80
  multivitamins and folic acid, 142
  prostate and ALA, 91–92
  and vitamin D, 144
canola, 88–90
carbohydrates, 94, 164, 165, 180
cardiac arrest, 89
Cardiazem, 46
Cardiolite scans, 25
cardiovascular disease. *See* heart disease
cardiovascular exercise, 223–25
catechins, 122, 123, 124, 126
cereals, 186–87
chest pain, 9
children
  and atherosclerosis, 138
  blood pressure measurements, 43
  body mass index for, 207
  calories, daily requirements, 193
  diabetes in, 48, 49
  diet of, xxiii
  fats, daily requirements, 193
  fatty acid intake, 85
  fish intake, 87
  high blood pressure in, 31
  "kid-friendly" meals, 193–94
  learning disabilities and mercury, 87
  obesity and overweight, xxii, 47–48
  sodium requirements, 74, 193
  statin therapy in, 32
  vitamin D deficiency, 144
chocolate, dark, 125–28
cholesterol
  and aging, 7

apo B, 38
content of selected foods, 69
dietary, 67–71, 180
effect of legumes on, 105
high, in children, 32
high, in youths, 31
levels and menopause, 34
listed on nutrition label, 180
lowering, 117, 118, 168–69
and nuts, 112
raising, 117
reducing dietary, 71
test for, 13
total, 16
circulatory system, 4–6
Clinton, Bill, 24
coenzyme Q10
food sources, 150
and heart disease, 150, 152
and hypertension, 151
recommended intake, 151
role of, 150
side effects of supplements, 151
supplements, 150–51
coffee, 124
computed tomography angiogram (CTA), 22–23
congestive heart failure. See heart failure
corn syrup
high fructose, 72
coronary angiography, 21–22
coronary artery disease. See heart disease
coronary catheterization, 22
Coumadin, 88, 151, 154
Cozaar, 46
C-reactive protein, 18, 100, 169
CRP. See C-reactive protein
CTA scan, 22–23

dairy products
purchasing, 184–85
and saturated fat, 61
DASH diet, 112, 159–63
DASH Sodium Trial, 76, 105, 116
DHA fatty acids
benefits of, 89
in fish, 84–85, 86
in fish oil supplements, 87

diabetes
and age, 49
in children, 49
and egg consumption, 67–68
and exercise, 49
and genetics, 50
gestational, 50
importance of exercise, 47
lowering triglycerides, 85
and magnesium, 145–46
magnesium loss, 148
men with, and egg consumption, 69
and overweight, 50
as risk factor, 30
risk factor for heart disease, 48–50
and sedentary lifestyle, 50
and soluble fibre intake, 102
statistics, xxi
test for control of, 20–21
type 2, xxii, 31, 48, 49–50, 72, 100, 101, 105–6, 112, 145–46
diet
ALA in, 90
children's, 32
and cholesterol, 36, 37–38, 39
and health claims on products, 183
and heart disease, 52, 58
and heart disease risk factors, 158–59
and hypertension, 44
indulging as treat, 215
losing weight, 210–16
lowering cholesterol, 58
and nutrition, 52
reducing saturated fat in, 63–64
reducing trans fats in, 65–67
and triglycerides, 39
vegetarian, 169
dietary cholesterol, 67–71
Diovan, 46
diuretics, 45, 148
Doppler ultrasound, 23

eating habits. See diet
ECG, 23–24
echocardiogram, 23
eggs
buying guide, 70
cholesterol in, 67

diabetes and, 67–68
and heart disease, 67
and omega-3 fatty acids, 69, 70
recommended intake, 68–69
EKG, 23–24
electrocardiogram (ECG, EKG), 23–24
environmental factors
and type 2 diabetes, 49
EPA fatty acid, 84
benefits of, 89
in fish, 84–85, 86
in fish oil supplements, 87
estrogen, 33
ethnic background
as risk factor, 35
event monitoring, 26
exercise
advantages of, 47
cardiovascular, 223–25
consulting with doctor, 230
and diabetes, 49
fitness journal, 229
flexibility, 227–28
and heart disease, 222
heart rate zone, 224–25
importance of, 38, 39
lack of and hypertension, 44
lifestyle approach, 228
maintaining, 228–30
with partner, 229
personal trainer, 229
scheduling, 229
strength, 225–27
and weight loss, 47, 218–19, 222
exercise electrocardiogram, 24

family history
and hypertension, 44
as risk factor, 34–35
fast food restaurants. See restaurants
fats. (See also monounsaturated fats;
saturated fats; trans fats; unsaturated
fats)
calories in, 96
chemical structure, 59
children's requirements, 193
in diet, 52
intake, xxiii

listed on nutrition label, 179–80
lowering intake, 181
monounsaturated, 93–98
polyunsaturated, 84
recommended intake, 96, 191
replacing saturated and trans, 93
in restaurant meals, 190–94, 195–96
saturated, 36
trans, 64–67
visceral, 47
fatty acids, 59
fibrates, 40
fibre
foods containing, 101
increasing, 181
lack in juices, 120
listed on nutrition label, 180
soluble, 100, 101–4, 117
fibrinogen, 19
fish
fatty acids in, 84–85
and mercury, 86–87
purchasing, 185–86
recommended intake, 85–86
fish oil supplements
contraindications, 87–88
flavonoids, 122, 126, 127
flaxseed
ALA in, 88–90
oil, 92
flexibility exercise, 227–28
folate, 107, 138–43
food sources, 140
in fruit and vegetables, 117
recommended intake, 139
folic acid, 19. (See also folate)
contraindications for, 142, 143
and multivitamins, 142
supplements, 143
food journal, 214–15
food labels, 175–76
expiration date, 185
nutrition and health claims, 182–83
foods. (See also diet)
ALA in, 90–91
calories in selected, 217
on grocery list, 174
monounsaturated fats in, 97

saturated fats in, 59, 60, 62
soluble fibre in, 101, 102, 103
sugars in, 71–74
whole grains in, 99
Framingham Risk Score, 14–15, 23
free radicals, 95, 109, 118, 133, 150
fructose, 72
fruit
  daily servings, xxi, 119–20
  and heart disease, 116–22
  increasing intake, 121
  juice, 120–21
  nutrients in, 117
  purchasing, 183–84
  serving size, 120
  vitamin E and, 132

garlic
  and atherosclerosis, 153
  and blood cholesterol, 152–53
  contraindications, 154
  nutrients in, 152
  side effects, 154
  supplements, 152–53, 154
Gelok, Michelle, xxiii
gender
  as risk factor, 32–34
General Mills Goodness Corner, 175, 177
genetics
  and cholesterol, 37–38
  and diabetes, 50
  and homocysteine, 139
  and hypertension, 44
  and type 2 diabetes, 49
gestational diabetes, 50
glycemic index
  legumes, 106
  of sugars, 72
  and whole-grain foods, 101
"good" cholesterol. See HDL cholesterol
grapefruit juice
  danger of, 46
greens, leafy, 118
grocery shopping
  bread and crackers, 186
  cereals, 186–87
  dairy case, 184–85
  fish counter, 185–86

  healthy food symbols, 175–78
  making a list, 174
  meat counter, 185–86
  produce section, 183–84
  store layout, 175
  tips, 174–75, 183–87

HDL cholesterol
  alcohol and, 79
  desirable ranges, 16
  and diet, 52
  and eggs, 67
  and estrogen, 33
  and exercise, 47
  and fats, 58, 60
  and heart disease, 13, 38–39
  increasing, 94–95
  measurement of, 36–37
  and monounsaturated fats, 93
  and protein in diet, 94
  and risk of atherosclerosis, 15
  and smoking, 35
  and stearic acid, 61
  and trans fats, 64
Health Check program, 176–77
healthy food symbols, 175–78
heart, 4–6
Heart and Stroke Foundation of Canada,
  xxi, 10, 31, 33, 34, 46, 61, 65, 68, 80,
  85, 138, 140, 176–77
heart attack, 8–13
  and CRP, 18, 100, 169
  and homocysteine, 19
  in men, 32
  risk factors, 30–52
  silent, 33
  surgery, 11–12
  symptoms, 9–10, 33
  treatment, 10–12
  in women, 32–34
heart disease
  and ALA fatty acids, 89
  and alcohol, 53, 79
  blood tests for, 13–21
  and body mass index, 207–8
  and cholesterol, 13, 15–16, 38–39,
  coenzyme Q10 and, 150, 152
  and CRP, 18

diabetes risk factor, 48-50
diet and, xxii, 52, 58, 59–64, 67, 111, 116–22, 158–59
and exercise, 222
and hemoglobin A1c, 20–21
and inflammation, 18
and lifestyle, 158–59
magnesium and, 146
overweight, 41, 47–48
risk factors, xxii, 21, 41, 52–53
and saturated fat, 59–64
screening procedures, 21–26
and sodium, 76–77
statistics, xxi
and trans fats, 64
types, 6–13
vitamins and, 132, 135–36, 137, 143
in youths, 31–32
heart rate zone, 224–25
heart valves, 13
hemoglobin A1c (HbA1c), 20–21
heparin, 11
heredity. (See also genetics)
and blood pressure, 77
high sensitivity C-reactive protein. See C-reactive protein
hip fracture, 34
Holter monitoring, 25–26
homocysteine, 19, 117, 124, 138–40
and folic acid, 142
hormone replacement therapy, 34
HS-CRP. See C-reactive protein
hunger level, 213–14
hypertension, 41–46
and caffeine, 124
and coenzyme Q10 supplements, 151
masked, 43
medications for, 45–46
risk factors for, 43–44
and salt, 76
treating, 44–46
white coat, 43

impaired fasting glucose, 48, 49, 50. (See also diabetes)
implantable cardioverter defibrillator (ICD), 13, 87–88, 92
Inderal, 45

indulging, 215
inflammation, 64, 80, 85, 113, 153
and atherosclerosis, 18
benefits of ALA, 89–90
and diet, 52
insulin and fat and, 47
ingredients lists, 79, 181–82, 183
insulin
and body fat, 47, 50
and diabetes, 48
effect of trans fats on, 64
resistance, 51, 72
INTERHEART, 30, 35
irregular heartbeats, 12. (See also arrhythmias)
ischemic heart disease. See heart disease
isoflavone, 109

Jack Astor's, 190, 192–93, 194
Jenkins, David, 168
juices, 120–21

The Keg, 190, 192, 194
Kelsey's, 190, 191, 193
Keys, Ancel, 58
"kid-friendly" meals, 193–94
kidneys, 44, 45
Kraft Canada, 175
Kraft's Sensible Solution, 177

labelling programs (food), 175–88
lauric acids, 60
LDL cholesterol, 14–15, 37–38
and coenzyme Q10, 150
and estrogen, 33
and fats, 58
and heart disease, 13, 15–16
high, and diet, 52
limiting dietary cholesterol, 67
link with sugars, 72
lipoprotein (a), 17
lowering, 39, 94–95, 102, 114–15
measurement of, 36
and monounsaturated fats, 93
and nuts, 114–15
and olive oil, 94–95
and protein in diet, 94
and saturated fat, 60

and stearic acid, 61
and trans fats, 64
and whole grains, 100
learning disabilities, 87
legumes
    cooking with, 107–8
    effect on blood pressure, 105
    effect on cholesterol, 105
    glycemic index and, 106
    increasing intake, 110–11
    nutrients in, 106–7
    preparation, 105
    and type 2 diabetes, 105–6
lifestyle
    risk factors and heart disease, 158–59
lipid profile, 13–17
lipoprotein (a), 17
liver
    and blood clots, 19
    triglyceride production in, 17, 39
Lopresor, 45
low-density lipoprotein cholesterol. See
    LDL cholesterol
lycopene, 117

magnesium, 107, 113
    and arrhythmia, 146
    deficiency, 148–49
    food sources, 146, 148
    in hard water, 146
    and heart disease, 146
    recommended intake, 147–48
    role of, 145
    side effects of supplements, 150
    supplement, 148–50
    and type 2 diabetes, 145–46
margarine
    made from olive oil, 98
    and plant sterols, 114–15
    soft, 96
    sterol-enriched, 169
meals
    planning, and weight loss, 212
meat
    purchasing, 185–86
    and saturated fat, 61
Medcan Clinic, 16
Mediterranean diet, 84

men
    ALA intake, 90
    and alcoholic intake, 53, 80
    with diabetes, egg consumption for, 69
    fat intake, recommended, 61
    fibre intake, recommended, 180
    folate intake, recommended, 139, 140
    fruit and vegetable intake, benefits of,
      116
    heart disease and vitamin E, 137
    hypertension in, 43
    lowering cholesterol, 102
    magnesium requirements, 107
    prostate cancer, 91–92
    sedentary lifestyle of, 46
    sodium intake, recommended, 74
    vitamin C intake, recommended, 133
    vitamin E requirements, 137
menopause, 33, 34, 43. (See also women,
    post-menopausal)
mercury, 86–87
metabolic syndrome, 50–52, 72, 100, 102
    and DASH diet, 160
Mevacor, 168, 169
Milestones, 190, 191
Monopril, 46
monounsaturated fats
    foods rich in, 97
    and heart health, 93–94
    increasing intake, 97–98
    listed on nutrition label, 179–80
    and olive oil, 94–95
    recommendations for, 95–98
    and weight gain, 96
multivitamins, 141, 142
myocardial infarction. See heart attack
myristic acids, 60

neural tube defects, 141–42
niacin, 38
    and cholesterol reduction, 41
nicotinic acid, 40
nitroglycerine, 8, 10, 11
Norvasc, 46
nutrition
    and diet, 52
    and health claims on products, 182–83
    labelling programs, 175–78, 178–82

serving size, 178–79
sodium, 180
Nutrition Facts boxes, 63, 64, 65, 66, 73, 74, 78, 178–81, 183, 184, 186
nutrition label, xxiii
    calories, 179
    carbohydrates, 180
    cholesterol, 180
    fats, 63, 65, 66, 179–80
    fibre, 180
    and health claims, 182–83
    percentage daily value, 181
    protein, 181
    in restaurants, 190
    serving size, 178–79
    sugars, 180
nuts
    and blood pressure, 112
    and cholesterol, 112
    and heart disease, 111
    increasing intake, 115
    nutritional content, 113–14
    plant sterols in, 114–15
    protein in, 113
    and type 2 diabetes, 112
    vitamins in, 113

oat bran, 58, 102
obesity, xxii
    abdominal, 51
    in children, 31
    and hypertension, 44
    as risk factor, 47–48
    and sugar intake, 72
oils
    ALA in, 90
    and cholesterol levels, 60
    olive, 94–95
    and omega-3 fats, 84
    omega-3 fatty acids in, 92
    in OmniHeart diet, 166
    and saturated fats, 59
olive oil, 94–95
    anti-inflammatory properties, 95
omega-3 fatty acids. (See also ALA fatty acid; DHA fatty acids; EPA fatty acid)
    in eggs, 69, 70
    increasing intake, 88–90, 92

in oils, 84
and triglycerides, 85
types, 84–85
in walnuts, 113
OmniHeart diet, 163–68
OmniHeart study, 93–94
osteoporosis, 34, 143, 145
overweight, xxii
    and diabetes, 50
    and health risks, 206
    and hypertension, 44
    as risk factor for heart disease, 41, 47–48
    and sugar intake, 72

palmitic oils, 60
peanut butter, 112
PepsiCo, 175
PepsiCo's Smart Spot, 176, 177–78
percentage daily value, 181
physical activity. (See also exercise)
    guidelines, 222–23
physical inactivity. See sedentary lifestyle
phytochemicals, 95, 99, 106, 109, 117, 126
phytosterols, 100
plant sterols, 114–15
plaque
    calcified, 153
    slowing buildup, 98
Plavix, 11
polyunsaturated fats, 84, 95. (See also fats)
    listed on nutrition label, 179–80
portfolio diet, 168–71
portion sizes, 212–13, 218
    in restaurant meals, 197
potassium, 44, 45, 77–78, 117
pre-diabetes, 48, 49
pregnancy
    ALA intake during, 90
    caffeine intake during, 124
    and folic acid, 141
    mercury exposure during, 87
President's Choice, 175
President's Choice Blue Menu, 177
processed meats, 78
prostate cancer, 91–92

protein
    and blood pressure, 94
    and cholesterol, 94
    C-reactive, 100
    in diet, 94, 164, 165, 166, 167
    listed on nutrition label, 181
    loss in grain refining, 99
    in nuts, 113
    in soy foods, 110
psyllium, 102

Red Lobster, 194
renin inhibitors, 46
resins, 39–40
restaurants
    breakfasts in, 202
    calories in meals, 190–94
    checking for trans fats, 66
    ethnic cuisines, 197–202
    fats in meals, 190–94, 195–96
    "kid-friendly" meals, 193–94
    low-fat cooking techniques, 194–95
    nutrition labelling and, 190
    portion sizes, 197
    sodium in meals, 75, 190–94, 196
    sugar in meals, 196
    tips for healthy meals in, 194–97
resveratrol, 80, 113
risk
    for atherosclerosis, 15–16
Russert, Tim, 24

salt. See sodium
saturated fats
    and blood cholesterol, 58
    in foods, 59, 60, 61, 62
    and heart disease, 59–64
    and LDL cholesterol, 60
    listed on nutrition label, 179–80
    in oils, 59
    reducing, 61–62, 63–64
    replacing, 93
    in soy foods, 109
sedentary lifestyle. (See also exercise)
    dangers of, 46–47
    and diabetes, 50
    and hypertension, 44

seniors
    and vitamin B12, 142
serving size, 178–79
Seven Countries Study, 58
shopping. See grocery shopping
shopping list, 174–75
shrimp, 68
side effects
    of medications, 40, 41
smoking
    cessation, 38
    contraindications for beta carotene,
        134
    and hypertension, 44
    as risk factor, 30, 35–36
    and vitamin C, 133
snacks, 212, 213, 218
Sobeys, 175, 176
Sobeys Compliments Balance-équilibre,
    177
sodium
    benefits of, 74
    and DASH diet, 160
    in diet, 52, 75
    in foods, 75
    and heart disease, 76–77
    and hypertension, 44, 58, 76
    in juices, 120–21
    listed on nutrition label, 180
    lowering intake, 78–79, 181
    and potassium, 77
    recommended intake, 74–75
    requirements, 74–75, 191, 193
    in restaurant meals, 190–94, 196
soy, 104–11
statins, 11
statin therapy, 39, 152
    for children, 32
    side effects, 40
stearic acid, 60–61
stenting, 11
strength exercise, 225–27
stress
    and caffeine, 124
    and elevated blood pressure, 43
    and heart attack, 53
    and weight loss, 47
stretching exercise, 227–28

stroke
  and atherosclerosis, 7
  and CRP, 18
  and estrogen, 34
  and homocysteine, 19
  prevention, 116
  statistics, xxi
sugars
  in foods, 71–74
  link with LDL cholesterol, 72
  listed on nutrition label, 180–81
  and obesity, 72
  and overweight, 72
  reducing in diet, 73–74
  refined, 58
  in restaurant meals, 196
  and triglycerides, 72
supermarkets. (*See also* grocery
    shopping)
  labelling programs, 176, 177
supplements
  antioxidant, 138
  beta carotene, 134
  coenzyme Q10, 150–51
  folic acid, 142, 143
  magnesium, 148–50
  vitamin, 132–34
  vitamin D, 144–45
  vitamin E, 135, 136
surgery
  for heart attack, 11–12

tea, 122–25
teenagers. *See* youths
Tekturna, 46
Tenormin, 45
thallium scans, 25
tomatoes, 117–18
trans fats
  and cholesterol levels, 64
  effect on insulin, 64
  and heart disease, 64
  listed on nutrition label, 65, 66,
    179–80
  reducing, 65–67
  replacing, 93
  in restaurant food, 66, 190, 195–96
treadmill stress test, 24

triglycerides, 7
  and alcohol intake, 80
  and heart disease, 39
  lowering, 69, 85
  measurement of, 36–37
  and omega-3 fish oils, 85
  production of, 17
  and protein in diet, 94
  and soy, 108
  sugar and, 72
  test for, 13

unsaturated fats, 59
  in diet, 164, 165, 166, 167–68

vascular dementia, 7
Vasotec, 46
vegetables
  daily servings, 119–20
  and heart disease, 116–22
  increasing intake, 121
  juice, 120–21
  nutrients in, 117
  purchasing, 183–84
  serving size, 120
  vitamin E and, 132
vegetarians
  diet for, 169
  vitamin B12 intake, 142
ventricular fibrillation, 12
ventricular tachycardia, 12
very low-density lipoproteins, 17
visceral fat, 47
vitamin B6, 19
  food sources, 141
  and homocysteine levels, 139
  recommended daily allowance, 141
vitamin B12, 19
  food sources, 141, 142
  and homocysteine levels, 139
  recommended daily allowance, 141
  for seniors, 142
vitamin C, 132
  in foods, 133–34
  in fruit and vegetables, 117
  and vitamin E, 133
vitamin D, 36
  and calcium, 143

and cancer, 144
daily dosage, 145
deficiency, 143, 144
food sources, 143
function of, 143
and heart disease, 143
supplements, 144–45
vitamin E
and coenzyme Q10, 150
foods containing, 137–38,
and heart disease, 132, 135–36
monounsaturated fats in, 94
for post-menopausal women, 137
supplements, 135–37
and vitamin C, 133,
vitamins
in nuts, 113
vitamin supplements
advantages and disadvantages, 132–34
VLDL. *See* very low-density lipoproteins

waist circumference, 51, 52, 208–9
waist-to-hip ratio, 209–10
walnuts, 88–90, 113
Wappell, Tom, 190
water, hard *vs.* soft, 146
water pills, 45
weighing in, 215, 218
weight, 206–8, 210–19
weight loss, 38, 39, 47, 49, 117. (*See also* diet)
weight-loss plateaus, 215–16
whole grains, 98–104

wine
red, 79–80
women
ALA intake, 90
and alcoholic intake, 53, 80
breastfeeding, 90
diabetes in, xxii
fat intake, recommended, 61
fibre intake, recommended,180
folate intake, recommended, 139, 140
fruit and vegetable intake, benefits of, 116
heart attack symptoms, 33
heart disease in, xxii
hypertension in, 43
lowering cholesterol, 102
magnesium requirements, 107
post-menopausal, 85, 98, 100–101, 102, 127, 137, 145–46
pregnancy, 87, 90
sedentary lifestyle of, 46
sodium intake, recommended, 74
and type 2 diabetes, 146
vitamin C intake, recommended, 133
vitamin E requirements, 137

youths
body mass index for, 207
diabetes in, 48
and heart disease, 31–32
sedentary lifestyle, 46–47
sodium requirements, 75

Recipe index

almond
  and berry yogurt parfait, 245
  and blueberry smoothie, 247
  strawberry oat bran cereal, 255
  toasted, with green beans, 284
  tofu, 307–8
apple
  baked, cinnamon pecan, 368
  blueberry muffins, 342–43
  chutney, 335
  and cinnamon hot oats, 246
  and raspberry crisp, 362–63
  and squash soup, 280
asparagus
  and red pepper frittata, 309
avocado
  lime dressing, 266

banana
  bread, chocolate, 356–57
  split, 250
barley
  and chicken soup, 271–72
basil
  and sautéed tomatoes, 291
beans
  black, and chickpea salad, 256
  black, and wild rice salad, 265
  black, spicy soup, 278–79
  green with toasted almonds, 284
  refried, baked tortilla, 315
  white, and vegetable soup, 281–82
beef
  stroganoff, 293–94
  and vegetable stew, slow cooker,
    337–38
beer bread, 350–51

beet
  salad, roasted, 263
berry
  and almond yogurt parfait, 245
  salad, 261
black beans. *See* beans
blueberry
  and almond smoothie, 247
  and apple muffins, 342–43
  maple pancakes, 248–49
breads. (*See also* sandwiches)
  carrot walnut, 344–45
  chocolate banana, 356–57
  easy beer, 350–51
  French toast, 251
  tuna bruschetta, 329
breakfast banana split, 250
breakfast recipes, 245–55
bruschetta
  tuna, 329
burgers
  turkey, 340–41

cake
  chocolate, with crystallized ginger,
    365–66
carrot
  ginger soup, 269–70
  and walnut bread, 344–45
cereals
  strawberry almond oat bran, 255
chard. *See* Swiss chard
cheese
  cottage, and fruit, 252
chicken
  barley soup, 271–72
  breasts, roasted, with curry sauce, 336
  citrus, with potatoes, slow cooker, 339

grilled, and mixed vegetable pasta, 296
lemon, 332
lemon sesame stir-fry, 299
mango stir-fry, 295
mustard-glazed, 334
chickpea
and black bean salad, 256
goulash, 310–11
chili
chipotle, 312
chocolate
banana bread, 356–57
cake, with crystallized ginger, 365–66
fruit fondue, 367
and zucchini muffins, 346–47
cilantro
and lime dressing, 265
sesame pesto, 320
cinnamon orange loaf, 348–49
cookies
ginger flax, 371–72
corn
grilled, on the cob, 286
cornmeal
jalapeno muffins, 352–53
cottage cheese
and fresh fruit, 252
crepes
dessert, 369–70

desserts, 362–77
dips
lemon pepper salmon, 321
dressings. (See also salad dressings)
ginger, 287

eggplant
grilled, 287
eggs
asparagus and red pepper frittata, 309
omelet, egg white, 254

fennel
and tomato sauce, 328
figs
and orange granola bars, 373–74
and walnut salad, 259
fish and seafood dishes, 320–29

flax
French toast, 251
and ginger cookies, 371–72
fondue
chocolate fruit, 367
French toast
cinnamon flax, 251
frittata
asparagus and red pepper, 309
fruit
fondue, chocolate, 367
fresh, and cottage cheese, 252

garlic
and orange sauce, 305–6
and sautéed tomatoes, 291
gazpacho, 274
ginger
carrot soup, 269–70
flax cookies, 371–72
glaze, 364
and orange glaze, 290
poppy dressing, 267
glazes
ginger, 364
orange ginger, 290
goat cheese
spinach and mushroom salad and, 264
granola
bars, orange fig, 373–74
grapefruit
broiled, with ginger glaze, 364
green beans. See beans

honey
balsamic dressing, 268
hot and sour soup, 275–76

lemon poppy seed loaf, 354–55
lentils
slow cooker stewed, 317
soup, curried, 273
lime
and avocado dressing, 266
and cilantro dressing, 265

main dishes, meatless, 307–19
main dishes, poultry and meat, 330–41

mango
    cashew salad, 260
    and chicken stir-fry, 295
meat loaf
    Moroccan turkey, 333
meatballs
    honey garlic soy, 313–14
miso soup, 276
muffins, 342–43, 346–47, 352–53,
    358–61
mushroom
    grilled balsamic portobello, 285
    and spinach salad, 264.
mussels
    in white wine sauce, 323–24

nuts
    cashew and mango salad, 260

oats
    apple and cinnamon, 246
    bran cereal, strawberry almond, 255
omelet
    egg white, 254
onions
    caramelized, 283
orange
    and cinnamon loaf, 348–49
    and fig granola bars, 373–74
    and garlic sauce, 305–6
    and ginger glaze, 290
    ginger smoothie, 253
    and squash, baked, 288

pancakes
    blueberry maple, 248–49
parsnip
    and pear soup, 277
pasta dishes, 293, 296, 300–2
pasta salad
    with tuna, capers, lemon, 300
pears
    and parsnip soup, 277
    poached in pomegranate juice, 375
peas
    snap, and salmon pasta, 301
pesto
    sesame cilantro, 320

pie
    pumpkin ginger, 376–77
pomegranate juice
    pears poached in, 375
poppy seeds
    and ginger dressing, 267
    and lemon loaf, 354–55
pork
    chops, honey garlic, 331
    loin chops, with apple chutney, 335
potatoes
    and citrus chicken, slow cooker, 339
pumpkin
    ginger pie, 376–77
    quinoa muffins, 358–59

quick breads, 344–45, 348–51, 354–57
quinoa
    and pumpkin muffins, 358–59
    spinach and sprouts salad, 257–58
    tabbouleh, 262

raspberry
    and apple crisp, 362–63
    and poached pears, 375
red peppers
    and asparagus frittata, 309
rhubarb
    and strawberry muffins, 360–61
rub
    Cajun and lime, 286

salad dressings, 256, 265–68
salads, 256–65, 300
salmon
    grilled with pesto, 320
    lemon pepper dip, 321
    pasta and snap peas, 301
    pepper-crusted, 324
    smoked, sandwich, 326
sandwiches
    roast vegetable, 316
    seared tuna, with caramelized onions,
        325
    smoked salmon, 326
sauces
    curry, 336
    orange garlic, 305–6

tomato fennel, 328
  white wine, 323–24
shrimp
  honey garlic stir-fry, 297–98
side dishes, 283–92
slow cooker
  beef and vegetable stew, 337–38
  citrus chicken with potatoes, 339
  stewed lentils, 317
smoked salmon sandwich, 326
smoothies
  blueberry almond, 247
  orange ginger, 253
sole
  with tomatoes and olives, 327
soups, 269–82
spinach
  and mushroom salad, 264
  and sprouts salad, 257–58
sprouts
  and spinach salad, 257–58
squash
  and apple soup, 280
  orange baked, 288
  roasted, with orange ginger glaze, 289
stir-fries, 295, 297–99, 303–6
strawberry
  almond oat bran cereal, 255
  and rhubarb muffins, 360–61
Swiss chard
  spicy sesame, 292

tabbouleh
  quinoa, 262
tempeh
  stir-fry, with orange garlic sauce,
    305–6
textured vegetable protein
  meatballs, 313–14
tilapia
  in tomato fennel sauce, 328
tofu
  almond-crusted, 307–8
  cutlets, 319

hot and sour soup, 275–76
  miso soup, 276
  spicy baked bites, 318
  sweet and sour stir-fry, 303–4
tomatoes
  cherry, sautéed, 291
  and fennel sauce, 328
  gazpacho, 274
  with sole and olives, 327
toppings
  maple oat, 362–63
tortilla
  refried bean, baked, 315
trout
  lemon thyme grilled, 322
tuna
  bruschetta, 329
  pasta salad, 300
  seared, sandwiches, 325
turkey
  burgers, 340–41
  grilled honey tarragon breasts, 330
  Moroccan meatloaf, 333

vegetables
  and beef stew, slow cooker, 337–38
  roasted, 290
  roasted, sandwich, 316
  roasted and pasta, 302
  and white bean soup, 281–82

walnut
  and carrot bread, 344–45
  and fig salad, 259
white beans. See beans
wild rice
  and black bean salad, 265

yogurt
  almond and berry parfait, 245
  mixed berry salad, 261

zucchini
  and chocolate muffins, 346–47